ORder

Goals of Lecture game
Disclamer on Page

Welcome Quotes

10 things money cannot

Buy

Personalized Treatment of Breast Cancer

Masakazu Toi • Eric Winer • John Benson •
Suzanne Klimberg
Editors

Personalized Treatment of Breast Cancer

Springer

Editors
Masakazu Toi
Department of Breast Surgery
Graduate School of Medicine
Kyoto University
Kyoto
Japan

Eric Winer
Dana-Farber Cancer Institute
Harvard Medical School
Boston
Massachusetts
USA

John Benson
Cambridge Breast Unit
Addenbrookes Hospital
Cambridge
UK

Suzanne Klimberg
University of Arkansas for Medical Sciences and the Winthrop P. Rockefeller Institute
Little Rock
Arkansas
USA

ISBN 978-4-431-55551-3 ISBN 978-4-431-55552-0 (eBook)
DOI 10.1007/978-4-431-55552-0

Library of Congress Control Number: 2016936781

Printed on acid-free paper

This Springer imprint is published by Springer Nature
The registered company is Springer Japan KK

Preface

A multidisciplinary and personalized approach is essential for the treatment of breast cancer, particularly for primary breast cancer. Recent cancer genome analysis has clarified a huge heterogeneity in the genomic profile of breast cancers and a dynamism in the progression and therapeutic selection. Therefore, multiple therapy modalities are indispensable for controlling such a dynamic disease, and personalization of the treatment in each therapeutic modality is required. This book covers current topics in the treatment of primary breast cancer from the personalization point of view. Not only locoregional treatment but also systemic therapy and other key components, necessary for the management, are contained in this project. The contributions of globally known cancer investigators has made it possible to present a broad view of the status and future perspectives. It will be absolutely helpful for young physicians, fellows, and researchers to learn the scientific background, treatment strategy, clinical practice and techniques, novel methodology, and therapeutic concept. There is also no doubt that the contents are useful for breast cancer physicians who are responsible for breast cancer patients as well. Finally, I believe this book encourages us to consider new therapeutic concepts and therapeutic tools.

Kyoto, Japan Masakazu Toi

Contents

Part I
Treatment for the Patients Having Breast Cancer High-Risk

Chapter 1
Risk-Reducing Surgery for Breast Cancer Patients with BRCA Mutations

Eun-Kyu Kim, Sung-Won Kim, and Dong-Young Noh

Abstract Women who carry a germ line mutation in either the BRCA1 or BRCA2 gene have a higher lifetime risk of developing breast and ovarian cancers, often at young ages. Moreover, women with BRCA-associated breast cancer develop second contralateral breast cancers (CBCs) and ovarian cancers at higher rates than those with sporadic breast cancer. Although intensified screening may help identify cancers at an early, favorable stage, it cannot prevent them. Therefore, BRCA1/2 mutation carriers with breast cancer may consider prophylactic surgical strategies such as contralateral prophylactic mastectomy (CPM) and bilateral prophylactic oophorectomy (BPO). There have been increasing interests in CPM, which has been reported to reduce the risk of future CBC by at least 90 %. BPO is the prevailing preventive choice for prophylactic treatment among BRCA mutation carriers, and it reduces the risk of ovarian cancer by about 90 % and breast cancer by about 50 %. Data on the survival of BRCA-associated breast cancer patients who opt for subsequent CPM are inconsistent, but BPO seems to be associated with improved breast- and ovarian cancer-specific mortality as well as improved all-cause mortality among BRCA1/2 mutation carriers. Although prophylactic surgery does not address the cause of these cancers, which is the gene mutations, it is highly effective for cancer prevention and survival.

Keywords Risk-reducing surgery • Contralateral prophylactic mastectomy • Bilateral prophylactic oophorectomy • Contralateral breast cancer • BRCA-associated breast cancer

---

E.-K. Kim
Department of Surgery, Seoul National University College of Medicine, Seoul National University Bundang Hospital, 82, Gumi-ro 173 beon-gil, Bundang gu, Seongnam-si 463-707, Gyeonggi-do, South Korea

S.-W. Kim
Department of Surgery, Daerim St. Mary's Hospital, 657, Siheung-daero, Yeongdeungpo-gu, Seoul 150-822, South Korea

D.-Y. Noh (✉)
Department of Surgery, Seoul National University College of Medicine, Seoul National University Hospital, 101 Daehak-ro, Jongno-gu, Seoul 110-744, South Korea
e-mail: dynoh@snu.ac.kr

M. Toi et al. (eds.), *Personalized Treatment of Breast Cancer*,
DOI 10.1007/978-4-431-55552-0_1

1.1 Subsequent Cancer Risk and Its Prevention in Patients with BRCA-Associated Breast Cancer

Women with BRCA1 or BRCA2 mutations have a higher lifetime risk of developing breast and ovarian cancers [1]. Meta-analyses indicate that BRCA1 and BRCA2 mutation carriers have a 57–65 % and a 45–49 % lifetime probability of developing breast cancer, respectively [2, 3]. The risk of ovarian cancer is also dependent on whether the mutation has occurred in BRCA1 or BRCA2; the lifetime risks of ovarian cancer were reported to be 36–54 % for BRCA1 and 10–27 % for BRCA2 mutation carriers [1, 2, 4, 5].

It is well established that women who have had breast cancer in the past are at an increased risk for contralateral breast cancer (CBC). The Surveillance, Epidemiology, and End Results (SEER) database reported a 4.2 % incidence of CBC from 1973 to 1996. The actuarial risk of developing CBC was 0.6 % per year; thus, the actuarial risk at 5, 10, 15, and 20 years was 3 %, 6.1 %, 9.1 %, and 12 %, respectively [6]. This represents an approximately 1.5-fold to two-fold increased risk for subsequent breast cancer compared with the general population [7, 8]. Compared to patients with sporadic breast cancer, women with BRCA1- and BRCA2-associated breast cancer are reported to have 4.5-fold (95 % confidence interval [CI] = 2.8-fold to 7.1-fold) and 3.4-fold (95 % CI = 2.0-fold to 5.8-fold) increased risks of CBC, respectively [9]. The risk of CBC in patients with BRCA-associated breast cancer is 1.5–3.1 % per year, with 10-year estimates of 25–38 % reported for mutation carriers from high-risk families, compared with rates of 3–7 % for women without mutations [9–16]. Metcalfe et al. reported that the 15-year actuarial risk of CBC was 36.1 % for BRCA1 mutation carriers and 28.5 % for BRCA2 mutation carriers [17]. At 25 years, the cumulative risk for CBC in patients with BRCA1/2 mutations was reported to be 47.4 % [18] (Table 1.1).

Several factors influence the risk of CBC in BRCA mutation carriers (Table 1.2). Younger age at the first breast cancer diagnosis is reported to be associated with a higher risk of CBC in patients with BRCA1 mutations [9, 10, 12, 17, 18]. In addition, several studies have found a 1.3–1.8-fold higher risk of CBC in BRCA1 mutation carriers compared with BRCA2 mutation carriers [9, 12, 18]. Data from

Table 1.1 Rates of contralateral breast cancer in BRCA1/2 mutation carriers with breast cancer

Study [reference]	Patients (n)		CBC (%)			
	BRCA1/2	Sporadic	BRCA1/2	Sporadic	P	F/U (years)
Haffty et al. [11]	22	105	42	9	0.001	12
Pierce et al. [14]	162	445	39	7	<0.0001	15
Metcalfe et al. [17]	810	–	31.6 (BRCA1) 28.5 (BRCA2)	–	–	15
Graeser et al. [18]	1042	–	47.4	–	–	25

Abbreviations: *CBC* contralateral breast cancer, *F/U* follow-up

Table 1.2 Factors that influence the risk of metachronous contralateral breast cancer in BRCA1/2 mutation carriers with breast cancer

Factor	Risk of metachronous contralateral breast cancer
Young age at diagnosis	Elevated
Mutated gene	BRCA1 > BRCA2
Estrogen receptor status	(+) < (−)/no effect[a]
Tamoxifen	Decreased/no effect[a]
Chemotherapy	Decreased/no effect[a]
Contralateral prophylactic mastectomy	Decreased (more than 90 %)
Bilateral prophylactic oophorectomy	Decreased (about 50 %)

[a]Risk reduction demonstrated in some studies but not confirmed in all studies

the German Consortium for Hereditary Breast and Ovarian Cancer show that the risk of CBC for BRCA1 mutation carriers diagnosed with their first breast cancer before the age of 40 is 62.9 % (95 % CI = 50.4–75.4 %) after 25 years, compared with only 19.6 % (95 % CI = 5.3–33.9 %) for patients who were older than 50 years at their first breast cancer diagnosis [18]. According to this report, family members of patients with BRCA1 mutations had a 1.6-fold (95 % CI = 1.2-fold to 2.3-fold) higher risk of CBC compared to those of patients with BRCA2 mutations. More recently, Metcalfe et al. reported the results of a prospective study on 810 BRCA1/2 mutation carriers with breast cancer [17]. In this study, women younger than 50 years at the time of their first breast cancer diagnosis were significantly more likely to develop CBC at 15 years, compared with those older than 50 years (37.6 % vs. 16.8 %, $P = 0.003$). Women younger than 50 years with two or more first-degree relatives with early-onset breast cancer were at high risk of CBC, compared to women with fewer or no first-degree relatives with breast cancer (50 % vs. 36 %, $P = 0.005$). The 15-year actuarial risk of CBC was 36.1 % for women with BRCA1 mutations and 28.5 % for women with BRCA2 mutations. Estrogen receptor status of the primary cancer, chemotherapy, and the use of tamoxifen were not associated with the risk of CBC.

The principal goal in the treatment of patients with breast cancer is to minimize their likelihood of dying from their primary breast cancer. For women with BRCA1/2-associated breast cancer, however, minimizing the incidence of and the mortality due to subsequent cancers, such as metachronous CBC and ovarian cancer, is just as important as treating a primary breast cancer. While intensified screening may help identify subsequent cancers at an early, favorable stage, it cannot prevent the development of such cancers. Therefore, BRCA1/2 mutation carriers with breast cancer may consider preventive strategies such as contralateral prophylactic mastectomy (CPM), bilateral prophylactic oophorectomy (BPO), or medical treatment with tamoxifen to reduce their risk for subsequent cancer development [19]. CPM has been reported to reduce the risk of future CBC by at least 90 % [20–23], similar to the risk reduction of breast cancer with bilateral prophylactic mastectomy among unaffected BRCA1/2 mutation carriers. BPO is the most effective option for the prevention of ovarian cancer [24, 25], and the incidence of

CBC is also reduced by BPO or tamoxifen [12, 26]. In this chapter, we review the literature regarding risk-reducing surgery for BRCA1/2 mutation carriers with breast cancer.

1.2 Contralateral Prophylactic Mastectomy

CPM refers to the removal of the normal intact contralateral breast among women with unilateral breast cancer. As previously described, the cumulative risk of CBC in patients with BRCA1/2 germ line mutations has been estimated to be up to 47.4 % at 25 years [18]. Given the substantial risk of CBC and the unsatisfactory benefits of other prophylactic modalities such as tamoxifen or BPO, some patients with BRCA1/2-associated breast cancer choose to undergo CPM following treatment of the initial breast cancer or opt to be treated initially with bilateral mastectomy if rapid genotyping analysis is made available [27, 28]. Among the available risk-reducing measures, the most effective option for CBC risk reduction is CPM. CPM decreases the risk of CBC by 90–95 % in women with a family history of breast cancer and in those with BRCA1/2 mutations [20–23]. This degree of risk reduction is similar to the reduction in the risk of breast cancer with bilateral prophylactic mastectomy among unaffected BRCA mutation carriers [29–31].

Historically, CPM has been recommended for high-risk patients, including breast cancer patients with BRCA mutations, as a means to reduce the development of CBC and the associated mortality. The ultimate goal of CPM is, indubitably, to improve the survival of breast cancer patients with BRCA1/2 mutations. However, even among these high-risk patients, the efficacy of CPM in improving long-term clinical outcomes is questionable. Despite the significant risk of CBC in patients with BRCA mutations and the obvious prophylactic effect of CPM, data on the survival of primary breast cancer patients who opt for subsequent CPM have been inconsistent. Whereas some studies showed improved survival following CPM [20, 22, 32–36], others showed no survival benefit with CPM [23, 37, 38] (Table 1.3).

In the Cancer Research Network study by Herrinton et al., patients in the CPM group experienced both lower breast cancer mortality and all-cause mortality than those in the non-CPM group (hazard ratio [HR] = 0.57, 95 % CI = 0.45–0.72 and HR = 0.60, 95 % CI = 0.50–0.72, respectively) [22]. Using the SEER data of 8902 women who underwent mastectomy for primary breast cancer and CPM, Bedrosian et al. also reported improved breast cancer-specific survival with CPM (HR = 0.63, 95 % CI = 0.57–0.69) [32]. In a retrospective single-center study by Boughey et al., 10-year overall and disease-free survival rates were better in the CPM group than in the mastectomy-only group (HR = 0.68, 95 % CI = 0.54–0.86 and HR = 0.66, 95 % CI = 0.53–0.82, respectively) [33]. In another retrospective single-center study, Peralta et al. reported a 27 % absolute improvement in disease-free survival and a 15 % absolute improvement in overall survival after 15 years following CPM [20]. In a recent retrospective multicenter study, Metcalfe et al. reported that

Table 1.3 Studies assessing the effect of contralateral prophylactic mastectomy on survival

Author [reference]	Year	Design	No. of patients	Follow-up	Survival benefit of CPM
Peralta et al. [20]	2000	R	CPM: 64 Non-CPM: 182	15 years	Associated with improved DFS (15-year DFS was 55 % for the CPM group and 28 % for the non-CPM group, P = 0.01)
Herrinton et al. [22]	2005	R	CPM: 908 Non-CPM: 46,368	5.7 years	Associated with improved BCSS and OS (HR = 0.57, 95 % CI = 0.45–0.72 and HR = 0.60, 95 % CI = 0.50–0.72, respectively)
Bedrosian et al. [32]	2010	R	CPM: 8748 Non-CPM: 95,283	47 months	Associated with improved BCSS (HR = 0.63, 95 % CI = 0.57–0.69)
Boughey et al. [33]	2010	CC	CPM: 385 Non-CPM: 385	17.3 years	Associated with improved OS and DFS (HR = 0.68, 95 % CI = 0.54–0.86 and HR = 0.66, 95 % CI = 0.53–0.82, respectively)
Evans et al. [34]	2013	R	CPM: 105 Non-CPM: 593	10 years	Associated with improved OS (HR = 0.37, 95 % CI = 0.17–0.80)
Metcalfe et al. [35]	2014	R	CPM: 181 Non-CPM: 209	14.3 years	Associated with improved BCSS (HR = 0.52, 95 % CI = 0.29–0.93)
Heemskerk-Gerritsen et al. [36]	2014	P	CPM: 242 Non-CPM: 341	11.4 years	Associated with improved OS (HR = 0.49, 95 % CI = 0.29–0.82)
van Sprundel et al. [23]	2005	R	CPM: 79 Non-CPM: 69	7.4 years	No association with improved OS
Chung et al. [37]	2012	CC	CPM: 177 Non-CPM: 178	61 months	No association with improved OS, DFS, or DMFS
Kurian et al. [46]	2014	R	BM: 11,692 BCT: 104,420 UM: 73,622	89.1 months	No significant difference in OS between BM and BCT groups but higher mortality rates in the UM group
Fayanju et al. [38]	2014	MA	14 studies CPM: 13,142 Non-CPM: 146,174	6.1 years	No association with improved OS or BCSS

Abbreviations: *R* retrospective cohort, *CC* case-control, *P* prospective cohort, *MA* meta-analysis, *CPM* contralateral prophylactic mastectomy, *BM* bilateral mastectomy, *BCT* breast-conserving treatment (breast-conserving surgery plus radiotherapy), *UM* unilateral mastectomy, *BCSS* breast cancer-specific survival, *OS* overall survival, *DFS* disease-free survival, *DMFS* distant metastasis-free survival, *HR* hazard ratio, *CI* confidence interval

BRCA mutation carriers with stage I or II breast cancer treated with bilateral mastectomy are less likely to die from breast cancer than those treated with unilateral mastectomy; the 20-year survival rate for women who underwent CPM was 88 % (95 % CI = 83–93 %), and the rate for those who did not undergo CPM was 66 % (95 % CI = 59–73 %) [35]. In the Metcalfe study, CPM was associated with a 48 % reduction in the risk of death from breast cancer after adjustment for age, year of diagnosis, treatment, and other prognostic features (HR = 0.52, 95 % CI = 0.29–0.93). Recently, Heemskerk-Gerritsen et al. reported the results of a prospective analysis of 583 BRCA-associated primary breast cancer patients (242 who underwent CPM and 341 under surveillance) in an ongoing nationwide Dutch study (HEBON study; Hereditary Breast and Ovarian cancer study, the Netherlands) [36]. In this study, the CPM group showed lower mortality than the surveillance group (9.6 and 21.6 per 1000 person-years of observation, respectively; adjusted HR = 0.49, 95 % CI = 0.29–0.82).

The CPM-associated survival benefit seems to be more evident in patients diagnosed with primary breast cancer at a young age, those with low-grade and/or non-triple-negative tumors, those not treated with adjuvant chemotherapy, and those with early-stage (I and II) tumors [32, 36]. Using Markov modeling, Schrag et al. estimated that CPM would increase life expectancy by 0.6–2.1 years in a 30-year-old early-stage breast cancer patient with a BRCA mutation [19]. In addition, the survival advantage from CPM seems to act independently of bilateral salpingo-oophorectomy, which substantially reduces the risk of CBC and ovarian cancer as well as the risk of relapse of primary breast cancer [34].

In contrast, some studies showed no survival benefit following CPM. A retrospective cohort study conducted by van Sprundel et al. showed no difference in overall survival between the group who underwent CPM and the surveillance group in Dutch patients with BRCA-associated breast cancer [23]. In a single-center study conducted by Chung et al., CPM did not improve overall, disease-free, or distant metastasis-free survival over a median follow-up period of 61 months [37]. Recently, Fayanju et al. conducted a meta-analysis of 14 studies and reported that both the relative and absolute risks of metachronous CBC were significantly decreased among CPM recipients compared with non-recipients (HR = 0.04, 95 % CI = 0.02–0.09), but there was no improvement in overall survival or breast cancer-specific mortality with CPM [38]. A recent Cochrane analysis also concluded that "there is insufficient evidence that CPM improves survival" [39].

Despite the conflicting data regarding its survival benefit, there is increasing interest in CPM for risk reduction among breast cancer patients [40–46]. Turtle et al. reviewed the SEER database and found an increase in the use of CPM from 4.3 to 11 % for the treatment of invasive disease and from 8.4 to 16.4 % for the treatment of noninvasive disease from 1998 to 2003 [40, 41]. Other studies using different databases have confirmed this finding. Using the American College of Surgeons' National Cancer Data Base, Yao et al. reported a similar increase in CPM rates from 1998 to 2007 with no plateau at the end of the study period [44]. Based on data from the New York State Cancer Registry, McLaughlin et al. reported that the number of women undergoing CPM more than doubled from 1995 to 2005

[45]. A recent large observational cohort study based on the population-based California Cancer Registry by Kurian et al. demonstrated a significantly increased rate of bilateral mastectomy, from 2.0 % in 1998 to 12.3 % in 2013, among 189,734 patients, and showed that its associated overall survival was comparable to that associated with breast-conserving surgery plus radiation, with a median follow-up period of 89.1 months [46]. The proposed explanations for the increased rates of CPM among patients with unilateral breast cancer include the increasing use of highly sensitive breast magnetic resonance imaging (MRI), which leads to increases in anxiety-producing recall and biopsy rates that may drive patients to choose preventive surgery, and the increasing use of genetic testing, which facilitates the identification of high-risk patients who benefit from risk-reducing surgery [46].

In BRCA1/2 mutation carriers with breast cancer, the rates of CPM have been reported to be 27–48 % [27, 47]. In a multinational cohort study reporting that 27 % of BRCA mutation carriers with unilateral breast cancer elected to undergo CPM, there were large differences in the adoption of CPM by country; 38 % of North American women (women in the United States or Canada) underwent CPM, whereas only 5 % of European women chose to undergo CPM [47]. However, some studies from Europe have reported much higher CPM rates, ranging from 51 to 65 %, among breast cancer survivors [48, 49]. To date, few studies have assessed the rate of CPM among Asian patients with BRCA-associated breast cancer. The Korean Hereditary Breast Cancer (KOHBRA) study group reported that only 6.4 % of women with BRCA-associated breast cancer opted to undergo subsequent CPM for CBC prevention [50]. In 2009, the Asian BRCA (ABRCA) consortium was launched to study hereditary breast and ovarian cancer in Asian patients, and 15 countries (Korea, Japan, China, Hong Kong, Indonesia, Malaysia, Singapore, India, the Philippines, Vietnam, Thailand, Pakistan, Bangladesh, Taiwan, and Australia) are now participating in this consortium. This international collaboration is expected to elucidate the utilization patterns of risk-reducing modalities in Asian BRCA mutation carriers.

For patients with BRCA-associated breast cancer, an important factor facilitating the decision regarding CPM is the fear of developing metachronous CBC [51]. Women choose to undergo CPM to take control of their cancer and manage their fear [52]. Although periodic surveillance (mammography and breast MRI) is a more noninvasive option than prophylactic mastectomy, patients' prior experiences of undergoing intensive treatments, such as chemotherapy and radiotherapy, underlie their pleas for a more efficacious remedy. Interestingly, pathologic examination of CPM specimens, especially from women older than 40 years of age, revealed high-risk histopathologic lesions, such as atypical lobular hyperplasia, atypical ductal hyperplasia, lobular carcinoma in situ, and ductal carcinoma in situ, in 3–57 % of patients [53–55]. Younger age, high cancer-specific distress, mastectomy for primary breast cancer treatment, and prophylactic oophorectomy are suggested to influence opting for CPM among women with BRCA-associated breast cancer [27, 47].

Most patients are satisfied with their decision to undergo CPM. The greatest reported benefit contributing to patient satisfaction is a reduction in breast cancer-related concerns [56]. Mutation carriers often report decreased anxiety about developing cancer following prophylactic mastectomy. According to Frost et al., 83 % of patients reported satisfaction with their decision to undergo CPM at a mean of 10 years after surgery [57]. Studies examining psychosocial and quality of life outcomes after prophylactic mastectomy have reported generally high levels of satisfaction, little distress, and overall quality of life comparable to that of women who chose not to undergo prophylactic mastectomy [57–59]. However, some women experience negative psychosocial outcomes following CPM, most often related to high levels of psychological distress, issues with sexual function or body image, and poor cosmetic outcome [59–61].

In an effort to improve cosmetic results and to increase the acceptance rate of prophylactic surgery, there is increasing interest in the use of nipple-sparing mastectomy (NSM), which combines skin-sparing mastectomy with preservation of the nipple-areola complex (NAC) [62]. Whereas classic subcutaneous mastectomy has been criticized because the 5–10 % of breast tissue that remains under the flaps and the NAC increases the risk of cancer at these sites [63], NSM results in thinner skin flaps and a 2- to 3-mm-thick nipple-areolar flap, with the goal of leaving less remaining breast tissue and thus reducing the risk of subsequent cancer development [62]. Currently, total (simple) mastectomy is generally recommended over classic subcutaneous mastectomy or NSM. However, technical advances in skin-sparing techniques and the availability of approaches such as muscle-containing flaps or implantable prostheses have broadened the surgical options available to women considering these procedures [64]. In a report on prophylactic NSM, in which the retroareolar ducts (nipple core) were removed, breast cancer developed in 2 of 55 patients during a median follow-up period of 24.6 months: in the upper outer quadrant in one patient and in the axillary tail in the other patient, but none at the NAC [62]. Another study on a series of 397 NSMs performed at two different institutions on 201 BRCA1/2 mutation carriers reported only four (2.0 %) cancer events: three in cancer patients and one in a patient undergoing NSM for risk reduction, but none at the NAC [65]. Prospective comparative studies with long-term follow-up are needed to precisely establish the risks of cancer after NSM.

1.3 Bilateral Prophylactic Oophorectomy

In 2002, two large case series demonstrated the efficacy of BPO for the prevention of both breast and gynecologic (ovarian, fallopian tube, and primary peritoneal) cancers in BRCA mutation carriers [24, 25], and subsequent reports have also provided strong evidence that BPO is highly protective against BRCA-associated cancers [5, 66–69]. BPO reduces the risk of ovarian cancer by about 90 % and that of breast cancer by about 50 %. In the largest of these studies, Eisen et al. performed an international case-control study on 1439 patients with BRCA-associated breast cancer and 1866 matched controls without breast cancer [67]. BPO was associated with a significant reduction in breast cancer risk among BRCA1 mutation carriers by 56 % (odds ratio [OR] = 0.44, 95 % CI = 0.29–0.66). For BRCA2 mutation carriers, however, the difference in risk was not statistically significant. The risk reduction was greater if the oophorectomy was performed before age 40 (OR = 0.36, 95 % CI = 0.20–0.64) rather than after age 40 (OR = 0.53, 95 % CI = 0.30–0.90). The protective effect was evident for 15-years post-BPO among BRCA1/2 mutation carriers (OR = 0.39, 95 % CI = 0.26–0.57). In another retrospective analysis of 551 BRCA mutation carriers, BPO reduced the risk of ovarian cancer by 96 % (HR = 0.04, 95 % CI = 0.01–0.16) and that of breast cancer by 53 % (HR = 0.47, 95 % CI = 0.29–0.77) at a mean follow-up time of 8.8 years [25]. A prospective multicenter study also reported that the risk of both breast and ovarian cancers was significantly lower in BRCA mutation carriers who underwent BPO than in those who did not [68, 69]. Recently, Rebbeck et al. conducted a meta-analysis of 10 studies and showed that BPO is strongly associated with reductions in the risk of breast and gynecologic cancers [5]. BPO was associated with a significant reduction in the risk of breast cancer in BRCA1/2 mutation carriers (HR = 0.49; 95 % CI = 0.37–0.65), and similar risk reductions were observed in BRCA1 mutation carriers (HR = 0.47; 95 % CI = 0.35–0 64) and in BRCA2 mutation carriers (HR = 0.47; 95 % CI = 0.26–0.84). BPO was also associated with a significant reduction in the risk of BRCA1/2-associated ovarian or fallopian tube cancer (HR = 0.21; 95 % CI = 0.12–0.39).

The risk of CBC in patients with BRCA-associated breast cancer was also reported to be lower after oophorectomy when it was performed in a premenopausal carrier, presumably because of the induction of premature menopause [12, 14, 17]. By assessing 810 patients with BRCA-associated breast cancer, Metcalfe et al. reported that the strongest predictor of CBC in women with BRCA mutations is oophorectomy [17]. Patients who underwent oophorectomy had a significantly lower risk of CBC than those who did not undergo oophorectomy (relative risk [RR] = 0.48, 95 % CI = 0.27–0.82, $P = 0.002$). This effect was observed in women who were diagnosed with their initial breast cancer under the age of 50 years (RR = 0.39, 95 % CI = 0.23–0.67, $P = 0.0006$) and was significant for those with BRCA1 mutations (RR = 0.48, 95 % CI = 0.27–0.84, $P = 0.01$). In patients with BRCA2 mutations, oophorectomy was associated with a 51 % reduction in CBC risk, but this finding was not statistically significant ($P = 0.11$). Among young (<50 years) patients with two intact ovaries, the 15-year cumulative incidence of CBC was 58 %, and if a woman in this subgroup also had two or more first-degree relatives with breast cancer, the 15-year risk was elevated to 68 %. A recent meta-analysis also indicates that BPO is associated with a decreased risk of CBC in patients with BRCA1/2-associated breast cancer (RR = 0.52, 95 % CI = 0.37–0.74) [70]. Despite its apparent protective effect, the risk of CBC in patients with BRCA-associated breast cancer after oophorectomy was still higher than that seen in a control group of women with sporadic breast cancer [14]. For women with hereditary breast and ovarian cancer syndrome, the National Comprehensive Cancer Network (NCCN) guidelines recommend risk-reducing salpingo-oophorectomy (BPO), ideally performed between ages 35 and 40, and upon completion of childbearing or on an individualized basis based on the earliest age of onset of ovarian cancer in the family [71].

Recently, Domchek et al. reported the results of a prospective multicenter cohort study of 2482 BRCA1/2 mutation carriers performed to estimate the reduction in risk and mortality with BPO [72]. In this study, women who underwent BPO experienced lower all-cause mortality (HR = 0.40, 95 % CI = 0.26–0.61), breast cancer-specific mortality (HR = 0.44, 95 % CI = 0.26–0.76), and ovarian cancer-specific mortality (HR = 0.21, 95 % CI = 0.06–0.80) than those who did not undergo BPO. Moreover, in mutation carriers with prior breast cancer, BPO was associated with significantly lower all-cause mortality (HR = 0.30, 95 % CI = 0.17–0.52) and breast cancer-specific mortality (HR = 0.35, 95 % CI = 0.19–0.67). However, studies with larger datasets and longer follow-up periods are needed to define more precisely the reduction in mortality conferred by BPO.

Currently, BPO is the prevailing choice for risk-reducing treatment among BRCA mutation carriers in the United States and Canada [73, 74]. In some ways, BPO may be superior to prophylactic mastectomy, because it reduces the risk of both breast and ovarian cancer, and there are now data to indicate that BPO also reduces both overall mortality and cancer-specific mortality. In addition, BPO is associated with lower morbidity than prophylactic mastectomy as well as a superior side effect profile [75]. Considering the later diagnosis and the higher mortality of ovarian cancer compared to breast cancer, BPO is currently recommended by most experts in the field of prevention of hereditary breast and ovarian cancer syndrome [74, 75]. In a North American survey of women who had recently received a positive BRCA test result, 60 % underwent BPO and 25 % opted for prophylactic mastectomy, whereas only 12 % chose to take tamoxifen [73]. BRCA1 mutation carriers are more likely to opt for BPO than are BRCA2 mutation carriers [76, 77]. As is the case for CPM, few studies have assessed the rate of BPO among Asian BRCA mutation carriers with breast cancer. In a single-center study conducted by the KOHBRA study group, 22.4 % of BRCA1/2 mutation carriers with breast cancer underwent BPO to prevent subsequent ovarian cancer, whereas 66.7 % opted for intensive surveillance [50].

A few studies have evaluated psychosocial outcomes and quality of life following BPO. In 2005, Madalinska et al. performed a nationwide, multicenter, cross-sectional, observational study comparing psychosocial and quality of life outcomes among high-risk women who had undergone BPO and those who had opted for screening to manage their increased ovarian cancer risk [78]. In this study, there were no differences in overall quality of life between the two groups. Patients who opted for BPO reported experiencing less worry about breast and ovarian cancers than those who opted for screening. However, women who underwent BPO reported significantly more endocrine symptoms and worse sexual functioning than those who did not undergo BPO.

1.4 In-Breast Tumor Recurrence-Reducing Surgery in Patients with BRCA-Associated Breast Cancer

Breast-conserving treatment (BCT), defined as breast-conserving surgery combined with radiotherapy, is a standard treatment for early-stage breast cancer and results in survival equivalent to that following mastectomy in women with sporadic breast cancer [79, 80]. However, in women with BRCA-associated breast cancer, outcomes of mastectomy and BCT have not yet been directly compared. Thus, the equivalence of the rates of local control, disease-free survival, and overall survival with the two treatments is not yet proven.

Several studies have shown a higher risk of ipsilateral in-breast events, including the recurrence of the initial tumor and the development of a second primary tumor, in patients with BRCA-associated breast cancer treated with BCT than in sporadic controls who received BCT [11, 14, 81–83]. In a multi-institutional study by Pierce et al., the rate of in-breast tumor recurrence at 10 years was twice as high among BRCA1/2 mutation carriers treated with BCT compared with sporadic controls who received BCT [14]. Moreover, another multi-institutional study demonstrated that BRCA mutation carriers who underwent BCT to treat their breast cancer have an elevated risk of local failure in the ipsilateral breast, most occurrences of which appeared to be second primary cancers rather than failure to control the primary tumor, compared with carriers treated with mastectomy (23.5 % vs. 5.5 %, respectively; $P < 0.0001$) [84]. Although patients with BRCA-associated breast cancer have similar survival whether treated with BCT or mastectomy [84], these findings suggest that, for patients with BRCA-associated breast cancer in whom BCT is possible, mastectomy may be an alternative treatment option from the viewpoint of preventing subsequent ipsilateral in-breast events.

If rapid presurgical BRCA testing is possible, women with breast cancer who are confirmed to carry BRCA mutations may consider more extensive surgery, such as mastectomy with or without CPM, to reduce the risk of ipsilateral in-breast events instead of choosing BCT. Recent studies have examined the impact of genetic assessment on surgical choices at the time of diagnosis of breast cancer: breast cancer patients who received positive results for BRCA mutation prior to surgery are more likely to undergo bilateral mastectomy than BCT, with rates ranging from 42 to 100 % [27, 28, 85, 86]. However, the genotyping test for BRCA1/2 mutation is time consuming, and patients may undergo BCT before receiving their BRCA1/2 test results. In addition, for the past decade, BRCA testing has usually been offered after treatment of breast cancer [87]. With respect to the prevention of future in-breast events, an ipsilateral prophylactic completion mastectomy can also be considered for patients with BRCA-associated breast cancer previously treated with BCT.

References

1. Ford D, Easton DF, Stratton M, Narod S, Goldgar D, Devilee P, Bishop DT, Weber B, Lenoir G, Chang-Claude J, Sobol H, Teare MD, Struewing J, Arason A, Scherneck S, Peto J, Rebbeck TR, Tonin P, Neuhausen S, Barkardottir R, Eyfjord J, Lynch H, Ponder BA, Gayther SA, Zelada-Hedman M et al (1998) Genetic heterogeneity and penetrance analysis of the BRCA1 and BRCA2 genes in breast cancer families. The breast cancer linkage consortium. Am J Hum Genet 62(3):676–689
2. Antoniou A, Pharoah PD, Narod S, Risch HA, Eyfjord JE, Hopper JL, Loman N, Olsson H, Johannsson O, Borg A, Pasini B, Radice P, Manoukian S, Eccles DM, Tang N, Olah E, Anton-Culver H, Warner E, Lubinski J, Gronwald J, Gorski B, Tulinius H, Thorlacius S, Eerola H, Nevanlinna H, Syrjakoski K, Kallioniemi OP, Thompson D, Evans C, Peto J, Lalloo F, Evans DG, Easton DF (2003) Average risks of breast and ovarian cancer associated with BRCA1 or BRCA2 mutations detected in case series unselected for family history: a combined analysis of 22 studies. Am J Hum Genet 72(5):1117–1130. doi:10.1086/375033
3. Chen S, Parmigiani G (2007) Meta-analysis of BRCA1 and BRCA2 penetrance. J Clin Oncol Off J Am Soc Clin Oncol 25(11):1329–1333. doi:10.1200/JCO.2006.09.1066
4. King MC, Marks JH, Mandell JB, New York Breast Cancer Study G (2003) Breast and ovarian cancer risks due to inherited mutations in BRCA1 and BRCA2. Science 302(5645):643–646. doi:10.1126/science.1088759
5. Rebbeck TR, Kauff ND, Domchek SM (2009) Meta-analysis of risk reduction estimates associated with risk-reducing salpingo-oophorectomy in BRCA1 or BRCA2 mutation carriers. J Natl Cancer Inst 101(2):80–87. doi:10.1093/jnci/djn442
6. Gao X, Fisher SG, Emami B (2003) Risk of second primary cancer in the contralateral breast in women treated for early-stage breast cancer: a population-based study. Int J Radiat Oncol Biol Phys 56(4):1038–1045
7. Kurian AW, McClure LA, John EM, Horn-Ross PL, Ford JM, Clarke CA (2009) Second primary breast cancer occurrence according to hormone receptor status. J Natl Cancer Inst 101 (15):1058–1065. doi:10.1093/jnci/djp181
8. Saltzman BS, Malone KE, McDougall JA, Daling JR, Li CI (2012) Estrogen receptor, progesterone receptor, and HER2-neu expression in first primary breast cancers and risk of second primary contralateral breast cancer. Breast Cancer Res Treat 135(3):849–855. doi:10.1007/s10549-012-2183-5
9. Malone KE, Begg CB, Haile RW, Borg A, Concannon P, Tellhed L, Xue S, Teraoka S, Bernstein L, Capanu M, Reiner AS, Riedel ER, Thomas DC, Mellemkjaer L, Lynch CF, Boice JD Jr, Anton-Culver H, Bernstein JL (2010) Population-based study of the risk of second primary contralateral breast cancer associated with carrying a mutation in BRCA1 or BRCA2. J Clin Oncol Off J Am Soc Clin Oncol 28(14):2404–2410. doi:10.1200/JCO.2009.24.2495
10. Verhoog LC, Brekelmans CT, Seynaeve C, Meijers-Heijboer EJ, Klijn JG (2000) Contralateral breast cancer risk is influenced by the age at onset in BRCA1-associated breast cancer. Br J Cancer 83(3):384–386. doi:10.1054/bjoc.2000.1239
11. Haffty BG, Harrold E, Khan AJ, Pathare P, Smith TE, Turner BC, Glazer PM, Ward B, Carter D, Matloff E, Bale AE, Alvarez-Franco M (2002) Outcome of conservatively managed early-onset breast cancer by BRCA1/2 status. Lancet 359(9316):1471–1477. doi:10.1016/S0140-6736(02)08434-9
12. Metcalfe K, Lynch HT, Ghadirian P, Tung N, Olivotto I, Warner E, Olopade OI, Eisen A, Weber B, McLennan J, Sun P, Foulkes WD, Narod SA (2004) Contralateral breast cancer in BRCA1 and BRCA2 mutation carriers. J Clin Oncol Off J Am Soc Clin Oncol 22 (12):2328–2335. doi:10.1200/JCO.2004.04.033
13. Brekelmans CT, Seynaeve C, Menke-Pluymers M, Bruggenwirth HT, Tilanus-Linthorst MM, Bartels CC, Kriege M, van Geel AN, Crepin CM, Blom JC, Meijers-Heijboer H, Klijn JG (2006) Survival and prognostic factors in BRCA1-associated breast cancer. Ann Oncol Off J Eur Soc Med Oncol ESMO 17(3):391–400. doi:10.1093/annonc/mdj095

14. Pierce LJ, Levin AM, Rebbeck TR, Ben-David MA, Friedman E, Solin LJ, Harris EE, Gaffney DK, Haffty BG, Dawson LA, Narod SA, Olivotto IA, Eisen A, Whelan TJ, Olopade OI, Isaacs C, Merajver SD, Wong JS, Garber JE, Weber BL (2006) Ten-year multi-institutional results of breast-conserving surgery and radiotherapy in BRCA1/2-associated stage I/II breast cancer. J Clin Oncol Off J Am Soc Clin Oncol 24(16):2437–2443. doi:10.1200/JCO.2005.02.7888
15. Brekelmans CT, Tilanus-Linthorst MM, Seynaeve C, vd Ouweland A, Menke-Pluymers MB, Bartels CC, Kriege M, van Geel AN, Burger CW, Eggermont AM, Meijers-Heijboer H, Klijn JG (2007) Tumour characteristics, survival and prognostic factors of hereditary breast cancer from BRCA2-, BRCA1- and non-BRCA1/2 families as compared to sporadic breast cancer cases. Eur J Cancer 43(5):867–876. doi:10.1016/j.ejca.2006.12.009
16. van der Kolk DM, de Bock GH, Leegte BK, Schaapveld M, Mourits MJ, de Vries J, van der Hout AH, Oosterwijk JC (2010) Penetrance of breast cancer, ovarian cancer and contralateral breast cancer in BRCA1 and BRCA2 families: high cancer incidence at older age. Breast Cancer Res Treat 124(3):643–651. doi:10.1007/s10549-010-0805-3
17. Metcalfe K, Gershman S, Lynch HT, Ghadirian P, Tung N, Kim-Sing C, Olopade OI, Domchek S, McLennan J, Eisen A, Foulkes WD, Rosen B, Sun P Narod SA (2011) Predictors of contralateral breast cancer in BRCA1 and BRCA2 mutation carriers. Br J Cancer 104 (9):1384–1392. doi:10.1038/bjc.2011.120
18. Graeser MK, Engel C, Rhiem K, Gadzicki D, Bick U, Kast K, Froster UG, Schlehe B, Bechtold A, Arnold N, Preisler-Adams S, Nestle-Kraemling C, Zaino M, Loeffler M, Kiechle M, Meindl A, Varga D, Schmutzler RK (2009) Contralateral breast cancer risk in BRCA1 and BRCA2 mutation carriers. J Clin Oncol Off J Am Soc Clin Oncol 27 (35):5887–5892. doi:10.1200/JCO.2008.19.9430
19. Schrag D, Kuntz KM, Garber JE, Weeks JC (2000) Life expectancy gains from cancer prevention strategies for women with breast cancer and BRCA1 or BRCA2 mutations. JAMA 283(5):617–624
20. Peralta EA, Ellenhorn JD, Wagman LD, Dagis A, Andersen JS, Chu DZ (2000) Contralateral prophylactic mastectomy improves the outcome of selected patients undergoing mastectomy for breast cancer. Am J Surg 180(6):439–445
21. McDonnell SK, Schaid DJ, Myers JL, Grant CS, Donohue JH, Woods JE, Frost MH, Johnson JL, Sitta DL, Slezak JM, Crotty TB, Jenkins RB, Sellers TA, Hartmann LC (2001) Efficacy of contralateral prophylactic mastectomy in women with a personal and family history of breast cancer. J Clin Oncol Off J Am Soc Clin Oncol 19(19):3938–3943
22. Herrinton LJ, Barlow WE, Yu O, Geiger AM, Elmore JG, Barton MB, Harris EL, Rolnick S, Pardee R, Husson G, Macedo A, Fletcher SW (2005) Efficacy of prophylactic mastectomy in women with unilateral breast cancer: a cancer research network project. J Clin Oncol Off J Am Soc Clin Oncol 23(19):4275–4286. doi:10.1200/JCO.2005.10.080
23. van Sprundel TC, Schmidt MK, Rookus MA, Brohet R, van Asperen CJ, Rutgers EJ, Van't Veer LJ, Tollenaar RA (2005) Risk reduction of contralateral breast cancer and survival after contralateral prophylactic mastectomy in BRCA1 or BRCA2 mutation carriers. Br J Cancer 93 (3):287–292. doi:10.1038/sj.bjc.6602703
24. Kauff ND, Satagopan JM, Robson ME, Scheuer L, Hensley M, Hudis CA, Ellis NA, Boyd J, Borgen PI, Barakat RR, Norton L, Castiel M, Nafa K, Offit K (2002) Risk-reducing salpingo-oophorectomy in women with a BRCA1 or BRCA2 mutation. N Engl J Med 346 (21):1609–1615. doi:10.1056/NEJMoa020119
25. Rebbeck TR, Lynch HT, Neuhausen SL, Narod SA, Van't Veer L, Garber JE, Evans G, Isaacs C, Daly MB, Matloff E, Olopade OI, Weber BL, Prevention, Observation of Surgical End Points Study G (2002) Prophylactic oophorectomy in carriers of BRCA1 or BRCA2 mutations. N Engl J Med 346(21):1616–1622. doi:10.1056/NEJMoa012158
26. Narod SA, Brunet JS, Ghadirian P, Robson M, Heimdal K, Neuhausen SL, Stoppa-Lyonnet D, Lerman C, Pasini B, de los Rios P, Weber B, Lynch H, Hereditary Breast Cancer Clinical Study G (2000) Tamoxifen and risk of contralateral breast cancer in BRCA1 and BRCA2

mutation carriers: a case-control study. Hereditary Breast Cancer Clinical Study Group. Lancet 356(9245):1876–1881

27. Schwartz MD, Lerman C, Brogan B, Peshkin BN, Halbert CH, DeMarco T, Lawrence W, Main D, Finch C, Magnant C, Pennanen M, Tsangaris T, Willey S, Isaacs C (2004) Impact of BRCA1/BRCA2 counseling and testing on newly diagnosed breast cancer patients. J Clin Oncol Off J Am Soc Clin Oncol 22(10):1823–1829. doi:10.1200/JCO.2004.04.086
28. Smith KL, Isaacs C (2011) BRCA mutation testing in determining breast cancer therapy. Cancer J 17(6):492–499. doi:10.1097/PPO.0b013e318238f579
29. Hartmann LC, Sellers TA, Schaid DJ, Frank TS, Soderberg CL, Sitta DL, Frost MH, Grant CS, Donohue JH, Woods JE, McDonnell SK, Vockley CW, Deffenbaugh A, Couch FJ, Jenkins RB (2001) Efficacy of bilateral prophylactic mastectomy in BRCA1 and BRCA2 gene mutation carriers. J Natl Cancer Inst 93(21):1633–1637
30. Meijers-Heijboer H, van Geel B, van Putten WL, Henzen-Logmans SC, Seynaeve C, Menke-Pluymers MB, Bartels CC, Verhoog LC, van den Ouweland AM, Niermeijer MF, Brekelmans CT, Klijn JG (2001) Breast cancer after prophylactic bilateral mastectomy in women with a BRCA1 or BRCA2 mutation. N Engl J Med 345(3):159–164. doi:10.1056/NEJM200107193450301
31. Rebbeck TR, Friebel T, Lynch HT, Neuhausen SL, Van't Veer L, Garber JE, Evans GR, Narod SA, Isaacs C, Matloff E, Daly MB, Olopade OI, Weber BL (2004) Bilateral prophylactic mastectomy reduces breast cancer risk in BRCA1 and BRCA2 mutation carriers: the PROSE Study Group. J Clin Oncol Off J Am Soc Clin Oncol 22(6):1055–1062. doi:10.1200/JCO.2004.04.188
32. Bedrosian I, Hu CY, Chang GJ (2010) Population-based study of contralateral prophylactic mastectomy and survival outcomes of breast cancer patients. J Natl Cancer Inst 102 (6):401–409. doi:10.1093/jnci/djq018
33. Boughey JC, Hoskin TL, Degnim AC, Sellers TA, Johnson JL, Kasner MJ, Hartmann LC, Frost MH (2010) Contralateral prophylactic mastectomy is associated with a survival advantage in high-risk women with a personal history of breast cancer. Ann Surg Oncol 17 (10):2702–2709. doi:10.1245/s10434-010-1136-7
34. Evans DG, Ingham SL, Baildam A, Ross GL, Lalloo F, Buchan I, Howell A (2013) Contralateral mastectomy improves survival in women with BRCA1/2-associated breast cancer. Breast Cancer Res Treat 140(1):135–142. doi:10.1007/s10549-013-2583-1
35. Metcalfe K, Gershman S, Ghadirian P, Lynch HT, Snyder C, Tung N, Kim-Sing C, Eisen A, Foulkes WD, Rosen B, Sun P, Narod SA (2014) Contralateral mastectomy and survival after breast cancer in carriers of BRCA1 and BRCA2 mutations: retrospective analysis. BMJ 348: g226. doi:10.1136/bmj.g226
36. Heemskerk-Gerritsen BA, Rookus MA, Aalfs CM, Ausems MG, Collee JM, Jansen L, Kets CM, Keymeulen KB, Koppert LB, Meijers-Heijboer HE, Mooij TM, Tollenaar RA, Vasen HF, Hebon, Hooning MJ, Seynaeve C (2014) Improved overall survival after contralateral risk-reducing mastectomy in BRCA1/2 mutation carriers with a history of unilateral breast cancer: a prospective analysis. Int J Cancer J Int Cancer. doi:10.1002/ijc.29032
37. Chung A, Huynh K, Lawrence C, Sim MS, Giuliano A (2012) Comparison of patient characteristics and outcomes of contralateral prophylactic mastectomy and unilateral total mastectomy in breast cancer patients. Ann Surg Oncol 19(8):2600–2606. doi:10.1245/s10434-012-2299-1
38. Fayanju OM, Stoll CR, Fowler S, Colditz GA, Margenthaler JA (2014) Contralateral prophylactic mastectomy after unilateral breast cancer: a systematic review and meta-analysis. Ann Surg 260(6):1000–1010. doi:10.1097/SLA.0000000000000769
39. Lostumbo L, Carbine NE, Wallace J (2010) Prophylactic mastectomy for the prevention of breast cancer. Cochrane Database Syst Rev 11:CD002748. doi:10.1002/14651858.CD002748.pub3
40. Tuttle TM, Habermann EB, Grund EH, Morris TJ, Virnig BA (2007) Increasing use of contralateral prophylactic mastectomy for breast cancer patients: a trend toward more

aggressive surgical treatment. J Clin Oncol Off J Am Soc Clin Oncol 25(33):5203–5209. doi:10.1200/JCO.2007.12.3141

41. Tuttle TM, Jarosek S, Habermann EB, Arrington A, Abraham A, Morris TJ, Virnig BA (2009) Increasing rates of contralateral prophylactic mastectomy among patients with ductal carcinoma in situ. J Clin Oncol Off J Am Soc Clin Oncol 27(9):1362–1367. doi:10.1200/JCO.2008.20.1681
42. King TA, Sakr R, Patil S, Gurevich I, Stempel M, Sampson M, Morrow M (2011) Clinical management factors contribute to the decision for contralateral prophylactic mastectomy. J Clin Oncol Off J Am Soc Clin Oncol 29(16):2158–2164. doi:10.1200/JCO.2010.29.4041
43. Guth U, Myrick ME, Viehl CT, Weber WP, Lardi AM, Schmid SM (2012) Increasing rates of contralateral prophylactic mastectomy – a trend made in USA? Eur J Surg Oncol J Eur Soc Surg Oncol Br Assoc Surg Oncol 38(4):296–301. doi:10.1016/j.ejso.2011.12.014
44. Yao K, Stewart AK, Winchester DJ, Winchester DP (2010) Trends in contralateral prophylactic mastectomy for unilateral cancer: a report from the National Cancer Data Base, 1998–2007. Ann Surg Oncol 17(10):2554–2562. doi:10.1245/s10434-010-1091-3
45. McLaughlin CC, Lillquist PP, Edge SB (2009) Surveillance of prophylactic mastectomy: trends in use from 1995 through 2005. Cancer 115(23):5404–5412. doi:10.1002/cncr.24623
46. Kurian AW, Lichtensztajn DY, Keegan TH, Nelson DO, Clarke CA, Gomez SL (2014) Use of and mortality after bilateral mastectomy compared with other surgical treatments for breast cancer in California, 1998–2011. JAMA 312(9):902–914. doi:10.1001/jama.2014.10707
47. Metcalfe KA, Lubinski J, Ghadirian P, Lynch H, Kim-Sing C, Friedman E, Foulkes WD, Domchek S, Ainsworth P, Isaacs C, Tung N, Gronwald J, Cummings S, Wagner T, Manoukian S, Moller P, Weitzel J, Sun P, Narod SA, Hereditary Breast Cancer Clinical Study G (2008) Predictors of contralateral prophylactic mastectomy in women with a BRCA1 or BRCA2 mutation: the Hereditary Breast Cancer Clinical Study Group. J Clin Oncol Off J Am Soc Clin Oncol 26(7):1093–1097. doi:10.1200/JCO.2007.12.6078
48. Meijers-Heijboer EJ, Verhoog LC, Brekelmans CT, Seynaeve C, Tilanus-Linthorst MM, Wagner A, Dukel L, Devilee P, van den Ouweland AM, van Geel AN, Klijn JG (2000) Presymptomatic DNA testing and prophylactic surgery in families with a BRCA1 or BRCA2 mutation. Lancet 355(9220):2015–2020
49. Evans DG, Lalloo F, Hopwood P, Maurice A, Baildam A, Brain A, Barr L, Howell A (2005) Surgical decisions made by 158 women with hereditary breast cancer aged <50 years. Eur J Surg Oncol J Eur Soc Surg Oncol Br Assoc Surg Oncol 31(10):1112–1118. doi:10.1016/j.ejso.2005.05.007
50. Koo DH, Chung IY, Kang E, Han SA, Kim SW (2011) Usage patterns of surveillance, chemoprevention and risk-reducing surgery in Korean BRCA mutation carriers: 5 years of experience at a single institution. J Breast Cancer 14(S):S17–S23. doi:10.4048/jbc.2011.14.S.S17
51. Kwong A, Chu AT (2012) What made her give up her breasts: a qualitative study on decisional considerations for contralateral prophylactic mastectomy among breast cancer survivors undergoing BRCA1/2 genetic testing. Asian Pac J Cancer Prev APJCP 13(5):2241–2247
52. Covelli AM, Baxter NN, Fitch MI, McCready DR, Wright FC (2014) 'Taking Control of Cancer': understanding women's choice for mastectomy. Ann Surg Oncol. doi:10.1245/s10434-014-4033-7
53. Hoogerbrugge N, Bult P, de Widt-Levert LM, Beex LV, Kiemeney LA, Ligtenberg MJ, Massuger LF, Boetes C, Manders P, Brunner HG (2003) High prevalence of premalignant lesions in prophylactically removed breasts from women at hereditary risk for breast cancer. J Clin Oncol Off J Am Soc Clin Oncol 21(1):41–45
54. Goldflam K, Hunt KK, Gershenwald JE, Singletary SE, Mirza N, Kuerer HM, Babiera GV, Ames FC, Ross MI, Feig BW, Sahin AA, Arun B, Meric-Bernstam F (2004) Contralateral prophylactic mastectomy. Predictors of significant histologic findings. Cancer 101(9):1977–1986. doi:10.1002/cncr.20617

55. Leunen K, Drijkoningen M, Neven P, Christiaens MR, Van Ongeval C, Legius E, Amant F, Berteloot P, Vergote I (2008) Prophylactic mastectomy in familial breast carcinoma. What do the pathologic findings learn us? Breast Cancer Res Treat 107(1):79–86. doi:10.1007/s10549-007-9525-8
56. Tuttle TM, Abbott A, Arrington A, Rueth N (2010) The increasing use of prophylactic mastectomy in the prevention of breast cancer. Curr Oncol Rep 12(1):16–21. doi:10.1007/s11912-009-0070-y
57. Frost MH, Slezak JM, Tran NV, Williams CI, Johnson JL, Woods JE, Petty PM, Donohue JH, Grant CS, Sloan JA, Sellers TA, Hartmann LC (2005) Satisfaction after contralateral prophylactic mastectomy: the significance of mastectomy type, reconstructive complications, and body appearance. J Clin Oncol Off J Am Soc Clin Oncol 23(31):7849–7856. doi:10.1200/JCO.2005.09.233
58. Geiger AM, Nekhlyudov L, Herrinton LJ, Rolnick SJ, Greene SM, West CN, Harris EL, Elmore JG, Altschuler A, Liu IL, Fletcher SW, Emmons KM (2007) Quality of life after bilateral prophylactic mastectomy. Ann Surg Oncol 14(2):686–694. doi:10.1245/s10434-006-9206-6
59. Brandberg Y, Sandelin K, Erikson S, Jurell G, Liljegren A, Lindblom A, Linden A, von Wachenfeldt A, Wickman M, Arver B (2008) Psychological reactions, quality of life, and body image after bilateral prophylactic mastectomy in women at high risk for breast cancer: a prospective 1-year follow-up study. J Clin Oncol Off J Am Soc Clin Oncol 26(24):3943–3949. doi:10.1200/JCO.2007.13.9568
60. Montgomery LL, Tran KN, Heelan MC, Van Zee KJ, Massie MJ, Payne DK, Borgen PI (1999) Issues of regret in women with contralateral prophylactic mastectomies. Ann Surg Oncol 6 (6):546–552
61. Altschuler A, Nekhlyudov L, Rolnick SJ, Greene SM, Elmore JG, West CN, Herrinton LJ, Harris EL, Fletcher SW, Emmons KM, Geiger AM (2008) Positive, negative, and disparate–women's differing long-term psychosocial experiences of bilateral or contralateral prophylactic mastectomy. Breast J 14(1):25–32. doi:10.1111/j.1524-4741.2007.00521.x
62. Sacchini V, Pinotti JA, Barros AC, Luini A, Pluchinotta A, Pinotti M, Boratto MG, Ricci MD, Ruiz CA, Nisida AC, Veronesi P, Petit J, Arnone P, Bassi F, Disa JJ, Garcia-Etienne CA, Borgen PI (2006) Nipple-sparing mastectomy for breast cancer and risk reduction: oncologic or technical problem? J Am Coll Surg 203(5):704–714. doi:10.1016/j.jamcollsurg.2006.07.015
63. Hartmann LC, Schaid DJ, Woods JE, Crotty TP, Myers JL, Arnold PG, Petty PM, Sellers TA, Johnson JL, McDonnell SK, Frost MH, Jenkins RB (1999) Efficacy of bilateral prophylactic mastectomy in women with a family history of breast cancer. N Engl J Med 340(2):77–84. doi:10.1056/NEJM199901143400201
64. Levine DA, Gemignani ML (2003) Prophylactic surgery in hereditary breast/ovarian cancer syndrome. Oncology 17(7):932–941; discussion 946-938, 950-932
65. Yao K, Liederbach E, Tang R, Lei L, Czechura T, Sisco M, Howard M, Hulick PJ, Winchester DJ, Coopey SB, Smith BL (2014) Nipple-sparing mastectomy in BRCA1/2 mutation carriers: an interim analysis and review of the literature. Ann Surg Oncol. doi:10.1245/s10434-014-3883-3
66. Kramer JL, Velazquez IA, Chen BE, Rosenberg PS, Struewing JP, Greene MH (2005) Prophylactic oophorectomy reduces breast cancer penetrance during prospective, long-term follow-up of BRCA1 mutation carriers. J Clin Oncol Off J Am Soc Clin Oncol 23 (34):8629–8635. doi:10.1200/JCO.2005.02.9199
67. Eisen A, Lubinski J, Klijn J, Moller P, Lynch HT, Offit K, Weber B, Rebbeck T, Neuhausen SL, Ghadirian P, Foulkes WD, Gershoni-Baruch R, Friedman E, Rennert G, Wagner T, Isaacs C, Kim-Sing C, Ainsworth P, Sun P, Narod SA (2005) Breast cancer risk following bilateral oophorectomy in BRCA1 and BRCA2 mutation carriers: an international case-control study. J Clin Oncol Off J Am Soc Clin Oncol 23(30):7491–7496. doi:10.1200/JCO.2004.00.7138

68. Domchek SM, Friebel TM, Neuhausen SL, Wagner T, Evans C, Isaacs C, Garber JE, Daly MB, Eeles R, Matloff E, Tomlinson GE, Van't Veer L, Lynch HT, Olopade OI, Weber BL, Rebbeck TR (2006) Mortality after bilateral salpingo-oophorectomy in BRCA1 and BRCA2 mutation carriers: a prospective cohort study. Lancet Oncol 7(3):223–229. doi:10.1016/S1470-2045(06)70585-X
69. Kauff ND, Domchek SM, Friebel TM, Robson ME, Lee J, Garber JE, Isaacs C, Evans DG, Lynch H, Eeles RA, Neuhausen SL, Daly MB, Matloff E, Blum JL, Sabbatini P, Barakat RR, Hudis C, Norton L, Offit K, Rebbeck TR (2008) Risk-reducing salpingo-oophorectomy for the prevention of BRCA1- and BRCA2-associated breast and gynecologic cancer: a multicenter, prospective study. J Clin Oncol Off J Am Soc Clin Oncol 26(8):1331–1337. doi:10.1200/JCO.2007.13.9626
70. Valachis A, Nearchou AD, Lind P (2014) Surgical management of breast cancer in BRCA-mutation carriers: a systematic review and meta-analysis. Breast Cancer Res Treat 144 (3):443–455. doi:10.1007/s10549-014-2890-1
71. National Comprehensive Cancer Network (2014) Genetic/familial high-risk assessment: breast and ovarian (version 2. 2014). NCCN clinical practice guidelines in oncology. http://www.nccn.org. Accessed 19 Nov 2014
72. Domchek SM, Friebel TM, Singer CF, Evans DG, Lynch HT, Isaacs C, Garber JE, Neuhausen SL, Matloff E, Eeles R, Pichert G, Van t'veer L, Tung N, Weitzel JN, Couch FJ, Rubinstein WS, Ganz PA, Daly MB, Olopade OI, Tomlinson G, Schildkraut J, Blum JL, Rebbeck TR (2010) Association of risk-reducing surgery in BRCA1 or BRCA2 mutation carriers with cancer risk and mortality. JAMA 304(9):967–975. doi:10.1001/jama.2010.1237
73. Narod SA, Foulkes WD (2004) BRCA1 and BRCA2: 1994 and beyond. Nat Rev Cancer 4 (9):665–676. doi:10.1038/nrc1431
74. Rubinstein WS (2005) Surgical management of BRCA1 and BRCA2 carriers: bitter choices slightly sweetened. J Clin Oncol Off J Am Soc Clin Oncol 23(31):7772–7774. doi:10.1200/JCO.2005.07.906
75. Fatouros M, Baltoyiannis G, Roukos DH (2008) The predominant role of surgery in the prevention and new trends in the surgical treatment of women with BRCA1/2 mutations. Ann Surg Oncol 15(1):21–33. doi:10.1245/s10434-007-9612-4
76. Schwartz MD, Kaufman E, Peshkin BN, Isaacs C, Hughes C, DeMarco T, Finch C, Lerman C (2003) Bilateral prophylactic oophorectomy and ovarian cancer screening following BRCA1/BRCA2 mutation testing. J Clin Oncol Off J Am Soc Clin Oncol 21(21):4034–4041. doi:10.1200/JCO.2003.01.088
77. Manchanda R, Burnell M, Abdelraheim A, Johnson M, Sharma A, Benjamin E, Brunell C, Saridogan E, Gessler S, Oram D, Side L, Rosenthal AN, Jacobs I, Menon U (2012) Factors influencing uptake and timing of risk reducing salpingo-oophorectomy in women at risk of familial ovarian cancer: a competing risk time to event analysis. BJOG 119(5):527–536. doi:10.1111/j.1471-0528.2011.03257.x
78. Madalinska JB, Hollenstein J, Bleiker E, van Beurden M, Valdimarsdottir HB, Massuger LF, Gaarenstroom KN, Mourits MJ, Verheijen RH, van Dorst EB, van der Putten H, van der Velden K, Boonstra H, Aaronson NK (2005) Quality-of-life effects of prophylactic salpingo-oophorectomy versus gynecologic screening among women at increased risk of hereditary ovarian cancer. J Clin Oncol Off J Am Soc Clin Oncol 23(28):6890–6898. doi 10.1200/JCO.2005.02.626
79. Fisher B, Anderson S, Bryant J, Margolese RG, Deutsch M, Fisher ER, Jeong JH, Wolmark N (2002) Twenty-year follow-up of a randomized trial comparing total mastectomy, lumpectomy, and lumpectomy plus irradiation for the treatment of invasive breast cancer. N Engl J Med 347(16):1233–1241. doi:10.1056/NEJMoa022152
80. Veronesi U, Cascinelli N, Mariani L, Greco M, Saccozzi R, Luini A, Aguilar M, Marubini E (2002) Twenty-year follow-up of a randomized study comparing breast-conserving surgery with radical mastectomy for early breast cancer. N Engl J Med 347(16):1227–1232. doi:10.1056/NEJMoa020989

81. Seynaeve C, Verhoog LC, van de Bosch LM, van Geel AN, Menke-Pluymers M, Meijers-Heijboer EJ, van den Ouweland AM, Wagner A, Creutzberg CL, Niermeijer MF, Klijn JG, Brekelmans CT (2004) Ipsilateral breast tumour recurrence in hereditary breast cancer following breast-conserving therapy. Eur J Cancer 40(8):1150–1158. doi:10.1016/j.ejca.2004.01.017
82. Turner BC, Harrold E, Matloff E, Smith T, Gumbs AA, Beinfield M, Ward B, Skolnick M, Glazer PM, Thomas A, Haffty BG (1999) BRCA1/BRCA2 germline mutations in locally recurrent breast cancer patients after lumpectomy and radiation therapy: implications for breast-conserving management in patients with BRCA1/BRCA2 mutations. J Clin Oncol Off J Am Soc Clin Oncol 17(10):3017–3024
83. Garcia-Etienne CA, Barile M, Gentilini OD, Botteri E, Rotmensz N, Sagona A, Farante G, Galimberti V, Luini A, Veronesi P, Bonanni B (2009) Breast-conserving surgery in BRCA1/2 mutation carriers: are we approaching an answer? Ann Surg Oncol 16(12):3380–3387. doi:10.1245/s10434-009-0638-7
84. Pierce LJ, Phillips KA, Griffith KA, Buys S, Gaffney DK, Moran MS, Haffty BG, Ben-David M, Kaufman B, Garber JE, Merajver SD, Balmana J, Meirovitz A, Domchek SM (2010) Local therapy in BRCA1 and BRCA2 mutation carriers with operable breast cancer: comparison of breast conservation and mastectomy. Breast Cancer Res Treat 121(2):389–398. doi:10.1007/s10549-010-0894-z
85. Weitzel JN, McCaffrey SM, Nedelcu R, MacDonald DJ, Blazer KR, Cullinane CA (2003) Effect of genetic cancer risk assessment on surgical decisions at breast cancer diagnosis. Arch Surg 138(12):1323–1328. doi:10.1001/archsurg.138.12.1323; discussion 1329
86. Cortesi L, Razzaboni E, Toss A, De Matteis E, Marchi I, Medici V, Tazzioli G, Andreotti A, De Santis G, Pignatti M, Federico M (2014) A rapid genetic counselling and testing in newly diagnosed breast cancer is associated with high rate of risk-reducing mastectomy in BRCA1/2-positive Italian women. Ann Oncol Off J Eur Soc Med Oncol ESMO 25(1):57–63. doi:10.1093/annonc/mdt422
87. Trainer AH, Lewis CR, Tucker K, Meiser B, Friedlander M, Ward RL (2010) The role of BRCA mutation testing in determining breast cancer therapy. Nat Rev Clin Oncol 7 (12):708–717. doi:10.1038/nrclinonc.2010.175

Chapter 2
Prophylactic Risk-Reducing Surgery for Breast Cancer

Mihir M. Shah, Holly J. Pederson, Risal Djohan, Joseph P. Crowe, and Stephen R. Grobmyer

Abstract Advances in the understanding of the genetics and biology of breast cancer are defining patients at increased risk for the development of breast cancer. Prophylactic risk-reducing mastectomy and bilateral salpingo-oophorectomy are very good options for reducing breast cancer risk in selected patients with elevated breast cancer risk. Technical approaches to prophylactic surgery are evolving and are leading to improved patient cosmetic outcomes and lower morbidity. Decisions regarding utilization of these procedures for patients should take into account a specific patient's risk for developing breast cancer based on genetic, family, and personal medical history; patient age; and comorbid conditions. Limitations of prophylactic surgical approaches, alternatives, and side effects of prophylactic operations should also be considered carefully with patients who are considering these surgical interventions for breast cancer risk reduction.

Keywords Breast cancer • Prophylactic surgery • Mastectomy • Risk reducing • Salpingo-oophorectomy • Genetic mutation • BRCA1 • BRCA2 • LCIS

M.M. Shah • H.J. Pederson • J.P. Crowe
Section of Surgical Oncology, Cleveland Clinic, 9500 Euclid Ave./A81, Cleveland, OH 44118, USA

Breast Services, Cleveland Clinic, Cleveland, OH, USA

R. Djohan
Division of Plastic and Reconstructive Surgery, Cleveland Clinic, Cleveland, OH, USA

S.R. Grobmyer (✉)
Section of Surgical Oncology, Cleveland Clinic, 9500 Euclid Ave./A81, Cleveland, OH 44118, USA

Breast Services, Cleveland Clinic, Cleveland, OH, USA

Division of Plastic and Reconstructive Surgery, Cleveland Clinic, Cleveland, OH, USA
e-mail: grobmys@ccf.org

M. Toi et al. (eds.), *Personalized Treatment of Breast Cancer*,
DOI 10.1007/978-4-431-55552-0_2

2.1 Introduction

Patients diagnosed with specific genetic mutations, including BRCA1 and BRCA2, are known to be at significantly elevated risk for developing breast cancer [1, 2]. Other patients without known genetic mutations including those with personal history of breast cancer, a strong family history of breast cancer, a history of high-risk atypical lesions of the breast, or a history of chest wall irradiation prior to age 30 [3] have also elevated risk for developing breast cancer. Options for managing risk in these patients include intensive radiographic surveillance with mammography and MRI [4], chemoprophylaxis [5], and risk-reducing surgical procedures [6].

Surgical prophylaxis is the most effective strategy for reducing risk for subsequent development of breast cancer in patients with elevated risk [7]. This chapter will focus on indications for considering prophylactic risk-reducing breast surgery in patients at elevated risk for breast cancer, surgical options, impact of surgery on breast cancer risk reduction, and factors associated with patient's selection of risk-reducing breast surgery. In addition, attention will be given to the impact of prophylactic surgery on quality of life in patients who have undergone prophylactic risk-reducing breast surgery.

2.2 Patients at Elevated Risk for Development of Breast Cancer

2.2.1 BRCA Gene Mutation Carriers and Breast Cancer Risk

Hereditary breast and ovarian cancer syndrome is caused by mutations in the BRCA1 [1] or BRCA2 gene [2]. BRCA1 and BRCA2 mutations have been estimated to be present in 1:300–1:800 members of the general population. Among patients of Ashkenazi Jewish ancestry, the frequency of BRCA1 and BRCA2 mutations has been estimated to be 1:40 [8].

Lifetime risk estimates for the development of breast cancer in BRCA1 patients have been estimated to be between 40 and 87 %, and in BRCA2 patients, the risk has been estimated to be between 40 and 84 % [7]. Risk of breast cancer substantially increases beginning at age 30 in BRCA1 and BRCA2 mutation carriers [9] (Fig. 2.1).

Newly diagnosed breast cancer patients who have a mutation in BRCA1 or BRCA2 genes are at significantly elevated risk for the development of contralateral breast cancer (RR 3.56, CI 2.5–5.08, $p < 0.001$) [10]. The 10-year risk of contralateral breast cancer development has been estimated to range between 20 and 30 % [11, 12]. Specifically, patients with BRCA1 mutation have a higher risk of contralateral breast cancer compared to patients with BRCA2 mutation (RR 1.42, CI 1.01–1.99, $p = 004$) [10]. Among patients with BRCA1 and BRCA2 mutations and a new diagnosis of breast cancer, older age at breast cancer diagnosis and the use of chemoprophylaxis have been associated with a lower risk of contralateral breast cancer [10, 13].

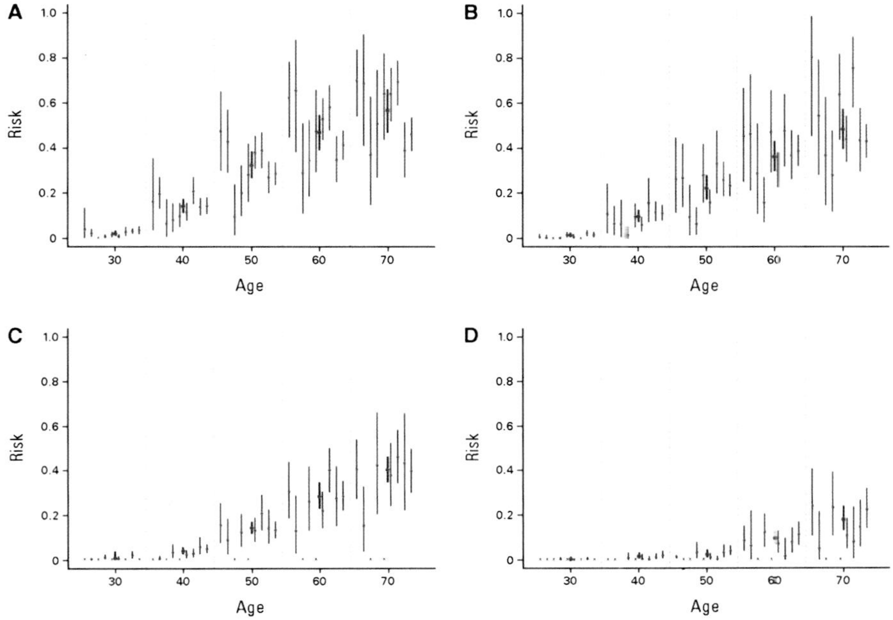

Fig. 2.1 (**a**) Breast cancer risk as a function of age for BRCA1 mutation carriers. (**b**) Breast cancer risk as a function of age for BRCA2 mutation carriers. (**c**) Ovarian cancer risk as a function of age for BRCA1 mutation carrier. (**d**) Ovarian cancer risk as a function of age for BRCA2 mutation carriers [9] (Reprinted with permission. © (2007) American Society of Clinical Oncology. All rights reserved. The authors, editors, and ASCO are not responsible for errors or omissions in the translation)

2.2.2 *Other Genetic Mutations and Breast Cancer*

Other genetic syndromes that have been associated with high risk for developing breast cancer include PTEN hamartoma tumor syndrome (PTEN) [14], Peutz-Jeghers syndrome (STK11) [15], Li-Fraumeni syndrome (TP53) [16], and hereditary diffuse gastric cancer (CDH1).

Other less common mutations have been associated with elevated breast cancer risk including CHEK2, ATM, BRIP1, PALB2, and RAD51C [8]. The breast cancer risk estimates associated with these less common mutations are highly variable (Table 2.1). When assessing risk for breast cancer (and appropriate screening or prophylactic strategies) in an individual patient with these less common mutations, strong consideration should be given to an individual's three-generation family history [17].

Table 2.1 Breast cancer risk among patients with high/moderate-risk genetic mutations [17, 77–81]

Genetic mutation	Breast cancer risk (%)
CHEK2	20–44
PALB2	33–58
ATM	16–60
CDH1	39–52
TP53	50–85
RAD51C	10–20
PTEN	67–85
STK11	8–45

2.2.3 *Lobular Neoplasia and Breast Cancer Risk*

Lobular neoplasia including atypical lobular hyperplasia (ALH) and lobular carcinoma in situ (LCIS) represents a spectrum of lesions that are associated with increased breast cancer risk [18]. ALH and LCIS are associated with a three- to fourfold and eight- to tenfold elevated risk of developing breast cancer, respectively [19, 20]. A recently reported large series of 646 patients with LCIS (median follow-up of 41.5 months) demonstrated that the risk of cancer development was 13.7 % [21]. Patients with ALH or LCIS have an elevated risk of developing breast cancer, and risk is not limited to the side of the initial diagnosis of lobular neoplasia.

2.2.4 *Patients with Unilateral Breast Cancer*

Among patients without a known genetic mutation or other high-risk history, a personal history of breast cancer is a well-established risk factor for synchronous and metachronous breast cancers. Patients with a newly diagnosed unilateral breast cancer have a 1–6 % chance of a synchronous contralateral breast cancer [22–24]. Patients with a personal history of breast cancer have an approximately 0.25–0.70 % risk per year of a metachronous contralateral breast cancer [25, 26].

2.3 Use of Prophylactic Mastectomy for Risk Reduction

Patients considering prophylactic mastectomy should receive multidisciplinary evaluation and risk assessment including genetic counseling where appropriate to clearly define the risks of breast cancer and discuss alternatives to prophylactic surgery. It has been observed that many women overestimate their true risk for breast cancer highlighting the importance of accurate and clear communication between physicians and patients [27, 28]. Decisions regarding prophylactic mastectomy should be made in the context of shared decision-making between the patient and provider [29].

2.3.1 Gene Mutation Carriers and Prophylactic Mastectomy

The use of prophylactic mastectomy for BRCA mutations has been observed to differ significantly by country [30]. Election of prophylactic mastectomy is related to age and is most common in women between 35 and 60 years old [31]. There is also international variation in the rate of contralateral prophylactic mastectomy in BRCA1 and BRCA2 mutation carriers following diagnosis of unilateral breast cancer with the highest rates observed in the United States (36.2 %) and lowest rates in Poland (2.7 %) and Israel (4.2 %) [32]. Predictors of prophylactic surgery among BRCA1 and BRCA2 mutation carriers include age <60, breast cancer history, and utilization of other risk-reducing operations [33].

2.3.2 Lobular Neoplasia and Bilateral Prophylactic Mastectomy

Historically, bilateral prophylactic mastectomy was the treatment of choice for LCIS [34]. Presently, bilateral prophylactic mastectomy is much less commonly used and is not the recommended approach for patients with LCIS for prophylaxis [35]. Prophylactic mastectomy may be a reasonable consideration for selected patients with LCIS and a strong family history or patients with a history of other high-risk breast lesions. A large SEER database study in 2009 demonstrated that ~18 % of patients with LCIS in the United States undergo prophylactic mastectomy [36].

2.3.3 Unilateral Breast Cancer and Contralateral Prophylactic Mastectomy

Concerns over risk of subsequent cancer development and other factors including cosmesis have led many patients in the United States to elect contralateral prophylactic mastectomy (CPM) in the setting of therapeutic unilateral mastectomy for breast cancer [37]. The rate of contralateral prophylactic mastectomy has been demonstrated to have increased dramatically in the last 10 years in the United States [38]. Factors associated with choice of CPM are young age at diagnosis, white race, higher education level, private insurance, preoperative MRI, care at an academic center, family history of breast cancer, and the decision to undergo breast reconstruction [35, 39]. Interestingly, the rate of CPM has not been observed to rise in other parts of the world [40]. International variation in physician attitudes toward prophylactic mastectomy has also been observed [41].

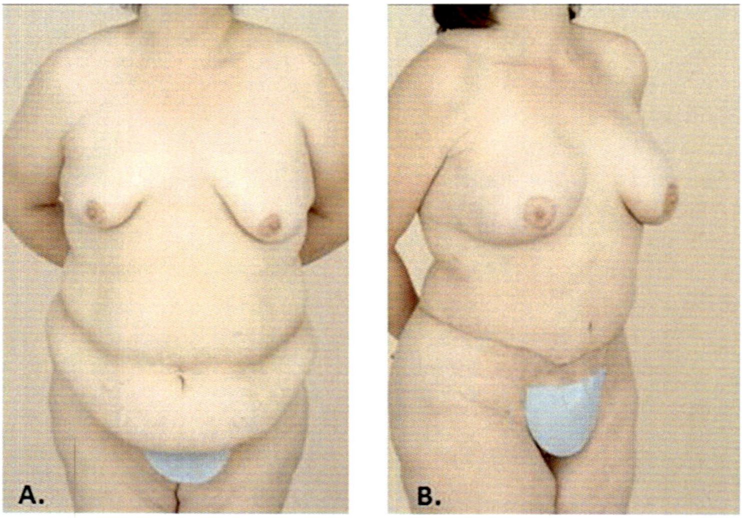

Fig. 2.2 (**a**) Preoperative photo of a patient with hereditary predisposition to breast cancer. (**b**) Postoperative photo following bilateral prophylactic mastectomy with deep inferior epigastric perforator (DIEP) flap (reconstruction)

2.4 Operative Considerations of Prophylactic Mastectomy

Traditionally, mastectomy procedures involved removal of a portion of the breast skin envelope as well as the nipple-areolar complex. Traditional approaches to mastectomy are currently performed in patients who do not desire breast reconstruction following mastectomy or in patients who prefer delayed reconstruction. In recent years, techniques have evolved to allow removal of the breast parenchyma without sacrifice of the skin envelope and/or nipple-areolar complex (i.e., nipple-sparing mastectomy or total skin-sparing mastectomy) [42]. Performance of nipple-sparing mastectomy facilitates subsequent immediate or delayed immediate breast reconstruction [43] (Fig. 2.1). Rates of breast reconstruction in BRCA1 and BRCA2 mutation carriers have been observed to vary by country [44]. Several recent series have demonstrated that nipple-sparing mastectomy is not associated with increased rate of recurrence in patients with BRCA1 and BRCA2 mutations, although oncologic follow-up in these series is relatively short [45–47].

Consideration for prophylactic mastectomy should begin at approximately age 30 in BRCA1 and BRCA2 mutation carriers as this is the time at which breast cancer risk steeply increases (Fig. 2.1).

Sentinel node biopsy is not routinely indicated in patients undergoing prophylactic mastectomy as the rates of finding histologically positive sentinel nodes associated with prophylactic mastectomy is ~1 % [22, 48, 49]. Some authors have advocated the use of preoperative breast MRI to exclude the presence of invasive

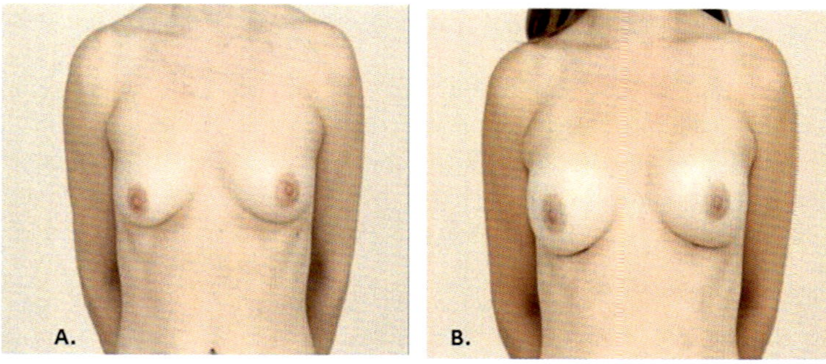

Fig. 2.3 (**a**) Preoperative photo of a patient with hereditary predisposition to breast cancer. (**b**) Postoperative photo following bilateral prophylactic mastectomy with immediate implant-based reconstruction

disease in the prophylactic mastectomy breast and hence exclude the need for sentinel node biopsy [48].

In patients undergoing prophylactic nipple-sparing mastectomy, nipple duct biopsies are helpful in evaluating the remaining nipple for the presence of any cancer or atypia [50]. However, studies have demonstrated that the incidence of a positive nipple duct biopsy in patients having prophylactic mastectomy is 1–4 % [47, 50]. BRCA1 and BRCA2 mutation patients do not have higher rates of pathologically positive nipple duct biopsies compared to non-mutation patients [47].

Overall complication rate with bilateral mastectomy with reconstruction is 10–20 % [51, 52]. Approximately half of the observed complications occur in the prophylactic mastectomy side [53]. Most common complications are hematoma, skin necrosis, cellulitis, and seroma [53]. Complications may lead to need for additional operations and loss of breast implant or even may delay delivery of necessary adjuvant therapies [54, 55]. The increased rate of complications associated with performing contralateral prophylactic mastectomy and associated potential delays in adjuvant therapy should be discussed with patients considering this option for breast cancer risk reduction [56].

2.5 Cancer Risk Reduction and Survival Associated with Prophylactic Mastectomy

Prophylactic surgery in BRCA1/2 patients reduces breast cancer risk in patients without previous breast cancer by >90 % [6, 57]. Kaas et al. have estimated that the risk of subsequent breast cancer in BRCA1 and BRCA2 mutation carriers following bilateral prophylactic mastectomy is <0.2 %/woman/year [58]. In patients without known genetic mutations determined to be at moderate to high risk for developing breast cancer, breast cancer risk reduction has similarly been reported to be ~90 % [59, 60].

In BRCA1 and BRCA2 mutation carriers with breast cancer, prophylactic surgery reduces incidence of breast cancer and may be associated with improvement in overall survival [61, 62]. Other studies have suggested that contralateral prophylactic mastectomy in BRCA1 and BRCA2 breast cancer patients has no impact on survival though follow-up in many of these studies is short and must be interpreted with caution [63].

In patients without a known genetic mutation who have unilateral mastectomy for breast cancer, contralateral prophylactic mastectomy has not been associated with improved survival, although, as expected, reduced rates of new primary metachronous breast cancer have been observed [63, 64].

2.6 Quality of Life Following Prophylactic Mastectomy

Studies have demonstrated that most high-risk women are generally satisfied with the decision to undergo bilateral prophylactic mastectomy [65, 66]. The greatest positive impact on patients undergoing prophylactic mastectomy is related to reduction in concerns over subsequent breast cancer events [67]. Negative effects on body image, sexual function, and depression in patients undergoing prophylactic mastectomy are well documented [65, 68, 69]. Others have reported patients' concerns regarding breast reconstruction, adverse body image, and insufficient information or support as common concerns among women who were dissatisfied or very dissatisfied with prophylactic mastectomy. Physician's advice as the primary reason for choosing prophylactic mastectomy has been associated with patient dissatisfaction [70, 71]. These adverse symptoms should be considered in the management of patients choosing prophylactic mastectomy. Support systems for women before, during, and after surgery are recommended for managing potential distress related to decision for prophylactic mastectomy [70, 72].

2.7 Oophorectomy and Breast Cancer Risk Reduction

Patients with BRCA1 and BRCA2 mutations are at elevated risk for the development of ovarian cancer, and prophylactic bilateral salpingo-oophorectomy (BSO) is commonly performed as it reduces the risk of developing ovarian cancer in these patients [73]. BSO also reduces the risk of breast cancer development in patients with BRCA1 and BRCA2 mutations [74, 75]. The benefit in terms of breast cancer risk reduction is related the patient age at the time of BSO, with the greatest breast cancer risk reduction observed in patients undergoing BSO before the age of 40. In patients <40 years, BSO is associated with a 64 % and 31 % breast cancer risk reduction in BRCA1 and BRCA2 mutation patients, respectively [76]. As breast cancer risk reduction is not complete with BSO, many patients in the United States with BRCA1 and BRCA2 mutations opt also for risk-reducing prophylactic mastectomy.

References

1. Miki Y, Swensen J, Shattuck-Eidens D et al (1994) A strong candidate for the breast and ovarian cancer susceptibility gene BRCA1. Science 266:66–71
2. Wooster R, Bignell G, Lancaster J et al (1995) Identification of the breast cancer susceptibility gene BRCA2. Nature 378:789–792
3. Janjan NA, Zellmer DL (1992) Calculated risk of breast cancer following mantle irradiation determined by measured dose. Cancer Detect Prev 16:273–282
4. Warner E, Hill K, Causer P et al (2011) Prospective study of breast cancer incidence in women with a BRCA1 or BRCA2 mutation under surveillance with and without magnetic resonance imaging. J Clin Oncol 29:1664–1669
5. Fisher B, Costantino JP, Wickerham DL et al (1998) Tamoxifen for prevention of breast cancer: report of the National Surgical Adjuvant Breast and Bowel Project P-1 study. J Natl Cancer Inst 90:1371–1388
6. Rebbeck TR, Friebel T, Lynch HT et al (2004) Bilateral prophylactic mastectomy reduces breast cancer risk in BRCA1 and BRCA2 mutation carriers: the PROSE Study Group. J Clin Oncol 22:1055–1062
7. Narod SA (2010) BRCA mutations in the management of breast cancer: the state of the art. Nat Rev Clin Oncol 7:702–707
8. Filippini SE, Vega A (2013) Breast cancer genes: beyond BRCA1 and BRCA2. Front Biosci (Landmark Ed) 18:1358–1372
9. Chen S, Parmigiani G (2007) Meta-analysis of BRCA1 and BRCA2 penetrance. J Clin Oncol 25:1329–1333
10. Valachis A, Nearchou AD, Lind P (2014) Surgical management of breast cancer in BRCA-mutation carriers: a systematic review and meta-analysis. Breast Cancer Res Treat 144:443–455
11. Verhoog LC, Brekelmans CT, Seynaeve C et al (2000) Contralateral breast cancer risk is influenced by the age at onset in BRCA1-associated breast cancer. Br J Cancer 83:384–386
12. Metcalfe K, Lynch HT, Ghadirian P et al (2004) Contralateral breast cancer in BRCA1 and BRCA2 mutation carriers. J Clin Oncol 22:2328–2335
13. Green L, Meric-Bernstam F (2011) Risk of ipsilateral and contralateral cancer in BRCA mutation carriers with breast cancer. Curr Breast Cancer Rep 3 151–155
14. Tan MH, Mester JL, Ngeow J et al (2012) Lifetime cancer risks in individuals with germline PTEN mutations. Clin Cancer Res 18:400–407
15. Boardman LA, Thibodeau SN, Schaid DJ et al (1998) Increased risk for cancer in patients with the Peutz-Jeghers syndrome. Ann Intern Med 128:896–899
16. Sidransky D, Tokino T, Helzlsouer K et al (1992) Inherited p53 gene mutations in breast cancer. Cancer Res 52:2984–2986
17. Euhus D (2014) Genetic testing today. Ann Surg Oncol 21:3209–3215
18. Oppong BA, King TA (2011) Recommendations for women with lobular carcinoma in situ (LCIS). Oncology (Williston Park) 25:1051-6–1058
19. Chuba PJ, Hamre MR, Yap J et al (2005) Bilateral risk for subsequent breast cancer after lobular carcinoma-in-situ: analysis of surveillance, epidemiology, and end results data. J Clin Oncol 23:5534–5541
20. Haagensen CD, Lane N, Lattes R et al (1978) Lobular neoplasia (so-called lobular carcinoma in situ) of the breast. Cancer 42:737–769

21. Oskar S, Muhsen S, Sung J et al (2011) Chemoprevention among women with lobular carcinoma in situ. Ann Surg Oncol 18:S59
22. Bunting PW, Cyr AE, Gao F et al (2014) Sentinel lymph node biopsy during prophylactic mastectomy: is there a role? J Surg Oncol 109:747–750
23. Grobmyer SR, Mortellaro VE, Marshall J et al (2008) Is there a role for routine use of MRI in selection of patients for breast-conserving cancer therapy? J Am Coll Surg 206:1045–1050; discussion 1050–2
24. King TA, Gurevich I, Sakr R et al (2011) Occult malignancy in patients undergoing contralateral prophylactic mastectomy. Ann Surg 254:2–7
25. Nichols HB, Berrington de Gonzalez A, Lacey JV Jr et al (2011) Declining incidence of contralateral breast cancer in the United States from 1975 to 2006. J Clin Oncol 29:1564–1569
26. Broet P, de la Rochefordiere A, Scholl SM et al (1995) Contralateral breast cancer: annual incidence and risk parameters. J Clin Oncol 13:1578–1583
27. Black WC, Nease RF Jr, Tosteson AN (1995) Perceptions of breast cancer risk and screening effectiveness in women younger than 50 years of age. J Natl Cancer Inst 87:720–731
28. Alexander NE, Ross J, Sumner W et al (1996) The effect of an educational intervention on the perceived risk of breast cancer. J Gen Intern Med 11:92–97
29. Rosenberg SM, Partridge AH (2014) Contralateral prophylactic mastectomy: an opportunity for shared decision making. JAMA Surg 149(6):589–590
30. Wainberg S, Husted J (2004) Utilization of screening and preventive surgery among unaffected carriers of a BRCA1 or BRCA2 gene mutation. Cancer Epidemiol Biomarkers Prev 13:1989–1995
31. Skytte AB, Gerdes AM, Andersen MK et al (2010) Risk-reducing mastectomy and salpingo-oophorectomy in unaffected BRCA mutation carriers: uptake and timing. Clin Genet 77:342–349
32. Metcalfe KA, Birenbaum-Carmeli D, Lubinski J et al (2008) International variation in rates of uptake of preventive options in BRCA1 and BRCA2 mutation carriers. Int J Cancer 122:2017–2022
33. Beattie MS, Crawford B, Lin F et al (2009) Uptake, time course, and predictors of risk-reducing surgeries in BRCA carriers. Genet Test Mol Biomarkers 13:51–56
34. Goldschmidt RA, Victor TA (1996) Lobular carcinoma in situ of the breast. Semin Surg Oncol 12:314–320
35. Burke EE, Portschy PR, Tuttle TM (2014) Prophylactic mastectomy: who needs it, when and why. J Surg Oncol 111(1):91–95
36. Portschy PR, Marmor S, Nzara R et al (2013) Trends in incidence and management of lobular carcinoma in situ: a population-based analysis. Ann Surg Oncol 20:3240–3246
37. Newman LA (2014) Contralateral prophylactic mastectomy: is it a reasonable option? JAMA 312:895–897
38. Kurian AW, Lichtensztajn DY, Keegan TH et al (2014) Use of and mortality after bilateral mastectomy compared with other surgical treatments for breast cancer in California, 1998–2011. JAMA 312:902–914
39. King TA, Sakr R, Patil S et al (2011) Clinical management factors contribute to the decision for contralateral prophylactic mastectomy. J Clin Oncol 29:2158–2164
40. Guth U, Myrick ME, Viehl CT et al (2012) Increasing rates of contralateral prophylactic mastectomy – a trend made in USA? Eur J Surg Oncol 38:296–301
41. Den Heijer M, van Asperen CJ, Harris H et al (2013) International variation in physicians' attitudes towards prophylactic mastectomy – comparison between France, Germany, the Netherlands and the United Kingdom. Eur J Cancer 49:2798–2805
42. Crowe JP Jr, Kim JA, Yetman R et al (2004) Nipple-sparing mastectomy: technique and results of 54 procedures. Arch Surg 139:148–150
43. Kronowitz SJ (2010) Delayed-immediate breast reconstruction: technical and timing considerations. Plast Reconstr Surg 125:463–474

44. Semple J, Metcalfe KA, Lynch HT et al (2013) International rates of breast reconstruction after prophylactic mastectomy in BRCA1 and BRCA2 mutation carriers. Ann Surg Oncol 20:3817–3822
45. Garcia-Etienne CA, Cody Iii HS 3rd, Disa JJ et al (2009) Nipple-sparing mastectomy: initial experience at the Memorial Sloan-Kettering Cancer Center and a comprehensive review of literature. Breast J 15:440–449
46. Reynolds C, Davidson JA, Lindor NM et al (2011) Prophylactic and therapeutic mastectomy in BRCA mutation carriers: can the nipple be preserved? Ann Surg Oncol 18:3102–3109
47. Peled AW, Irwin CS, Hwang ES et al (2014) Total skin-sparing mastectomy in BRCA mutation carriers. Ann Surg Oncol 21:37–41
48. McLaughlin SA, Stempel M, Morris EA et al (2008) Can magnetic resonance imaging be used to select patients for sentinel lymph node biopsy in prophylactic mastectomy? Cancer 112:1214–1221
49. Czyszczon IA, Roland L, Sahoo S (2012) Routine prophylactic sentinel lymph node biopsy is not indicated in women undergoing prophylactic mastectomy. J Surg Oncol 105:650–654
50. Camp MS, Coopey SB, Tang R et al (2014) Management of positive sub-areolar/nipple duct margins in nipple-sparing mastectomies. Breast J 20:402–407
51. Goldflam K, Hunt KK, Gershenwald JE et al (2004) Contralateral prophylactic mastectomy. Predictors of significant histologic findings. Cancer 101:1977–1986
52. Lostumbo L, Carbine NE, Wallace J (2010) Prophylactic mastectomy for the prevention of breast cancer. Cochrane Database Syst Rev 11:CD002748
53. Eck DL, Perdikis G, Rawal B et al (2014) Incremental risk associated with contralateral prophylactic mastectomy and the effect on adjuvant therapy. Ann Surg Oncol 21 3297–3303
54. Miller ME, Czechura T, Martz B et al (2013) Operative risks associated with contralateral prophylactic mastectomy: a single institution experience. Ann Surg Oncol 20:4113–4120
55. Osman F, Saleh F, Jackson TD et al (2013) Increased postoperative complications in bilateral mastectomy patients compared to unilateral mastectomy: an analysis of the NSQIP database. Ann Surg Oncol 20:3212–3217
56. Contant CM, Menke-Pluijmers MB, Seynaeve C et al (2002) Clinical experience of prophylactic mastectomy followed by immediate breast reconstruction in women at hereditary risk of breast cancer (HB(O)C) or a proven BRCA1 and BRCA2 germ-line mutation. Eur J Surg Oncol 28:627–632
57. Domchek SM, Friebel TM, Singer CF et al (2010) Association of risk-reducing surgery in BRCA1 or BRCA2 mutation carriers with cancer risk and mortality. JAMA 304:967–975
58. Kaas R, Verhoef S, Wesseling J et al (2010) Prophylactic mastectomy in BRCA1 and BRCA2 mutation carriers: very low risk for subsequent breast cancer. Ann Surg 251:488–492
59. Hartmann LC, Schaid DJ, Woods JE et al (1999) Efficacy of bilateral prophylactic mastectomy in women with a family history of breast cancer. N Engl J Med 340:77–84
60. McDonnell SK, Schaid DJ, Myers JL et al (2001) Efficacy of contralateral prophylactic mastectomy in women with a personal and family history of breast cancer. J Clin Oncol 19:3938–3943
61. Narod SA (2011) The impact of contralateral mastectomy on mortality in BRCA1 and BRCA2 mutation carriers with breast cancer. Breast Cancer Res Treat 128:581–583
62. Metcalfe K, Gershman S, Ghadirian P et al (2014) Contralateral mastectomy and survival after breast cancer in carriers of BRCA1 and BRCA2 mutations: retrospective analysis. BMJ 348: g226
63. Fayanju OM, Stoll CR, Fowler S et al (2014) Contralateral prophylactic mastectomy after unilateral breast cancer: a systematic review and meta-analysis. Ann Surg 260:1000–1010
64. Yao K, Winchester DJ, Czechura T et al (2013) Contralateral prophylactic mastectomy and survival: report from the National Cancer Data Base, 1998–2002. Breast Cancer Res Treat 142:465–476
65. Geiger AM, Nekhlyudov L, Herrinton LJ et al (2007) Quality of life after bilateral prophylactic mastectomy. Ann Surg Oncol 14:686–694

66. Altschuler A, Nekhlyudov L, Rolnick SJ et al (2008) Positive, negative, and disparate – women's differing long-term psychosocial experiences of bilateral or contralateral prophylactic mastectomy. Breast J 14:25–32
67. Tuttle TM, Abbott A, Arrington A et al (2010) The increasing use of prophylactic mastectomy in the prevention of breast cancer. Curr Oncol Rep 12:16–21
68. Montgomery LL, Tran KN, Heelan MC et al (1999) Issues of regret in women with contralateral prophylactic mastectomies. Ann Surg Oncol 6:546–552
69. Brandberg Y, Sandelin K, Erikson S et al (2008) Psychological reactions, quality of life, and body image after bilateral prophylactic mastectomy in women at high risk for breast cancer: a prospective 1-year follow-up study. J Clin Oncol 26:3943–3949
70. van Oostrom I, Meijers-Heijboer H, Lodder LN et al (2003) Long-term psychological impact of carrying a BRCA1/2 mutation and prophylactic surgery: a 5-year follow-up study. J Clin Oncol 21:3867–3874
71. Gahm J, Wickman M, Brandberg Y (2010) Bilateral prophylactic mastectomy in women with inherited risk of breast cancer–prevalence of pain and discomfort, impact on sexuality, quality of life and feelings of regret two years after surgery. Breast 19:462–469
72. Wasteson E, Sandelin K, Brandberg Y et al (2011) High satisfaction rate ten years after bilateral prophylactic mastectomy – a longitudinal study. Eur J Cancer Care (Engl) 20:508–513
73. Finch A, Beiner M, Lubinski J et al (2006) Salpingo-oophorectomy and the risk of ovarian, fallopian tube, and peritoneal cancers in women with a BRCA1 or BRCA2 Mutation. JAMA 296:185–192
74. Rebbeck TR, Levin AM, Eisen A et al (1999) Breast cancer risk after bilateral prophylactic oophorectomy in BRCA1 mutation carriers. J Natl Cancer Inst 91:1475–1479
75. Kauff ND, Domchek SM, Friebel TM et al (2008) Risk-reducing salpingo-oophorectomy for the prevention of BRCA1- and BRCA2-associated breast and gynecologic cancer: a multicenter, prospective study. J Clin Oncol 26:1331–1337
76. Eisen A, Lubinski J, Klijn J et al (2005) Breast cancer risk following bilateral oophorectomy in BRCA1 and BRCA2 mutation carriers: an international case-control study. J Clin Oncol 23:7491–7496
77. Antoniou AC, Casadei S, Heikkinen T et al (2014) Breast-cancer risk in families with mutations in PALB2. N Engl J Med 371:497–506
78. Goldgar DE, Healey S, Dowty JG et al (2011) Rare variants in the ATM gene and risk of breast cancer. Breast Cancer Res 13:R73
79. Lalloo F, Evans DG (2012) Familial breast cancer. Clin Genet 82:105–114
80. Mester J, Eng C (2015) Cowden syndrome: recognizing and managing a not-so-rare hereditary cancer syndrome. J Surg Oncol 111(1):125–130
81. Hearle N, Schumacher V, Menko FH et al (2006) Frequency and spectrum of cancers in the Peutz-Jeghers syndrome. Clin Cancer Res 12:3209–3215

Chapter 3
Merits and Demerits of Practice for Hereditary Breast and Ovarian Cancer Syndrome (Advices and Issues)

Hideko Yamauchi

Abstract Due to advancements of medical technology, medical management has been shifted from curative medicine to precision medicine. We could offer genetic test to estimate one's cancer risk and consider preemptive measures. There are many genetic cancer syndromes, and one of those is hereditary breast and ovarian cancer syndrome (HBOC). Practice for HBOC is required to offer medical choice for patients who have genetic mutations in BRCA1 and BRCA2. Each medical choice has merits and demerits. Those were summarized here for each process in practice for HBOC–BRCA counseling and testing, surveillance, risk reduction surgery, and chemoprevention. We, as medical professionals, should advice them those merits and demerits and support their decision-making process.

Keywords Breast cancer • BRCA • Hereditary • Genetic • Prophylactic surgery

3.1 Introduction

Hereditary breast and ovarian cancer syndrome (HBOC) is known as a syndrome that causes breast and ovarian cancer at exceptionally high rate in patients who have genetic mutations in BRCA1 and BRCA2. It is urgently required to recognize HBOC as a highly oncogenic genetic syndrome and necessary to intervene medically and socially to protect women with HBOC from its disastrous consequences. To protect the population from developing the disease, it is critical to distinguish this population and encourage them to be enrolled in regular screening and genetic counseling.

Whether people would like to know their risk, have genetic test, undergo intensive screening, or have protective strategies are their medical choice. We, as medical professionals, should offer them their medical choices and support their decision-making process. During this process, it is important to show merits and

H. Yamauchi (✉)
Department of Breast Surgical Oncology, St. Luke's International Hospital, 9-1 Akashi-cho, Chuo-ku, Tokyo 104-8560, Japan
e-mail: hideyama@luke.ac.jp

M. Toi et al. (eds.), *Personalized Treatment of Breast Cancer*,
DOI 10.1007/978-4-431-55552-0_3

demerits of BRCA testing and having advices to resolve issues during its counseling.

3.2 BRCA Counseling and Testing

Whether a client undergoes BRCA testing or not, it should be decided with well-informed process including merits and demerits of knowing test results. Counseling is very important to assess one's risk, provide information, and customize one's situation and needs.

3.2.1 Merits

It is very important to make one understand merits for knowing the information regarding HBOC and/or test result. We faced many patients who developed ovarian cancer after many years of diagnosis of breast cancer. We do not want to lose those patients without telling them the information regarding HBOC. There are clearly benefits to take the first step for HBOC management due to its high risks for developing breast and ovarian cancer [1].

Once the proband of the family is diagnosed, there is a possibility to find the carrier in other family member and save their life from preventive measures. The best merit of familiar cancer syndrome is to find all possible candidates in their family with genetic risks and place on appropriate management for preventing cancer.

3.2.2 Demerits

3.2.2.1 Analytical Validity

Test is always facing the limitation of analytical validity. One who decides to undergo test should understand the limitation of test. Studies from the European Molecular Genetics Quality Network showed that the overall error rate is 2.7 % (95 % CI 1.6–4.2 %) and analytic sensitivity is 97.1 % (95 % CI 95.2–98.5 %) [2].

For three common Ashkenazi Jewish founder mutations, the overall error rate is 0 %, and both analytical sensitivity and specificity are 100 % by the American College of Medical Genetics and Genomics and the College of American Pathologists Molecular Genetics Laboratory Survey [3].

Table 3.1 Rate of VUS (%)

Region	2002	2006	2008	2012
All	12.8	7.0	5.1	2.9
Western Europe	11.1	6.3	4.3	2.6
Central Europe	11.8	6.6	4.8	2.6
Native America	16.1	7.4	5.2	2.7
Latin America	26.1	11.2	6.6	3.9
Africa	38.6	21.0	10.9	5.0
Middle East	23.7	0.0	9.6	5.9
Asia	25.1	3.6	10.5	7.8

3.2.2.2 Variant Unknown Significance (VUS)

Result for BRCA1/2 test is qualitative, not quantitative. As a result, we receive three possible categories such as positive for deleterious mutation, negative for deleterious mutation, and genetic variant (suspected deleterious, favor polymorphism, and variant unknown significance). It is very confusing to have a result as a genetic variant, while rate of genetic variant is getting less frequent due to data accumulation [4]. We have to lead clients correctly for their clinical decision without cancer distress (Table 3.1).

3.2.2.3 Possible Risk for Negative Results

Even if BRCA test is negative, one always cannot deny the possibility of having unknown or very less frequent gene risk, and there are possible risks for breast cancer. One study from Canada showed that 1492 women who have strong family history and without BRCA mutation were followed at an average of 6.1 years and 65 women developed breast cancer [5]. The rate for developing breast cancer is four times higher than the general population in Canada. Therefore, we have to explain those limitations for the client.

3.2.2.4 Testing Cost

Cost for testing is not universal depending whether its patent is effective or not. Furthermore, its coverage is very varied depending on each countries or insurance carriers. In Japan, there is no coverage by insurance, and clients have to pay more than $3500 for BRCA testing out of their pockets. We have to advice them how effectively they can test if multiple family members are planning to have the test since single-site testing is much cheaper than initial test by full sequence.

3.2.2.5 Influence for Relatives

The one who decides to undergo test for BRCA status determination should consider influence for one's relatives. As a pretest counseling, we have to make them understand that this test result may have an impact for their relatives. BRCA genetic mutations penetrate as an autosomal dominant manner. Therefore, not all related relatives would carry this gene even if the one who tested carries this gene. After being well informed in this manner, we have to make sure how one will inform one's relatives if the result is positive and what are its barriers.

Parents who have a child with minor age should not force their child to undergo the test unless the child reaches the age when he or she can decide by himself/herself, since most related cancer will rarely occur before that age.

The result will affect also for male relatives though the data for male relatives is not well-established yet, especially for prostate and pancreatic cancer. The risk for breast cancer in BRCA-mutated male is higher than non-BRCA-mutated male [6]. BRCA2 mutation is related to higher risk for prostate (estimated relative risk: 4.65) and pancreatic cancer (estimated relative risk: 3.51) compared with non-mutated male [7, 8]. Among prostate cancer, BRCA-mutated prostate cancer had significantly higher Gleason score and more lymph node metastasis and distant metastasis [9, 10].

This may not be only for demerits since one may save their relative's life for knowing their risk. Therefore, it is very important to explain merits and demerits for relatives before a client undergoes the test.

3.2.2.6 Discriminations

There were huge anxieties for testing BRCA initially in the United States due to possibilities of discriminations for insurance and/or employment. Therefore, the Genetic Information Nondiscrimination Act (GINA) was established to protect people against discrimination in employment and health coverage {http://www.eeoc.gov/laws/types/genetic.cfm}. In Asia, while Korea provided already the system same as GINA, there is no such legal protection system yet in Japan.

3.3 Related Preventive Measures: Surveillance

- Surveillance is one of the major interventions to promote prevention. Especially for breast cancer prevention, there are mounting evidence to show improvement of survival if we can find breast cancer earlier. Same as in normal population, screening is one of the most accessible preventive measures for BRCA-mutated population. However, there are merits and demerits.

3.3.1 Merits

The benefit of screening should be survival benefit from early detection of the disease. Furthermore, screening is one of the well-accepted measures. The study showed also that surveillance by using MMG and MRI improved overall survival compared with no surveillance in BRCA1/2-mutated women [11]. For one who is diagnosed with HBOC, it is easier to accept compared with other preventive measures. Also, the cost is less compared with other preventive measures.

3.3.2 Demerits

3.3.2.1 For Ovarian Cancer Screening

While breast cancer has data for screening, there are no supporting data for ovarian cancer prevention. One study reported the clinical effectiveness of ovarian cancer screening among high-risk ovarian cancer women (BRCA-mutated women and/or family member) [12]. The combination of CA125 and transvaginal ultrasound revealed higher in the sensitivity, specificity, positive and negative predictive values (40 %, 99 %, 40 %, and 99 %, respectively), compared with each single modality by CA125 alone (50 %, 96 %, 13 %, and 99 %, respectively), pelvic exam (40 %, 98 %, 21 %, and 99 %, respectively), and transvaginal ultrasound (40 %, 90 %, 6 %, and 99 %, respectively). They concluded that it is very difficult to make the diagnosis before the advance stage. Especially ovarian cancer related with BRCA arises frequently from the epithelium of fallopian tube; it is too late even if enlarged ovary is detected by using transvaginal ultrasound. Therefore, screening of ovarian cancer for BRCA-mutated women is very limited.

3.3.2.2 Screening Modalities

Which modalities (i.e., mammogram, ultrasound, MRI) should be selected is still controversial. Studies showed that MRI has highest sensitivity compared with mammogram and US [13–16]. Therefore, MRI is recommended for screening among high-risk women in Western countries. While MRI is a well-accepted modality for high-risk screening especially in young age, data showed the effectiveness of ultrasound screening for dense breast [17]. The testing cost for ultrasound is much less compared with its for MRI and it required to consider the cost benefit.

3.3.2.3 Radiation Exposure Risk

Recently, data have proved the potential risk for cancer from radiation exposure for people who have BRCA mutation, especially for younger age, in two retrospective studies [18, 19]. Those studies collected history of past radiation exposure (i.e., diagnostic radiology including mammogram, chest X-ray) in BRCA-mutated women and concluded that women with history of radiation exposure have higher risk for developing breast cancer. On the other hand, two studies revealed that history of screening mammogram did not increase breast cancer risk [20, 21]. Theoretically, HBOC possibly increases risk for developing cancer from radiation. BRCA is a DNA repair gene such as p53. Li-Fraumeni syndrome is well known as sensitive to ionized radiation and has radiation exposure risk. Therefore, it is important to select modalities with consideration of starting age for planning screening in BRCA mutation carriers, at least until more data get accumulated.

3.4 Related Preventive Measures: Prophylactic Surgery

One of the strong preemptive strategies is prophylactic surgery. While other protective strategies for women with HBOC are chemoprevention with tamoxifen and oral contraceptives, prophylactic mastectomy or bilateral salpingo-oophorectomy is a strong strategy for women with mutated BRCA since the data confirmed the benefits.

3.4.1 Merits

Data for risk reduction mastectomy (RRM) showed clearly risk reduction in more than 90 % for breast cancer [22–29]. Survival improvement has been proven in women with BRCA1/2 mutation with prior history of unilateral breast cancer [25–27, 30–34].

Risk reduction for ovarian cancer by risk reducing salpingo-oophorectomy (RRSO) is also clear [29, 35, 36], while developing cancer after risk reduction surgery is more frequent than breast cancer since there is a peritoneal cancer incidence. Survival improvement is more prominent from ovarian cancer because ovarian cancer is very difficult to detect by surveillance and prognosis of ovarian cancer is poorer than breast cancer [29].

On the top of the risk reduction and survival benefit, there are huge advantages for psychological effect. Studies for 90 Swedish women who underwent bilateral mastectomy showed they experience no negative effect on anxiety and quality of life [37]. For analysis in Jewish women who are known to have high prevalence of BRCA, prophylactic surgery caused less distress [38].

3.4.2 Demerits

3.4.2.1 Physical Consequences (i.e., Artificial Menopause, Nipple Sensation)

Although surgery can reduce risk for developing cancer, there are several physical consequences, and women who consider these preventive measures have to be aware of those demerits. Postsurgical menopause is one of the significant consequences. Compared with breast, ovary is very important for producing hormone. Depending on the age, severity of menopausal symptoms may differ Hormone replacement therapy can be used for lowering symptoms [39]. One case control study showed that women with BRCA mutation did not have higher risk for developing breast cancer with hormone replacement therapy compared with control [40]. However, risks for breast cancer should be considered [41].

While breasts can be reconstructed, sensation of the skin and nipple would be diminished. Those consequences should be managed by team approach with gynecological physicians, nurse, psychologists, and others.

3.4.2.2 Psychological Influence

One's body image and esteem would be influenced from surgery.

One interesting study showed that women with RRSO had more physical morbidity and less psychological distress compared with controls [42].

3.4.2.3 Occult Cancer

Rates of occult cancer after risk-reducing mastectomy were reported and ranged from 5.0 to 25.6 % [43–46]. Range may differ whether lobular carcinoma in situ (LCIS) was included for occult cancer and subjects were limited only for BRCA-positive candidates. One paper examined the use of sentinel lymph node biopsy in case of prophylactic surgery [43]. We have to consider indication for axillary lymph node evaluation carefully because invasive cancer would be found in prophylactic specimens even if thorough radiological evaluations were done preoperatively (Table 3.2).

Occult cancer rate for ovarian cancer after RRSO was higher in BRCA1 compared with BRCA2 status since BRCA1 has higher prevalence for ovarian cancer [47–55]. Older age had risk for higher incidence for occult cancer, especially for ovarian cancer [47, 54]. Cancer is found not only in the ovary but also in tubal and peritoneal locations. Therefore, careful examination of the fallopian tube and peritoneum is required.

Data would be different how rigorously specimens after risk reduction surgery were examined. However, whether occult cancer would be diagnosed will affect treatment options, and one's prognosis is recommended for thorough pathological examination even for prophylactic specimens (Table 3.3).

Table 3.2 Rate of occult cancer after RRM

		Rate (%)	Total	Occult cancer	Subject
2003	Hoogerbrugge	25.6	1089	28 (IDC:1, DCIS:10, LCIS:17)	High risk including BRCA +(66 %)
2006	Boughey	5.0	436	22 (IDC:8, DCIS:14)	High risk including BRCA +(11 %)
2013	Evans	5.7	105	6 (IDC:4, DCIS:2)	BRCA+ with history of breast cancer
2013	Burger	5.0	83	4 (IDC:1, LCIS:3)	High risk including BRCA +(14 %)

Table 3.3 Rate of occult cancer after RRSO

		Rate	Total	Occult cancer	Subject
2002	Scheuer	2.2 %	90	2	BRCA+
2006	Finch	4.4 % (BRCA1:6.4, BRCA2:1.5)	159	7	BRCA +
2010	Domchek	2.5 %	647	16 (12BRCA1)	BRCA+
2011	Manvhanda	5.1 %	308	14	High risk including BRCA +(38 %)
2011	Powell	9.1 %	111	10	BRCA +
2011	Rabban	8.2 %	134	11	BRCA +
2011	Yates	7.9 %			BRCA +
2013	Reitsma	1.3 %	360		High risk including BRCA +(84 %)
2014	Sherman	2.6 % (BRCA1:4.6, BRCA2:3.5)	966	25	High risk including BRCA +

3.4.2.4 Community Consensus

While prophylactic surgery is one of the established options for high-risk women in Western countries, it is not accepted well in Asian communities, including Japan. It is urgently required to establish consensus and support system for risk reduction surgery in Asian communities.

3.5 Related Preventive Measures: Chemoprevention

Chemoprevention is one of the strategies to prevent cancer. Trials have been done for prevention in non-mutated populations. Currently, effectiveness of chemoprevention was 50 % of reduction as reported. Compred with the rate from risk-reducing surgery, this reduction rate is less. Due to advancement of medical technology, one can estimate one's risk and type of risk; we may be able to stratify chemoprevention measures in more personalized way.

3.5.1 *Merits*

- Data showed clearly the effectiveness for risk reduction. Tamoxifen is effective in 49 % reduction of breast cancer incidence in high-risk women [56]. A study showed that risk of contralateral breast cancer reduced more than 50 % in carriers when tamoxifen was given as treatment for initial breast cancer [57–59]. These data were confirmed also for BRCA-mutated candidates [60]. In the NSABP study of tamoxifen and raloxifene P-2 trial, same effect was confirmed by using raloxifene for chemoprevention [61].
- Oral contraceptives showed 40 % reduction in risk of ovarian cancer in the Cancer and Steroid Hormone Study [62]. For BRCA carriers, some reduction of ovarian cancer was noted, while there are concerns in the possibility of increased risk for breast cancer [63, 64].

3.5.2 *Demerits*

Drug administration would always have side effects from drug. It is required to give enough information for clients since medicine of chemoprevention is for prophylactic measure, not for curative measure.

3.6 Conclusion

Medicine has been advancing continuously. We hope that there would be better strategies for BRCA carriers to prevent cancer or cancer would be eliminated in the near future. In the meantime, physicians involved in women's health should discuss which strategies are best for women, and we should offer whichever best strategies to prevent the disastrous consequences.

References

1. Robson M, Offit K (2007) Clinical practice. Management of an inherited predisposition to breast cancer. N Engl J Med 357:154–162
2. Mueller CR, Kristoffersson U, Stoppa-Lyonnet D (2004) External quality assessment for mutation detection in the BRCA1 and BRCA2 genes: EMQN's experience of 3 years. Ann Oncol 15(Suppl 1):I14–I17
3. Tafe LJ, Datto MB, Palomaki GE, Lacbawan FL (2015) Molecular testing for the BRCA1 and BRCA2 Ashkenazi Jewish founder mutations: a report on the College of American Pathologists proficiency testing surveys. Genet Med 17:58–62

4. Eggington JM, Bowles KR, Moyes K, Manley S, Esterling L, Sizemore S et al (2014) A comprehensive laboratory-based program for classification of variants of uncertain significance in hereditary cancer genes. Clin Genet 86:229–237
5. Metcalfe KA, Finch A, Poll A, Horsman D, Kim-Sing C, Scott J et al (2009) Breast cancer risks in women with a family history of breast or ovarian cancer who have tested negative for a BRCA1 or BRCA2 mutation. Br J Cancer 100:421–425
6. Tai YC, Domchek S, Parmigiani G, Chen S (2007) Breast cancer risk among male BRCA1 and BRCA2 mutation carriers. J Natl Cancer Inst 99:1811–1814
7. Breast Cancer Linkage Consortium (1999) Cancer risks in BRCA2 mutation carriers. J Natl Cancer Inst 91:1310–1316
8. Liede A, Karlan BY, Narod SA (2004) Cancer risks for male carriers of germline mutations in BRCA1 or BRCA2: a review of the literature. J Clin Oncol 22:735–742
9. Thorne H, Willems AJ, Niedermayr E, Hoh IM, Li J, Clouston D et al (2011) Decreased prostate cancer-specific survival of men with BRCA2 mutations from multiple breast cancer families. Cancer Prev Res (Phila) 4:1002–1010
10. Castro E, Goh C, Olmos D, Saunders E, Leongamornlert D, Tymrakiewicz M, et al (2013) Germline BRCA mutations are associated with higher risk of nodal involvement, distant metastasis, and poor survival outcomes in prostate cancer. J Clin Oncol 31:1748–1757
11. Evans DG, Kesavan N, Lim Y, Gadde S, Hurley E, Massat NJ et al (2014) MRI breast screening in high-risk women: cancer detection and survival analysis. Breast Cancer Res Treat 145:663–672
12. Olivier RI, Lubsen-Brandsma MA, Verhoef S, van Beurden M (2006) CA125 and transvaginal ultrasound monitoring in high-risk women cannot prevent the diagnosis of advanced ovarian cancer. Gynecol Oncol 100:20–26
13. Sardanelli F, Podo F, Santoro F, Manoukian S, Bergonzi S, Trecate G et al (2010) Multicenter surveillance of women at high genetic breast cancer risk using mammography, ultrasonography, and contrast-enhanced magnetic resonance imaging (the high breast cancer risk italian 1 study): final results. Invest Radiol. 46:94–105
14. Kuhl C, Weigel S, Schrading S, Arand B, Bieling H, Konig R et al (2010) Prospective multicenter cohort study to refine management recommendations for women at elevated familial risk of breast cancer: the EVA trial. J Clin Oncol 28:1450–1457
15. Leach MO, Boggis CR, Dixon AK, Easton DF, Eeles RA, Evans DG et al (2005) Screening with magnetic resonance imaging and mammography of a UK population at high familial risk of breast cancer: a prospective multicentre cohort study (MARIBS). Lancet 365:1769–1778
16. Rijnsburger AJ, Obdeijn IM, Kaas R, Tilanus-Linthorst MM, Boetes C, Loo CE et al (2010) BRCA1-associated breast cancers present differently from BRCA2-associated and familial cases: long-term follow-up of the Dutch MRISC Screening Study. J Clin Oncol 28:5265–5273
17. Crystal P, Strano SD, Shcharynski S, Koretz MJ (2003) Using sonography to screen women with mammographically dense breasts. AJR Am J Roentgenol 181:177–182
18. Pijpe A, Andrieu N, Easton DF, Kesminiene A, Cardis E, Nogues C et al (2012) Exposure to diagnostic radiation and risk of breast cancer among carriers of BRCA1/2 mutations: retrospective cohort study (GENE-RAD-RISK). BMJ 345:e5660
19. Andrieu N, Easton DF, Chang-Claude J, Rookus MA, Brohet R, Cardis E et al (2006) Effect of chest X-rays on the risk of breast cancer among BRCA1/2 mutation carriers in the international BRCA1/2 carrier cohort study: a report from the EMBRACE, GENEPSO, GEO-HEBON, and IBCCS Collaborators' Group. J Clin Oncol 24:3361–3366
20. Narod SA, Lubinski J, Ghadirian P, Lynch HT, Moller P, Foulkes WD et al (2006) Screening mammography and risk of breast cancer in BRCA1 and BRCA2 mutation carriers: a case-control study. Lancet Oncol 7:402–406
21. Giannakeas V, Lubinski J, Gronwald J, Moller P, Armel S, Lynch HT et al (2014) Mammography screening and the risk of breast cancer in BRCA1 and BRCA2 mutation carriers: a prospective study. Breast Cancer Res Treat 147:113–118

22. Hartmann LC, Schaid DJ, Woods JE, Crotty TP, Myers JL, Arnold PG et al (1999) Efficacy of bilateral prophylactic mastectomy in women with a family history of breast cancer. N Engl J Med 340:77–84
23. Hartmann LC, Sellers TA, Schaid DJ, Frank TS, Soderberg CL, Sitta DL et al (2001) Efficacy of bilateral prophylactic mastectomy in BRCA1 and BRCA2 gene mutation carriers. J Natl Cancer Inst 93:1633–1637
24. Meijers-Heijboer H, van Geel B, van Putten WL, Henzen-Logmans SC, Seynaeve C, Menke-Pluymers MB et al (2001) Breast cancer after prophylactic bilateral mastectomy in women with a BRCA1 or BRCA2 mutation. N Engl J Med 345:159–164
25. Metcalfe K, Gershman S, Ghadirian P, Lynch HT, Snyder C, Tung N et al (2014) Contralateral mastectomy and survival after breast cancer in carriers of BRCA1 and BRCA2 mutations: retrospective analysis. BMJ 348:g226
26. Evans DG, Ingham SL, Baildam A, Ross GL, Lalloo F, Buchan I et al (2013) Contralateral mastectomy improves survival in women with BRCA1/2-associated breast cancer. Breast Cancer Res Treat 140:135–142
27. van Sprundel TC, Schmidt MK, Rookus MA, Brohet R, van Asperen CJ, Rutgers EJ et al (2005) Risk reduction of contralateral breast cancer and survival after contralateral prophylactic mastectomy in BRCA1 or BRCA2 mutation carriers. Br J Cancer 93:287–292
28. Kaas R, Verhoef S, Wesseling J, Rookus MA, Oldenburg HS, Peeters MJ et al (2010) Prophylactic mastectomy in BRCA1 and BRCA2 mutation carriers: very low risk for subsequent breast cancer. Ann Surg 251:488–492
29. Domchek SM, Friebel TM, Singer CF, Evans DG, Lynch HT, Isaacs C et al (2010) Association of risk-reducing surgery in BRCA1 or BRCA2 mutation carriers with cancer risk and mortality. JAMA 304:967–975
30. Heemskerk-Gerritsen BA, Rookus MA, Aalfs CM, Ausems MG, Collee JM, Jansen L et al (2015) Improved overall survival after contralateral risk-reducing mastectomy in BRCA1/2 mutation carriers with a history of unilateral breast cancer: a prospective analysis. Int J Cancer 136:668–677
31. Boughey JC, Hoskin TL, Degnim AC, Sellers TA, Johnson JL, Kasner MJ et al (2010) Contralateral prophylactic mastectomy is associated with a survival advantage in high-risk women with a personal history of breast cancer. Ann Surg Oncol 17:2702–2709
32. Bedrosian I, Hu CY, Chang GJ (2010) Population-based study of contralateral prophylactic mastectomy and survival outcomes of breast cancer patients. J Natl Cancer Inst 102:401–409
33. Herrinton LJ, Barlow WE, Yu O, Geiger AM, Elmore JG, Barton MB et al (2005) Efficacy of prophylactic mastectomy in women with unilateral breast cancer: a cancer research network project. J Clin Oncol 23:4275–4286
34. Peralta EA, Ellenhorn JD, Wagman LD, Dagis A, Andersen JS, Chu DZ (2000) Contralateral prophylactic mastectomy improves the outcome of selected patients undergoing mastectomy for breast cancer. Am J Surg 180:439–445
35. Rebbeck TR, Lynch HT, Neuhausen SL, Narod SA, Van't Veer L, Garber JE et al (2002) Prophylactic oophorectomy in carriers of BRCA1 or BRCA2 mutations. N Engl J Med 346:1616–1622
36. Kauff ND, Satagopan JM, Robson ME, Scheuer L, Hensley M, Hudis CA et al (2002) Risk-reducing salpingo-oophorectomy in women with a BRCA1 or BRCA2 mutation. N Engl J Med 346:1609–1615
37. Brandberg Y, Sandelin K, Erikson S, Jurell G, Liljegren A, Lindblom A et al (2008) Psychological reactions, quality of life, and body image after bilateral prophylactic mastectomy in women at high risk for breast cancer: a prospective 1-year follow-up study. J Clin Oncol 26:3943–3949
38. Metcalfe KA, Mian N, Enmore M, Poll A, Llacuachaqui M, Nanda S et al (2012) Long-term follow-up of Jewish women with a BRCA1 and BRCA2 mutation who underwent population genetic screening. Breast Cancer Res Treat 133:735–740

39. Finch A, Metcalfe KA, Chiang JK, Elit L, McLaughlin J, Springate C et al (2011) The impact of prophylactic salpingo-oophorectomy on menopausal symptoms and sexual function in women who carry a BRCA mutation. Gynecol Oncol 121:163–168
40. Eisen A, Lubinski J, Gronwald J, Moller P, Lynch HT, Klijn J et al (2008) Hormone therapy and the risk of breast cancer in BRCA1 mutation carriers. J Natl Cancer Inst 100:1361–1367
41. Finch A, Evans G, Narod SA (2012) BRCA carriers, prophylactic salpingo-oophorectomy and menopause: clinical management considerations and recommendations. Womens Health (Lond Engl) 8:543–555
42. Michelsen TM, Dorum A, Dahl AA (2009) A controlled study of mental distress and somatic complaints after risk-reducing salpingo-oophorectomy in women at risk for hereditary breast ovarian cancer. Gynecol Oncol 113:128–133
43. Boughey JC, Khakpour N, Meric-Bernstam F, Ross MI, Kuerer HM, Singletary SE et al (2006) Selective use of sentinel lymph node surgery during prophylactic mastectomy. Cancer 107:1440–1447
44. Evans DG, Howell A, Ingham SL, Buchan I (2013) Contralateral breast cancer risk in BRCA1/2-positive families needs to be adjusted for phenocopy rates particularly in second-degree untested relatives. Breast Cancer Res 15:401
45. Burger A, Thurtle D, Owen S, Mannu G, Pilgrim S, Vinayagam R et al (2013) Sentinel lymph node biopsy for risk-reducing mastectomy. Breast J. 19:529–532
46. Hoogerbrugge N, Bult P, de Widt-Levert LM, Beex LV, Kiemeney LA, Ligtenberg MJ et al (2003) High prevalence of premalignant lesions in prophylactically removed breasts from women at hereditary risk for breast cancer. J Clin Oncol 21:41–45
47. Finch A, Shaw P, Rosen B, Murphy J, Narod SA, Colgan TJ (2006) Clinical and pathologic findings of prophylactic salpingo-oophorectomies in 159 BRCA1 and BRCA2 carriers. Gynecol Oncol 100:58–64
48. Powell CB, Chen LM, McLennan J, Crawford B, Zaloudek C, Rabban JT et al (2011) Risk-reducing salpingo-oophorectomy (RRSO) in BRCA mutation carriers: experience with a consecutive series of 111 patients using a standardized surgical-pathological protocol. Int J Gynecol Cancer 21:846–851
49. Scheuer L, Kauff N, Robson M, Kelly B, Barakat R, Satagopan J et al (2002) Outcome of preventive surgery and screening for breast and ovarian cancer in BRCA mutation carriers. J Clin Oncol 20:1260–1268
50. Yates MS, Meyer LA, Deavers MT, Daniels MS, Keeler ER, Mok SC et al (2011) Microscopic and early-stage ovarian cancers in BRCA1/2 mutation carriers: building a model for early BRCA-associated tumorigenesis. Cancer Prev Res (Phila) 4:463–470
51. Rabban JT, Mackey A, Powell CB, Crawford B, Zaloudek CJ, Chen LM (2011) Correlation of macroscopic and microscopic pathology in risk reducing salpingo-oophorectomy: implications for intraoperative specimen evaluation. Gynecol Oncol 121:466–471
52. Domchek SM, Friebel TM, Garber JE, Isaacs C, Matloff E, Eeles R et al (2010) Occult ovarian cancers identified at risk-reducing salpingo-oophorectomy in a prospective cohort of BRCA1/2 mutation carriers. Breast Cancer Res Treat 124:195–203
53. Reitsma W, de Bock GH, Oosterwijk JC, Bart J, Hollema H, Mourits MJ (2013) Support of the 'fallopian tube hypothesis' in a prospective series of risk-reducing salpingo-oophorectomy specimens. Eur J Cancer 49:132–141
54. Sherman ME, Piedmonte M, Mai PL, Ioffe OB, Ronnett BM, Van Le L et al (2014) Pathologic findings at risk-reducing salpingo-oophorectomy: primary results from Gynecologic Oncology Group Trial GOG-0199. J Clin Oncol 32:3275–3283
55. Manchanda R, Abdelraheim A, Johnson M, Rosenthal AN, Benjamin E, Brunell C et al (2011) Outcome of risk-reducing salpingo-oophorectomy in BRCA carriers and women of unknown mutation status. BJOG 118:814–824
56. Fisher B, Costantino JP, Wickerham DL, Redmond CK, Kavanah M, Cronin WM et al (1998) Tamoxifen for prevention of breast cancer: report of the National Surgical Adjuvant Breast and Bowel Project P-1 Study. J Natl Cancer Inst 90:1371–1388

57. Phillips KA, Milne RL, Rookus MA, Daly MB, Antoniou AC, Peock S et al (2013) Tamoxifen and risk of contralateral breast cancer for BRCA1 and BRCA2 mutation carriers. J Clin Oncol 31:3091–3099
58. Pierce LJ, Levin AM, Rebbeck TR, Ben-David MA, Friedman E, Solin LJ et al (2006) Ten-year multi-institutional results of breast-conserving surgery and radiotherapy in BRCA1/2-associated stage I/II breast cancer. J Clin Oncol 24:2437–2443
59. Gronwald J, Tung N, Foulkes WD, Offit K, Gershoni R, Daly M et al (2006) Tamoxifen and contralateral breast cancer in BRCA1 and BRCA2 carriers: an update. Int J Cancer 118:2281–2284
60. King MC, Wieand S, Hale K, Lee M, Walsh T, Owens K et al (2001) Tamoxifen and breast cancer incidence among women with inherited mutations in BRCA1 and BRCA2: National Surgical Adjuvant Breast and Bowel Project (NSABP-P1) Breast Cancer Prevention Trial. JAMA 286:2251–2256
61. Vogel VG, Costantino JP, Wickerham DL, Cronin WM, Cecchini RS, Atkins JN et al (2010) Update of the National Surgical Adjuvant Breast and Bowel Project Study of Tamoxifen and Raloxifene (STAR) P-2 Trial: Preventing breast cancer. Cancer Prev Res (Phila) 3:696–706
62. The Cancer and Steroid Hormone Study of the Centers for Disease Control and the National Institute of Child Health and Human Development (1987) The reduction in risk of ovarian cancer associated with oral-contraceptive use. The Cancer and Steroid Hormone Study of the Centers for Disease Control and the National Institute of Child Health and Human Development. N Engl J Med 316:650–655
63. Narod SA, Dube MP, Klijn J, Lubinski J, Lynch HT, Ghadirian P et al (2002) Oral contraceptives and the risk of breast cancer in BRCA1 and BRCA2 mutation carriers. J Natl Cancer Inst 94:1773–1779
64. Narod SA, Risch H, Moslehi R, Dorum A, Neuhausen S, Olsson H et al (1998) Oral contraceptives and the risk of hereditary ovarian cancer. Hereditary Ovarian Cancer Clinical Study Group. N Engl J Med 339:424–428

Part II
Axillary Treatment

Chapter 4
Sentinel Lymph Node Biopsy and Neoadjuvant Chemotherapy in Breast Cancer Patients

John R. Benson

Abstract Patient selection and timing of sentinel lymph node (SLN) biopsy in the context of primary chemotherapy continues to evolve; there is some evidence that primary chemotherapy may modify lymphatic drainage patterns and cause differential downstaging between sentinel and non-sentinel lymph nodes. SLN biopsy undertaken prior to chemotherapy will minimise the risk of a false-negative result, may allow more accurate initial staging and provides important information on prognostication which can guide decisions about adjuvant radiotherapy. However, quantification of regional metastatic load is incomplete, and some advocate SLN biopsy after primary chemotherapy to take advantage of nodal downstaging and avoidance of axillary dissection in up to 40 % of patients. Initial reports on false-negative rates for SLN biopsy after primary chemotherapy in patients who had proven axillary node metastases at presentation based on needle core biopsy were relatively high and a cause for clinical concern. However, more recent data suggest that SLN biopsy is as accurate when performed post- as pre-neoadjuvant chemotherapy, and current practice incorporates both approaches.

Keywords Breast cancer • Neoadjuvant chemotherapy • Post-chemotherapy • Sentinel lymph node biopsy

4.1 Introduction

The technique of sentinel lymph node (SLN) biopsy is now widely practised in many centres around the world and has become standard of care with reduction of upper limb morbidity such as lymphoedema, shoulder stiffness and chronic pain which are commonly linked to axillary lymph node dissection [1, 2]. A review by the American Society of Clinical Oncology Technology Assessment panel reaffirmed that dual localisation techniques with a combination of blue dye and

J.R. Benson (✉)
Cambridge Breast Unit, Addenbrooke's Hospital and University of Cambridge, Hills Road, Cambridge CB2 0QQ, UK
e-mail: john.benson@addenbrookes.nhs.uk

M. Toi et al. (eds.), *Personalized Treatment of Breast Cancer*,
DOI 10.1007/978-4-431-55552-0_4

isotope maximise identification rates (>90 %) and are associated with high negative predictive values (>95 %) and a short learning curve [3]. Overall false-negative rates are between 5 and 10 % (mean 8.4 %) and are minimised by intraoperative digital examination and removal of nodes which are suspicious but neither hot nor blue. Though there is international consensus that a combination of dye and isotope is optimal for localisation of sentinel node(s), much variation exists in details of methodology, and there is an urgent need for standardisation of techniques to maximise sensitivity and specificity [4]. The NSABP B32 study is the largest of five randomised controlled trials comparing sentinel lymph node biopsy to conventional ALND in clinically node-negative breast cancer patients. With a mean follow-up of 96 months, no significant differences in the primary endpoints of overall survival, disease-free survival and regional control were reported, and SLN biopsy was declared a safe, accurate and effective method for staging clinically node-negative patients [5].

Patient selection and the timing of SLN biopsy in the context of primary chemotherapy continues to evolve as increasing numbers of patients undergo this modality sequence. Before the advent of SLN biopsy, all neoadjuvant chemotherapy patients had an ALND as definitive and standard treatment of regional nodes. The pretreatment status of axillary nodes was unknown, and it was recognised that some node-positive patients became node negative following primary chemotherapy consequent to nodal downstaging. Therefore, neoadjuvant therapy did not influence surgical treatment in terms of the axillary procedure as ALND remained standard of care irrespective of the primary treatment approach.

Following introduction of SLN biopsy, primary surgical patients could potentially avoid ALND, but neoadjuvant patients were obligated to undergo ALND despite a favourable breast tumour response which might render a patient suitable for breast-conserving surgery (BCS). A dichotomy of practice emerged in efforts to define how SLN biopsy should be optimally incorporated into the neoadjuvant setting. Some breast units opted for SLN biopsy in conjunction with completion ALND *after* chemotherapy. This practice was incorporated into prospective trials to assess the safety and accuracy of SLN biopsy following a period of induction chemotherapy which might potentially alter patterns of lymphatic drainage in the axilla and increase false-negative rates. These latter concerns led others to recommend an upfront SLN biopsy performed *prior* to initiation of chemotherapy. The intrinsic accuracy of this technique in terms of parameters such as SLN identification rates and false-negative rates would be no different to patients having primary surgical treatment.

Patients undergoing neoadjuvant chemotherapy now receive less extensive axillary surgery, and this is consistent with a shift in neoadjuvant strategy from inoperable to operable disease. No imaging modality can detect subclinical nodal involvement, but preoperative axillary ultrasound can identify suspicious nodes and in conjunction with percutaneous biopsy (core biopsy or fine needle aspiration) can detect up to 40 % of node-positive cases overall and in 75 % of cases with multiple (>4) involved nodes [6–8]. Neoadjuvant chemotherapy patients are more likely to be clinically node positive or clinically node negative with suspicious nodes sonographically. Therefore, preoperative axillary ultrasound (with or without node biopsy) is particularly important for this group of patients in terms of deselection for SLN biopsy.

4.2 Sentinel Lymph Node Biopsy Prior to Neoadjuvant Chemotherapy

Advantages – When SLN biopsy is undertaken prior to neoadjuvant chemotherapy, there will be minimal risk of an unacceptably high false-negative result, and information derived from SLN biopsy allows more accurate initial staging of patients [9–12]. Identification rates for an upfront approach are high and range from 98 to 100 % which is consistent with more extensive surgical experience of SLN biopsy pretreatment. Nodal positivity rates are variable (29–67 %) and reflect the heterogeneous nature of the primary tumours within most of these studies which confirm that SLN biopsy has satisfactory performance characteristics for larger tumours [13, 14]. A positive SLN biopsy result would prompt a subsequent ALND following neoadjuvant chemotherapy. By contrast, when the SLN is negative, no further axillary surgery is indicated, and completion ALND can be safely avoided at time of definitive surgery, be this wide local excision, simple mastectomy or mastectomy with immediate breast reconstruction [5]. Upfront SLN biopsy provides important information on prognostication and can guide treatment decisions for adjuvant radiotherapy, systemic therapy and axillary surgery. Although knowledge of the SLN status at presentation may influence decisions on irradiation of regional nodes, precise nodal quantification of axillary metastatic load with an upfront approach is limited; for example, a single positive node only may be retrieved at the time of SLN biopsy, but multiple nodes may be positive despite an innocent ultrasound examination of the axilla. This may be sufficient information alone to justify postmastectomy radiotherapy but not irradiation of the supraclavicular fossa which is presaged on involvement of at least four axillary nodes at presentation [15]. Any non-sentinel nodes containing tumour at the outset may be downstaged by chemotherapy and prior malignant involvement indicated by the presence of fibrosis on subsequent histopathological examination. Some advocate SLN biopsy after induction chemotherapy to take advantage of nodal downstaging and avoidance of ALND in some patients. Knowledge of pretreatment nodal status potentially influences the decision of whether or not to give chemotherapy if the primary tumour is relatively small and may also partly determine the type of chemotherapy and whether to include a taxane-based regimen (with or without an anthracycline). In addition to established clinicopathological factors, molecular tests can assess estimated risk of recurrence in patients with early stage breast cancer. Oncotype DX is one such prognostic test and is approved for clinical usage in many countries. This molecular test measures expression of a 21-gene profile with reverse transcriptase-polymerase chain reaction which does not require fresh frozen tissue and can be performed on paraffin-embedded tumour tissue [16]. Patients with larger tumours and a confirmed negative SLN biopsy but low score on Oncotype DX could be treated with neoadjuvant hormonal therapy rather than chemotherapy. However, although prognostic tests provide information about risk of recurrence and death, predictive markers are needed to select optimum therapy for individual patients.

Disadvantages – An upfront approach requires an additional operation for all patients undergoing neoadjuvant chemotherapy, irrespective of final nodal status. Nonetheless, it should be noted that selected node-positive patients will also need additional surgery when SLN biopsy follows chemotherapy and facilities for intraoperative node assessment are not available (completion ALND must then be carried out as a delayed procedure at a separate surgical sitting). Concerns have been expressed about possible delays in commencement of chemotherapy treatment when an upfront SLN biopsy policy is employed, with delays consequent to either scheduling issues or wound complications such as seromas and infection. In an audit undertaken in the author's unit of 24 clinically node-negative patients with tumours <5 cm undergoing SLN biopsy prior to chemotherapy, timeframes from diagnosis to SLN biopsy and start of chemotherapy were analysed [17]. The mean time from tissue diagnosis to SLN biopsy was 7.3 days [range 5–22 days], whilst the mean time from SLN biopsy to start of chemotherapy was 9.2 days [range 2–23 days]. The mean time interval from tissue diagnosis to start of chemotherapy was 16.5 days [range 13–25 days]. This time interval in excess of 2 weeks is significantly longer than the average time period of 8.3 days for the group of patients not undergoing SLN biopsy [t-Test, $p = 0.00002$]. However, such a delay is unlikely to be detrimental to outcome in the context of patients with clinically and sonographically node-negative disease. Amongst this group of 24 patients, one developed a wound infection subsequent to commencement of chemotherapy within 4 days of SLN biopsy. It may be prudent to wait at least 7 days from the time of SLN biopsy before starting chemotherapy and consider surgical antibiotic prophylaxis in this group of patients.

SLN biopsy undertaken prior to neoadjuvant therapy is helpful if negative as no further axillary treatment is necessary, and such a result can reinforce any decision to withhold subsequent supraclavicular irradiation. However, patients selected for neoadjuvant chemotherapy have a higher chance of nodal involvement and, in the event of a positive SLN biopsy, are then committed to completion ALND with no opportunity for nodal downstaging. An upfront SLN biopsy can be useful in patients who do not require chemotherapy if SLN biopsy negative, but often age, primary tumour size and information from core needle biopsy are sufficient to justify a recommendation for neoadjuvant chemotherapy.

4.3 Sentinel Lymph Node Biopsy After Neoadjuvant Chemotherapy

Advantages – Some advocate SLN biopsy after primary chemotherapy [18, 19] in order to take advantage of potential nodal downstaging and avoidance of ALND. Thus, rates of node positivity are reduced by 30 % for preoperative adriamycin and cyclophosphamide [18] and by up to 40 % for regimens incorporating a taxane with triple-negative and HER2-positive patients most likely to have a complete pathological nodal response [19]. A 'single' operation has the additional appeal of patient convenience and reduced costs when facilities for intraoperative node assessment are available. Early studies revealed that between 30 and 70 % of patients were committed to ALND with an upfront SLN biopsy. It should be noted however that many of these patients had relatively large primary tumours and few patients had preoperative axillary ultrasound which in conjunction with guided needle biopsy can deselect patients for SLN biopsy (who would then proceed directly to ALND). Hence, reports of higher rates of node positivity are not unexpected within this population of patients. Rates of complete pathological nodal response vary from 20 to 42 % in patients with needle biopsy-confirmed positive nodes pre-chemotherapy [20–23]. Most metastases diagnosed on needle biopsy are macrometastases (>2 mm), and it is conceivable that complete pathological response might be higher for nodes containing micrometastases only, though there is no current evidence to support this. There is a suggestion that knowledge of nodal response to chemotherapy is more relevant in terms of prognostication and decision-making for chest wall/supraclavicular radiotherapy than initial nodal status. In particular, those patients with a complete pathological response in both the breast and axilla appear to have a much better prognosis [24].

Disadvantages – It has been surmised that primary chemotherapy may modify lymphatic drainage patterns within the axilla where there is a degree of plasticity within the lymphatic network of vessels [25]. Distortion of lymphatics may occur secondary to tumour shrinkage with creation of aberrant lymphatic drainage patterns. This together with plugging of lymphatics by tumour emboli could increase false-negative rates. Moreover, induction chemotherapy could lead to differential downstaging between sentinel and non-sentinel nodes [26]. Notwithstanding these theoretical considerations, there is no conclusive evidence that such phenomena occur to any significant extent in neoadjuvant therapy patients, a fact which has encouraged a recent trend away from upfront SLN biopsy in neoadjuvant chemotherapy patients [27]. Interestingly, some have referred to a 'front to back, back to front' phenomenon in which chemotherapy is more likely to eradicate tumour within non-sentinel lymph nodes than the SLN in which the tumour cell burden is likely to be greater. Thus, although cancer cells spread first to the SLN and thereafter to the non-sentinel nodes, the inverse sequence applies to chemotherapy effect [28]. This would increase the negative predictive value of a negative SLN biopsy after chemotherapy. However, if tumour deposits responded earlier in the SLN than non-sentinel nodes, then a false-negative result would ensue.

4.4 Accuracy of Sentinel Lymph Node Biopsy After Chemotherapy

Node-negative patients – Single-institution studies have revealed sensitivity rates of 72–100 % with false-negative rates of 0–33 % when SLN biopsy follows neoadjuvant chemotherapy (NAC) [18, 26, 29–31]. However, most of these studies involved small numbers of patients, and a pooled analysis shows a false-negative rate of about 10 % with an identification rate of 89 %. Rates of identification in the NSABP B-27 study were 85 % using blue dye alone or a combination of blue dye and radioisotope with a reported false-negative rate of 11 % (the false-negative rate was higher for blue dye alone (14 %) compared with radioisotope with or without blue dye (8 %)) [26]. The French GANEA study also detected the SLN in 90 % of cases and reported an overall false-negative rate of 11 % (9.4 % for clinically node-positive cases, 11.6 % for clinically node-positive cases) [32]. An analysis by Hunt and colleagues revealed a false-negative rate of 5.9 % when SLN biopsy followed NAC and 4.1 % for upfront SLN biopsy ($p = 0.39$) [33]. Recent reports have shown false-negative rates in the region of 8–11 %; a meta-analysis of 21 single-institution studies involving more than 1200 patients undergoing post-chemotherapy SLN biopsy with completion ALND reported a pooled false-negative estimate of 12 % when SLN biopsy followed chemotherapy in clinically node-negative patients [34, 35]. A slightly lower figure of 9 % was calculated by Mamounas and Bellon when analysis was confined to studies published in the past 10 years, though values for false negativity ranged from 5 to 25 % [36].

These figures are similar to false-negative rates for primary surgery [3, 5, 37–39], but it should be noted that these two clinical scenarios may not be strictly comparable for several reasons – in the words of Michael Sabel, are we dealing here with 'apples and oranges' [27]. Firstly, only a subset of patients in these neoadjuvant studies had SLN biopsy post-chemotherapy with patient selection and surgeon experience introducing an element of bias. Thus, although standard ALND (level I/II) was a component of the trial protocol, a preliminary SLN biopsy could be undertaken before ALND at the discretion of the surgeon (approximately 20 % of patients) [26]. Secondly, there was much variation in the precise technique used for SLN biopsy (blue dye alone, isotope alone or a combination with dual localisation).

Node-positive patients – There have been mixed reports on false-negative rates when there is needle biopsy (cytology or core biopsy)-proven positive nodes pre-chemotherapy with a limited number of published studies relating specifically to this group of patients (see Table 4.1) [40–42]. Mamounas has recently cited an overall false-negative rate of 11.1 % for SLN biopsy post-neoadjuvant chemotherapy when there is confirmed nodal involvement at presentation [43]. These updated figures are reassuring and have led many experts to conclude that SLN biopsy is as accurate when performed post- as pre-neoadjuvant chemotherapy, but induction chemotherapy has the added advantage of potential downstaging of axillary nodes. However, a note of caution has been sounded by Alvarado and colleagues who

Table 4.1 False negative rates for SLN biopsy following primary chemotherapy in patients with biopsy-proven axillary nodal metastases

Author	No. of patients	False-negative rate (%)
Shen et al. [40]	69	25
Lee et al. [41]	238	5.6
Newman et al. [42]	54	10.7
Alvarado et al. [22]	150	16.1
Boughy et al. [23]	649	12.6

express concerns that false-negative rates can be unacceptably high when SLN biopsy follows neoadjuvant chemotherapy in patients presenting with node-positive disease [22]. They examined 150 patients with biopsy-proven axillary nodal metastases who proceeded to SLN biopsy after primary chemotherapy. Amongst 111 patients in whom ALND was performed, 15 had a false-negative result for an event rate of 20.8 % (15/72), and normalisation of nodes on ultrasound post-chemotherapy reduced this rate to 16.1 % (compared with 27.8 % for those with abnormal node morphology including size and cortical thickness). Furthermore, removal of a single SLN was associated with an even higher false-negative rate as was positivity for the HER2 receptor (33 % versus 18 %). The pathological complete nodal response in this study was 42 %, suggesting that a notable proportion of patients could have been spared the potential morbidity of an ALND [22].

There is a paucity of data on omission of completion ALND in needle biopsy-proven node-positive patients with a subsequent negative SLN biopsy after neoadjuvant chemotherapy (Table 4.1). In particular, it is unclear from some reports whether cited rates relate to patients with positive or negative initial nodal status, and there is confounding of studies due to some patients proceeding to ALND. For example, Hunt and colleagues reported recurrence rates of 1.2 % at a median follow-up of 55 months amongst a group of 575 patients undergoing SLN biopsy after primary chemotherapy, but almost one-third of patients had ALND either for SLN positivity (20.7 %) or as a planned procedure [33]. Further information is needed on rates of regional recurrence specifically in those patients with a negative SLN who did not have ALND. It is conceivable that axillary recurrence is higher when there is residual non-sentinel nodal disease after a false-negative SLN biopsy post-chemotherapy (no further chemotherapy routinely given) [44]. In a combined analysis of the NSABP B-27 and B-18 studies involving 3000 patients undergoing either mastectomy or breast conservation therapy, a total of 356 locoregional recurrence events were documented. The chance of recurrence was related to age, nodal status pre-chemotherapy and the breast/nodal pathological response rates, with low rates of recurrence for those patients achieving a complete pathological response. For those patients who were clinically node negative at the outset, rates of locoregional recurrence were low [45].

Boughy and colleagues have provided important information from the American College of Surgeons Oncology Group (ACOSOG) Z01071 trial which enrolled almost 700 patients and examined false-negative rates for patients with core biopsy-proven node-positive breast cancer (T0–T4, N1–2, M0) who underwent SLN biopsy and concomitant axillary lymph node dissection (ALND) after primary chemotherapy [23]. The primary endpoint for this study was the false-negative rate for clinically node-positive patients who have at least two SLNs removed for pathological examination. Though dual tracer techniques were recommended, this was not compulsory, and some patients underwent SLN biopsy with single tracer localisation (51 radioisotope only, 13 blue dye only). Rates of identification were 92.5 % overall (>90 % individually for both clinically N1 and N2 patients) with an accuracy of 84 % for assignment of correct nodal status. Forty percent of patients had a complete pathological nodal response with no evidence of any residual tumour on routine H&E staining (metastases >0.2 mm). Moreover, in 40 % of patients with nodal deposits, the sentinel node was the only positive node. Furthermore, the false-negative rate was almost 20 % when only a single tracer agent was employed compared with 12.6 % for dual tracer localisation and harvesting of a minimum of two nodes. It was recommended that at least three nodes be removed in this setting of SLN biopsy post-chemotherapy. Clips may be placed in the node at the time of initial core biopsy, and this will help to ensure that the correct node has been removed and confirm any pathological response to neoadjuvant chemotherapy. Results of this randomised study are consistent with the retrospective study of Alvarado although the latter provided no specific information on the technique of SLN localisation in relation to false-negative rates [22]. Park and colleagues likewise found a relatively high false-negative rate (22 %) when SLN biopsy was performed after neoadjuvant chemotherapy for locally advanced breast cancers. Radioisotope was employed as a sole tracer agent, and interestingly false-negative rates varied significantly between molecular tumour types with improved accuracy and lower false-negative rates for triple-negative breast cancer. These authors concluded that SLN biopsy post-chemotherapy should be restricted to this subgroup of triple-negative breast cancer [46].

On the basis of these Z1071 results, SLN biopsy after neoadjuvant chemotherapy for biopsy-proven nodal involvement at presentation can only be reliably used when dual localisation methods have been employed and at least two nodes have been removed and examined. Notwithstanding these findings on false-negative rates within the Z1071 study, which failed to reach a predefined upper threshold of 10 %, these may not necessarily translate into higher rates of locoregional recurrence. However, in contrast to patients undergoing SLN biopsy prior to any chemotherapy (be this neoadjuvant or adjuvant), this group of post-neoadjuvant patients will not receive any further chemotherapy that might eliminate tumour foci within 'non-sentinel' lymph nodes in the setting of false negativity. Longer-term follow-up will determine whether any change in performance parameters for SLN biopsy post-chemotherapy has any impact on clinical outcomes.

There is increasing evidence that decisions for radiotherapy (chest wall/supraclavicular) should be based on tumour response to chemotherapy rather than the status of the regional nodes per se at presentation. Knowledge of sentinel lymph node negativity from downstaging after neoadjuvant chemotherapy (when there were biopsy-confirmed nodal metastases at presentation) is very helpful when estimating benefit from radiotherapy. For clinically node-positive patients who become negative after neoadjuvant chemotherapy, there appears to be little benefit from radiotherapy. Hence, SLN biopsy after neoadjuvant chemotherapy allows assessment of specific response within the regional nodes to chemotherapy, whereas positive nodes might otherwise be removed with SLN biopsy and preclude any comment on nodal response following formal ALND after neoadjuvant chemotherapy [18, 26].

4.5 NSABP-51/RTOG-1304 Trial

Neoadjuvant chemotherapy can result in a significant downstaging of disease, such that patients presenting with extensive axillary lymph node involvement may have a complete pathological response with no evidence of axillary metastases following induction chemotherapy. Thus, the timing of SLN biopsy (before or after neoadjuvant chemotherapy) may significantly influence decisions concerning adjuvant radiotherapy. For instance, postmastectomy radiotherapy is generally recommended for patients who have metastases in >3 axillary nodes, but it is unclear if this decision should now be based on axillary status *before* or *after* administration of chemotherapy. If this should be based on nodal status at the time of initial presentation, then SLN biopsy prior to neoadjuvant chemotherapy should be urged. On the other hand, if nodal status after neoadjuvant chemotherapy provided sufficient basis for this decision on adjuvant radiotherapy, then SLN biopsy following chemotherapy would be the preferred option.

In an attempt to resolve this issue, a large randomised trial involving 1636 patients has been planned in the United States (NSABP-51/RTOG-1304 trial) [47]. This will be a phase III clinical trial evaluating postmastectomy chest wall and regional nodal radiotherapy and post-lumpectomy regional nodal radiotherapy in patients with positive axillary nodes before neoadjuvant chemotherapy who convert to pathologically negative axillary nodes after neoadjuvant chemotherapy. The study will recruit patients with T1–T3, N1 breast cancer, with documented positive axillary nodes by FNA or core biopsy. Following administration of neoadjuvant chemotherapy, those patients will undergo definitive surgery with histological documentation of negative axillary nodes (either by axillary dissection alone or SLN biopsy with or without axillary dissection). These patients who convert to node-negative status will then be randomised to receive either no regional nodal radiotherapy (and no chest wall radiotherapy for patients treated with mastectomy) or regional nodal radiotherapy (with chest wall radiotherapy for mastectomy patients). Thus, amongst node-positive patients who convert to node-negative status, this trial will determine whether or not decisions concerning adjuvant radiotherapy should be based on nodal status at the time of initial presentation. Ultimately, the results of this trial will be an important consideration in the decision-making process for recommending SLN biopsy either before or after administration of neoadjuvant chemotherapy.

4.6 SENTINA Trial

The German SENTINA trial addressed the role of repeat SLN biopsy in patients who had previously undergone the procedure prior to neoadjuvant chemotherapy [48]. Patients were allocated to one of four arms; initially clinically node-negative patients treated with upfront SLN biopsy were designated arms A and B; if the SLN was negative (arm A, 662 patients), then no further axillary surgery was undertaken. If the SLN was positive before chemotherapy, then repeat SLN biopsy with ALND was performed after chemotherapy (arm B, 360 patients). Patients who were initially clinically node positive were designated arms C and D; those who converted to clinically node-negative status after chemotherapy underwent SLN biopsy with ALND (arm C, 592 patients), whilst those who remained clinically node positive had a standard ALND (arm D, 123 patients). The sentinel node detection rates for arms A and B (pre-chemotherapy) were 99.1 %, 80.1 % for arm C and only 60.8 % for repeat SLN biopsy after chemotherapy (arm B). Moreover, the FNR for repeat SLN biopsy for arm B patients exceeded 50 % (51.6 %, 95 % CI 38.7–64.2 %), and sometimes only a single node was removed. The authors concluded that SLN biopsy is unacceptable as a repeat procedure following neoadjuvant chemotherapy. The FNR was noted to be relatively high for those patients in arm C who converted from clinically node positive to negative after chemotherapy (14.2 %, 95 % CI 9.9–19.4 %).

4.7 Conclusions

SLN biopsy can be performed either as an upfront procedure or following neoadjuvant chemotherapy with advantages and limitations of both approaches. A National Cancer Institute conference recommended SLN biopsy before or after chemotherapy for clinically node-negative disease which underlines the principle of multidisciplinary assessment and no single method applicable to all patients [49]. There is now greater confidence in declaration of a 'negative' SLN biopsy after primary chemotherapy for node-positive disease and withholding routine ALND in selected cases. False-negative results can be minimised by taking account of ultrasound characteristics post-chemotherapy and ensuring mandatory ALND when abnormal nodes persist sonographically [50]. Normal-appearing nodes are statistically more likely to be associated with a complete pathological nodal response than those with indeterminate features [22]. Nonetheless, the significance of micrometastases and isolated tumour cells in this setting is uncertain, and these may be of different biological consequence if they represent downstaged macrometastases. Ideally, there should be an 'all or none' response of nodes to chemotherapy, but it is conceded that in the 'post-Z0011 era', selected patients who are SLN biopsy positive pre-chemotherapy might avoid completion ALND as they will subsequently receive neoadjuvant/adjuvant therapies (including chemotherapy, hormonal therapy and breast radiotherapy). The use of a nomogram with a limited number of variables may have clinical utility for estimating the probability of residual disease in non-sentinel nodes [51]. This line of reasoning would not apply to SLN biopsy-positive patients *after* neoadjuvant chemotherapy who have residual disease post-chemotherapy and will receive no further chemotherapy (though possibly hormonal therapy/Herceptin). SLN biopsy should be considered post-chemotherapy in those patients for whom pretreatment nodal status would not impact on the choice of chemotherapy or radiotherapy. These recommendations can include selected cases of needle biopsy-proven node-positive cases at presentation that are clinically and sonographically node negative following chemotherapy with evidence of an excellent response in the breast and regional nodes to induction chemotherapy. Any evidence of sentinel node tumour deposits on H&E staining (including isolated tumour cells) should be followed by completion ALND irrespective of the type of breast surgery. Further information must be collected on outcomes in terms of both regional recurrence and overall survival for patients undergoing SLN biopsy after nodal downstaging with induction chemotherapy. In particular, sentinel lymph node-negative patients without completion ALND after neoadjuvant chemotherapy should be carefully monitored, and further axillary surgery for SLN-positive patients in this setting is mandatory at the present time.

Learning Points (Box 4.1)

1. There are advantages and limitations with both approaches to SLN biopsy in the context of neoadjuvant chemotherapy:
   - A National Cancer Institute conference in 2008 sanctioned SLN biopsy *before* or *after* neoadjuvant chemotherapy for clinically node-negative disease.
   - The National Comprehensive Cancer Network in 2011 recommended that SLN biopsy be performed prior to neoadjuvant chemotherapy.
2. There is now greater confidence in declaration of a 'negative' SLN biopsy after primary chemotherapy for node-positive disease and for withholding completion ALND in *selected* cases:
   - Two and possibly three sentinel nodes should be removed.
   - Dual localisation techniques should be employed with blue dye and isotope to minimise FNR.
   - Axillary nodes should be sonographically normal nodes following induction chemotherapy.
3. At the present time, routine SLN biopsy should be undertaken in conjunction with simultaneous completion ALND as a registration study to assess

(continued)

the accuracy of SLN biopsy after primary chemotherapy in terms of false-negative rates.

4. Any evidence of tumour deposits on H&E staining (including isolated tumour cells) should prompt a completion ALND *irrespective* of type of breast surgery.

   SLN biopsy post-chemotherapy should be considered in clinically/sonographically node-negative patients for whom pretreatment nodal status would *not* impact on choice of chemotherapy or radiotherapy.
5. The ongoing NSABP-51 trial is evaluating whether decisions for postmastectomy radiotherapy should be based on axillary status *before* or *after* chemotherapy.
6. If nodal status at presentation is deemed to be important, then upfront SLN biopsy should be urged but otherwise SLN biopsy post-chemotherapy preferred.

References

1. Mansel RE, Goyal A, Fallowfield L et al (2006) Sentinel node biopsy versus standard axillary treatment: results of the randomized multicentre UK ALMANAC trial. J Natl Cancer Inst 98:599–609
2. Purushotham AD, Upponi S, Klevesath MB, Bobrow L, Millar K, Myles JP et al (2005) Morbidity following sentinel lymph node biopsy in primary breast cancer – a randomized controlled trial. J Clin Oncol 23:4312–4321
3. Lyman GH, Guiliano AE, Somerfield MR et al (2005) The American Society of Clinical Oncology guideline recommendations for sentinel lymph node biopsy in early stage breast cancer. J Clin Oncol 23:7703–7720
4. Benson JR, Querci della Rovere G, and the Axilla Management Consensus Group (2007) Management of the axilla in women with breast cancer. Lancet Oncol 8:331–348
5. Krag D, Anderson SJ, Julian TB et al (2010) Sentinel lymph node resection compared with conventional axillary lymph node dissection in clinically node negative patients with breast cancer: overall survival findings from the NSABP B-32 randomised phase 3 trial. Lancet Oncol 11:927–933
6. Britton PD, Goud A, Godward S et al (2008) Use of ultrasound-guided axillary node core biopsy in staging of early breast cancer. Eur J Radiol 19:561–569
7. Mainiero MB, Cinelli CM, Koelliker SL et al (2010) Axillary ultrasound and fine-needle aspiration in the preoperative evaluation of the breast cancer patient: an algorithm based on tumor size and lymph node appearance. AJR Am J Roentgenol 195:1261–1267
8. Krishnamurthy S, Sneige N, Bedi DG et al (2002) Role of ultrasound-guided fine needle aspiration of indeterminate and suspicious axillary lymph nodes in the initial staging of breast carcinoma. Cancer 95:982–988
9. Schrenk P, Hochreiner G, Fridrik M et al (2003) Sentinel node biopsy performed before preoperative chemotherapy for axillary node staging in breast cancer. Breast J 9:282–287
10. Sabel MS, Schott AF, Kleer CG et al (2003) Sentinel node biopsy prior to neoadjuvant chemotherapy. Am J Surg 186:102–105
11. Menard J-P, Extra J-M, Jacquemier J et al (2009) Sentinel lymphadenectomy for the staging of clinical axillary node negative breast cancer before neoadjuvant chemotherapy. Eur J Surg Oncol 35:916–920

12. Straver ME, Rutgers EJT, Russel NS et al (2009) Towards rational axillary treatment in relation to neoadjuvant therapy in breast cancer. Eur J Cancer 45:2284–2292
13. Chung MH, Ye W, Giuliano AE (2001) Role for sentinel lymph node dissection in the management of large (>5cm) invasive breast cancer. Ann Surg Oncol 8:688–692
14. Bedrosian I, Reynolds C, Mick R et al (2000) Accuracy of sentinel lymph node biopsy in patients with large primary tumours. Cancer 88:2540–2545
15. Recht A, Edge SB, Solin LJ et al (2001) Post-mastectomy radiotherapy: clinical practice guidelines of the American Society of Clinical Oncology. J Clin Oncol 19:1539–1569
16. Paik S, Shak S, Tang G et al (2004) A multigene assay to predict recurrence of tamoxifen-treated, node negative breast cancer. N Eng J Med 35:2817–2826
17. Benson JR, Wishart GC, Ambler G, Provenzano E Sentinel lymph node biopsy before chemotherapy in breast cancer patients? 1st British Breast Cancer Research Meeting, September 2010
18. Fisher B, Brown A, Mamounas E et al (1997) Effect of preoperative chemotherapy on local-regional disease in women with operable breast cancer: findings from National Surgical Adjuvant Breast and Bowel Project B18. J Clin Oncol 15:2483–2493
19. Gianni L, Baselga J, Eirmann W et al (2002) First report of the European Cooperative Trial in operable breast cancer: effects of primary systemic therapy on local-regional disease. Proc Am Soc Clin Oncol 21:34a
20. Hennessy BT, Hortobagyi GN, Rouzier R et al (2005) Outcome after pathologic complete eradication of cytologically proven breast cancer axillary node metastases following primary chemotherapy. J Clin Oncol 23:9304–9311
21. Beatty JD, Precht LM, Lowe K et al (2009) Axillary conserving surgery is facilitated by neoadjuvant chemotherapy of breast cancer. Am J Surg 197:637–642
22. Alvarado R, Yi M, Le-Petross H et al (2012) The role for sentinel lymph node dissection after neoadjuvant chemotherapy in patients who present with node positive breast cancer. Ann Surg Oncol 19:3177–3184
23. Boughey JC, Suman VJ, Mittendorf EA et al (2013) Sentinel lymph node surgery after neoadjuvant chemotherapy in patients with node positive breast cancer. The ACOSOG Z1071 (Alliance) trial. JAMA 310(14):1455–1461
24. Klaube-Demore N, Ollia DW, Moore DT et al (2006) Size of residual lymph node metastasis after neoadjuvant chemotherapy in locally advanced breast cancer patients is prognostic. Ann Surg Oncol 13:685–691
25. Bleiweiss I (2007) Sentinel lymph nodes in breast cancer after 10 years: rethinking basic principles. Lancet Oncol 7:686–692
26. Mamounas EP, Brown A, Anderson et al (2005) Sentinel node biopsy after neoadjuvant chemotherapy in breast cancer: results from National Surgical Adjuvant Breast and Bowel Project. B-27. J Clin Oncol 23(12):2694–2702
27. Sabel M (2010) Sentinel lymph node biopsy before or after neoadjuvant chemotherapy: pros and cons. Surg Oncol Clin N Am 19:519–538
28. Torisu-Itakura H, Lee JH, Scheri RP et al (2007) Molecular characterization of inflammatory genes in sentinel and non-sentinel nodes in melanoma. Clin Cancer Res 13:3125–3132
29. Nason KS, Anderson BO, Byrd DR et al (2000) Increased false negative sentinel node biopsy rates after preoperative chemotherapy for invasive breast cancer. Cancer 89:2187–2194
30. Tafra L, Verbanac KM, Lannin DR (2001) Preoperative chemotherapy and sentinel lymphadenectomy for breast cancer. Am J Surg 182:312–315
31. Hino M, Sano M, Sato N et al (2008) Sentinel lymph node biopsy after neoadjuvant chemotherapy in a patient with operable breast cancer. Surg Today 38:585–591
32. Classe JM, Bordes V, Campion L et al (2009) Sentinel lymph node biopsy after neoadjuvant chemotherapy for advanced breast cancer: results of Ganglion Sentinelle et Chimiotherapie Neoadjuvante, A French prospective multicenter study (GANEA). J Clin Oncol 27:726–732
33. Hunt KK, Yi M, Mittendorf EA et al (2009) Sentinel lymph node surgery after neoadjuvant chemotherapy is accurate and reduces the need for axillary dissection in breast cancer patients. Ann Surg 250:558–566

34. Xing Y, Foy M, Cox DD et al (2006) Meta-analysis of sentinel lymph node biopsy after preoperative chemotherapy in patients with breast cancer. Br J Surg 93:539–546
35. van Deurzen CH, Vriens BE, Tjan-Heijnen VC et al (2009) Accuracy of sentinel lymph node biopsy after neoadjuvant chemotherapy in breast cancer patients: a systematic review. Eur J Cancer 45:3124–3130
36. Mamounas EP, Bellon JR (2010) Local-regional therapy considerations in patients receiving preoperative chemotherapy. In: Harris JR, Lippman MER, Morrow M (eds) Diseases of the breast, 4th edn. Lippincott Williams & Wilkins, Philadelphia, pp 730–744
37. Krag D, Weaver D, Ashikaga T et al (1998) The sentinel node in breast cancer – a multicenter validation study. N Eng J Med 229:941–946
38. Giuliano AE, Haigh PI, Brennan MB et al (2000) Prospective observational study of sentinel lymphadenectomy without further axillary dissection in patients with sentinel node negative breast cancer. J Clin Oncol 18:2553–2559
39. Veronesi U, Paganelli G, Viale G et al (2003) A randomized comparison of sentinel lymph node biopsy with routine axillary dissection in breast cancer. N Eng J Med 349:546–553
40. Shen J, Gilcrease MZ, Babiera GV et al (2007) Feasibility and accuracy of sentinel lymph node biopsy after preoperative chemotherapy in breast cancer patients with documented axillary metastases. Cancer 109:1255–1263
41. Lee S, Kim EY, Kang SH et al (2007) Sentinel node identification rate, but not accuracy, is significantly decreased after pre-operative chemotherapy in axillary node positive breast cancer patients. Breast Cancer Res Treat 102:283–288
42. Newman EA, Sabel MS, Nees AV et al (2007) Sentinel lymph node biopsy performed after neoadjuvant chemotherapy is accurate in patients with documented node positive breast cancer at presentation. Ann Surg Oncol 14:2946–2952
43. Mamounas EP (2012) Sentinel node biopsy in breast cancer: before or after neoadjuvant chemotherapy. Cancer Res 72(24 Suppl): Abstract nr ES6-1
44. Sabel MS (2007) Locoregional therapy of breast cancer: maximizing control, minimizing morbidity. Expert Rev Anticancer Ther 6:1261–1279
45. Mamounas E, Anderson S, Bear H et al (2012) Predictors of loco-regional failure in patients receiving neoadjuvant chemotherapy: results from combined analysis of NSABP B-27. J Clin Oncol 30(10):3916–3920
46. Park S, Park JM, Cho JH et al (2013) Sentinel node biopsy after neoadjuvant chemotherapy in patients with cytologically proven node positive breast cancer at diagnosis. Ann Surg Oncol 20:2858–2865
47. NSABP B-51/RTOG 1304. A randomized phase III clinical trial evaluating post-mastectomy chest wall and regional nodal XRT and post-lumpectomy regional nodal XRT in patients with positive axillary nodes before neoadjuvant chemotherapy who convert to pathologically negative axillary nodes after chemotherapy. www.med.wright.edu/dcop/schemas/B51
48. Kuehn T, Bauerfeind IGP, Fehm T, et al (2012) Sentinel lymph node biopsy results before or after neoadjuvant chemotherapy – final results from the prospective German multi-institutional SENTINA Trial. Cancer Res 72(24 Suppl): abstract nr S2-2
49. Bucholtz TA, Lehman CD, Harris JR et al (2008) Statement of the science concerning locoregional treatments after preoperative chemotherapy for breast cancer: a National Institute Conference. J Clin Oncol 26(5):791–797
50. Kang E, Chung IY, Han SA et al (2011) Feasibility and accuracy of sentinel lymph node biopsy in breast cancer patients with initial axillary lymph node metastasis after primary systemic therapy. J Breast Cancer 14:147–152
51. Jeruss JS, Winchester DJ, Sener SF et al (2005) Axillary recurrence after sentinel lymph node biopsy. Ann Surg Oncol 12:34–40

Chapter 5
Axillary Reverse Mapping (ARM) as a Means to Reduce Lymphedema During Sentinel Lymph Node or Axillary Node Dissection

V. Suzanne Klimberg and Michael Douek

Abstract Our group has hypothesized that variations in the anatomical location of the arm lymphatic drainage system within the axilla put the arm lymphatics at risk for disruption during an SLNB and/or ALND. Therefore, mapping and protecting the drainage of the arm versus that of the breast within the axilla by split mapping using blue dye to identify and protect the lymphatics draining from the arm (axillary reverse mapping (ARM)) and radioactivity to map those draining from the breast would decrease the likelihood of inadvertent disruption during lymphadenectomy. Mapping and sparing the lymphatics draining the arm during SLNB or ALND decrease the subsequent development of lymphedema as compared to SLN mapping alone.

Keywords Breast • Axillary reverse mapping • Lymphedema • Breast cancer

5.1 Background

Lymph node status is a key prognostic variable, and therapeutic decisions are based on the presence or absence of breast cancer cells metastatic to the axillary lymph node(s). The results of randomized prospective clinical trials, which guide current

---

Supported by a grant from the Arkansas Breast Cancer Research Program and the University of Arkansas for Medical Sciences Translational Research Institute (CTSA Grant Award #1UL1RR029884)
Supported by a grant from the Fashion Footwear Association of New York
Financial disclosures: medical director and stock in Ascendant Diagnostics (not relevant to paper)

V.S. Klimberg (✉)
Departments of Surgery and Pathology, University of Arkansas for Medical Sciences, Little Rock, AR, USA

Winthrop P. Rockefeller Cancer Institute, University of Arkansas for Medical Sciences, Slot 725, 4301 West Markham Street, Little Rock, AR 72212, USA
e-mail: klimbergsuzanne@uams.edu

M. Douek
Research Oncology, Division of Cancer Studies, King's College London, London, UK

M. Toi et al. (eds.), *Personalized Treatment of Breast Cancer*,
DOI 10.1007/978-4-431-55552-0_5

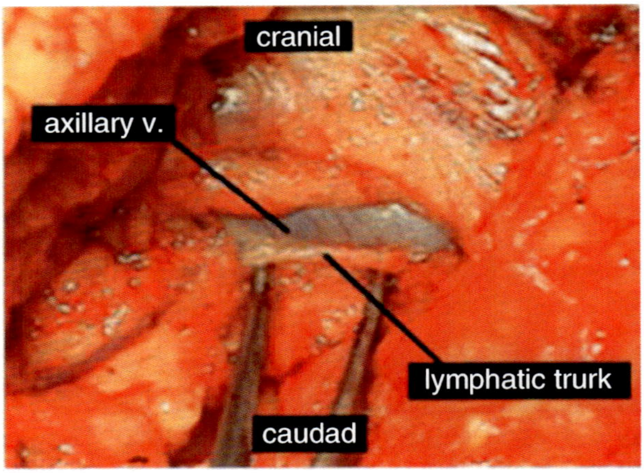

Fig. 5.1 Lymphatic trunk draining the arm is demonstrated just below the axillary vein

therapy, have been based on the pathologic status of the axillary lymph nodes. Although newer markers of oncogene expression show promise with respect to the treatment of breast cancer, the status of the axillary nodes remains the most important prognostic criteria and will continue to have direct impact on clinical decisions.

When necessary, the prescribed technique for axillary lymph node dissection (ALND) has changed little over the last several decades. The principal features include removal of the axillary tissue inferior to the axillary vein, lateral to the serratus, and anterior to the teres major [1]. The standard teaching was that the lymphatic ran along the inferior side of the axillary vein (Fig. 5.1), and avoiding skeletonizing the vein would prevent lymphedema. The morbidity and risks of an ALND include the risk of general anesthesia, permanent hypesthesia and/or dysesthesia at the posterior aspect of the arm [2], painful neuroma, postoperative seroma formation [3], and lymphedema of the arm [4]—the risk of which increases with greater extent of axillary node resection as well as breast surgery [5, 6]. It has been reported that 82 % of women experience at least one arm problem following ALND. Patients often have decreased mobilization of the shoulder and require physical therapy to regain full function of the upper extremity. Associated psychological distress ranges from 17 to 50 % [7, 8]. Depending on how it is defined, lymphedema alone has been reported to be as high as 77 % (Table 5.1 [9–18]). Routine use of sentinel lymph node biopsy (SLNB) has drastically reduced this risk but is still quite variable (0–13 %). The wide variability with both SLNB and ALND indicates a concomitant wide variation in technique in performance of these procedures. Therefore, there should be a modification of surgical technique that can reproducibly reduce lymphedema (LE). The following discussion attempts to establish the safety and efficacy of this new procedure, axillary reverse mapping (ARM), to identify and prevent one of the major surgical side effects of lymphadenectomy—lymphedema.

Table 5.1 Lymphedema in studies comparing SLNB and ALND

Study	SLNB (#)	ALND (#)	Lymphedema SLNB (%)	Lymphedema ALND (%)
Schrenk 2000	35	35	0	17
Haid 2002	57	140	4	27
Swenson 2002	169	78	4	14
Blanchard 2003	683	91	6	34
Schijven 2003	180	213	1	7
Ronka 2005	43	40	13	77
Leidenius 2005	92	47	5	28
Mansel 2006	515	516	5	13
McLaughlin 2008	600	336	5	16
B32	2008	1975	8	14

5.2 Surgical Lymphadenectomy and LE

Present-day sentinel lymph node biopsy (SLNB) or ALND does not take into account the anatomical drainage from the breast versus that of the arm because drainage from the arm into the axilla has only recently been published by our group [19–24]. Yet, lymphedema likely results from transection of lymph vessels from the arm coursing through the axilla and is the most prominent complication resulting from SLNB or ALND [22]. From its inception, SLNB, developed to prevent the high morbidity seen with ALND (Table 5.1), has been assumed to be less morbid, but until recently, few objective data existed. Because of the long-term sequelae of lymphedema, this surgical outcome is an important measurement when a replacement procedure for ALND is evaluated. Several cooperative group trials have shown lymphedema rates in approximately the 5–7 % range with SLN biopsy alone [16, 18, 25]. In the American College of Surgeons Oncology Group Z0010 prospective observational study [25], 2904 patients had arm circumference data recorded, both before surgery and 6 months after SLNB. Lymphedema was defined in this study as a change in arm circumference of >2 cm when compared with the contralateral or control arm and with baseline measurements. Nearly 7 % of the patients had a change in arm circumference >2 cm at 6 months. Multiple comparison studies, several of which were randomized, have confirmed that SLNB consistently has lower morbidity and lymphedema rates than ALND (Table 5.1). Lymphedema in ALND groups has been reported to range from 13 % to 77 %, varying with how closely lymphedema was monitored, the length of follow-up [4, 26], questionably the number of positive lymph nodes [27], the postoperative irradiation [5, 28], the extent of surgery and body habitus, and a number of other patient characteristics [26, 29]. Although the lymphedema rate was much lower with the SLNB, it was still clinically significant with a range of 0–13 % (Table 5.1).

Existing studies of LE are complicated by inconsistent relationships in a number of personal, disease, and treatment-related risk factors [26, 30] that include having more than five and in another study ten positive lymph nodes removed, postoperative infection, radiation to the axilla, younger age at diagnosis, history of hypertension, body mass index >30 kg/m^2, and length of follow-up. The evidence-based risk reduction for breast cancer-related secondary lymphedema is scant and contradictory, with most studies in the area limited by small numbers, retrospective design, and other methodological deficiencies [31]. Further, congenital hypoplasia of lymphatics can predispose patients to surgical lymphedema [32, 33]. In defining the "functional" anatomy of the axilla by using the methodology of ARM, we may be able to not only predict risk but potentially prevent lymphedema during SLNB±ALND.

Conventional wisdom teaches that the lymphatics reside juxtaposed to the vein, and if the surgeon can avoid skeletonizing the vein, then the risk of lymphedema could be minimized or avoided (Fig. 5.1). If this was the case, then SLNB should have mitigated the problem of surgical lymphedema. In fact, lymphatics with this positioning are rarely visible or recognized at the time of surgery. Therefore, we hypothesized that lymphedema is related to disruption of the virtually unknown arm lymphatic drainage during surgery. Foldi and others have carefully catalogued the drainage of the various parts of the arm, but once identified as a lymph node in the axilla, lymph nodes are categorized only as an axillary lymph node not distinguished from where it drains but by where it is positioned in the axillary bed (e.g., central) [20, 32]. Traditional lymphatic drainage of the arm is based on extensive lymphatic mapping of the arm but not the axilla.

Our group developed the concept of axillary reverse mapping (ARM) that utilizes a simple method, namely, blue dye injected into the upper volar subcutaneous tissue of the arm to map the lymphatic drainage of the arm in order to determine the in vivo anatomical variation in the axillary lymphatics, providing a road map to preserving them (Fig. 5.2). If arm lymphedema is caused by cutting lymphatics, then being able to see and identify them represents the first surgical procedure designed to preserve them. In effect, ARM is the reverse of SLN mapping that serves to map the lymph nodes draining the breast and then remove them; ARM is mapping the arm drainage in order to preserve it.

The most significant per person benefit gained by the ARM procedure is in ALND. If ALND is performed after SLNB, the SLNB must also use the ARM procedure as the low-lying lymphatics can otherwise be damaged during the initial staging procedure. A possible drawback to the ARM approach is that at present, about half of SLN mapping is done with blue dye or radioactivity alone, and the remaining uses dual mapping with both radioactivity and blue dye especially when learning the technique. In inexperienced hands, dual mapping may be more successful. To use ARM, surgeons would have to use radioactivity alone in the breast and reserve the blue dye for the ARM procedure or another or addition dye or procedure such as green dye or magnetic particles.

Our preliminary data focused on the development and safety of the ARM procedure and has demonstrated our ability to identify and preserve the ARM

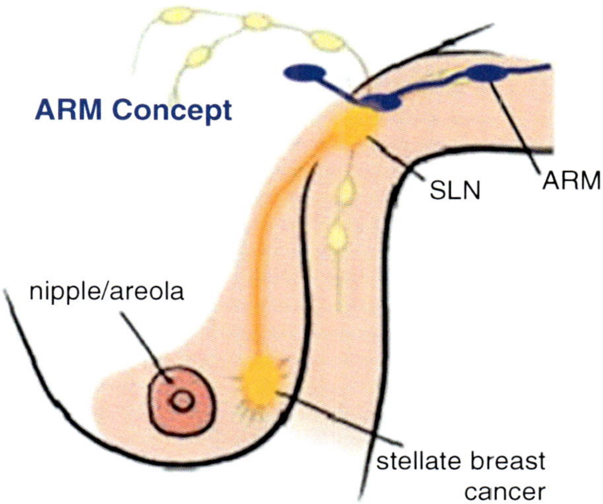

Fig. 5.2 Diagram of concept of axillary reverse mapping. Radioactive drainage from the breast SLN (*yellow*) can be identified and removed for examination, while the *blue* lymphatics (ARM) draining the arm can be identified and protected

lymphatics in most, but not all, patients and that there is little crossover (<4 %) between breast and arm lymphatics [19–24]. We have demonstrated safety in a small cohort of patients by removing the ARM identified node during ALND and demonstrating the absence of metastases even in clinically positive axillae.

5.3 Optimizing Breast Cancer Staging

According to the World Health Organization, as many as 170 million people worldwide and 3–5 million people in the United States suffer from secondary lymphedema. As many and varied procedures have failed to resolve lymphedema, it is our estimation that prevention is the key to avoiding lymphedema and further optimizing breast cancer staging. Axillary reverse mapping may be one tool to help us further refine the technique of axillary staging whether performing SLNB and/or ALND. As practiced around the world, the technique of ALND and even SLNB is not standardized, compromising the staging of and recurrence in the axilla and risk of lymphedema. Some might say the risk from SLNB is low already (0–13 %, Table 5.1). However, remember most lymphedema after an SLNB occurs from a negative SLNB. We should strive to lower the risk toward zero of a procedure that ultimately has no benefit to the patient. In addition, ARM may help identify patients who are at risk for LE early on and may benefit from early intervention. The ARM procedure is easy to learn and apply. Thus, any surgeon practicing could apply this technique to their present practice of lymphadenectomy with minimal training and cost with a potential huge benefit to the patient in the prevention or mitigation of surgical lymphedema. The preliminary data below outlines the methodical development of expertise in breast cancer surgery, development of SLNB, and evolution of our novel but elegantly simple idea, ARM. Future studies may use the knowledge gained to determine who is at risk for lymphedema and guide therapeutic surgical interventions for secondary lymphedema.

Even in the molecular age, the status of the axillary lymph nodes remains the most important predictor of outcome in breast cancer and, thus, continues to direct therapy [1]. The technique for axillary lymph node dissection (ALND), although supplanted by sentinel lymph node (SLN) for the majority of patients, has changed little since its inception being purely an anatomical dissection. Axillary lymph node dissection does not distinguish the breast from arm lymphatics as the possibility of mapping the drainage from the arm into the axilla has only recently been published by our group and questioned as well as confirmed by others using variations of the technique we developed [19–24, 34–42]. Transection of the major arm lymphatics during an ALND in patients without significant collaterals most likely is the root cause of lymphedema and arguably the most widely published complication of SLN or ALND. Table 5.1 demonstrates the wide variability in LE rates with SLNB or ALND highlighting the lack of standardization of these widely utilized procedures.

5.4 SLNB Reduces LE

Probe-guided and/or visual resection of radioactive sentinel nodes (the first nodes that receive drainage from tumors) can accurately identify regional metastases in patients with breast cancer. Multiple studies confirmed this including the definitive NSABP-32 trial which compared LE assessed by volume displacement of SLNB (n = 2006) versus SLNB+ALND (n = 1975) and demonstrated arm volume difference of 7.5 % versus 14 %, respectively [18]. Many other studies including the ACOSOG trials have confirmed that institution of SLNB for breast cancer patients reduces the risk of lymphedema of the affected arm ([42], Table 5.1). The literature to date supports injection with blue dye alone, radioactivity alone, or in combination (reviewed in [43]). The best method of injection to localize the SLN remains controversial even today, but a majority of surgeons use subareolar injection [44]. Although beginning surgeons find it easier to use dual mapping and that it may be more accurate, approximately 50 % of experienced mappers use single-agent localization with high efficacy.

5.5 Axillary Reverse Mapping (ARM): A New Concept to Identify and Enhance Lymphatic Preservation

Although SLN clearly reflects the status of the axillary lymph node basin and is less morbid, it has reduced but not prevented lymphedema. There can be no doubt that lymphedema is minimized with SLN in comparison to ALND as seen in eight clinical trials comparing the two (Table 5.1). Rates of lymphedema with SLN were much lower than those of ALND in the range of 0–13 % compared with 7–77 % for ALND. Several cooperative group trials have shown lymphedema rates in approximately the 5–7 % range with SLN biopsy alone [16–18, 25]. We hypothesized that this higher-than-expected rate of lymphedema may be secondary to disruption of low-lying arm lymphatics during an SLN biopsy procedure [19–24]. After sentinel lymph node (SLN) localization with subareolar technetium was assured, 5 mL of dermal blue dye was injected in the upper inner arm for localization of lymphatics draining the arm (axillary reverse mapping, ARM). The SLNB was then performed through an incision in the axilla. Data were collected on identification rates of hot versus blue nodes, variations in arm lymphatic drainage that might impact SLNB, crossover between the hot and the blue lymphatics, and final pathologic nodal diagnosis. Lymphatics draining the arm were near or in the SLN field in 40.6 % (87 of 241) of the patients, placing the patient at risk for disruption if not identified and preserved during an SLNB or an axillary lymph node dissection. ARM demonstrated that arm lymphatics do not cross over with the SLN drainage of the breast 97.2 % of the time and that none of the ARM lymph nodes removed were positive, even when the SLN was (5 of 12). We identified multiple variations of the arm lymphatics with some being as much as 4 cm below the vein (Fig. 5.3) [21]. Some ARM lymphatics were as large as 6 mm. Variations from the traditionally taught position just below the vein were seen as a medial or lateral apron and a sling low in the axilla. Another variation was blue lymphatics above the vein. Another variation was a complex of smaller lymphatics entwined as a cord. ARM lymphatics were juxtaposed to the hot SLNBs but separable. Disruption of the blue ARM node because of proximity to the hot SLN may explain the surprisingly high rate of lymphedema seen after SLNB. Identifying and preserving the blue ARM nodes

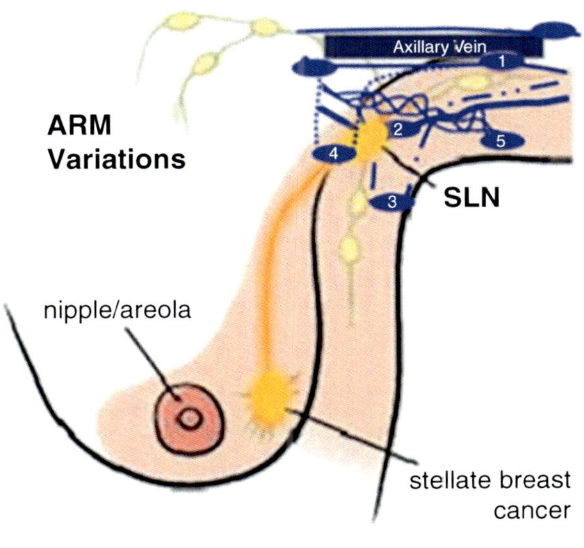

Fig. 5.3 Lymphatic variations. The diagram demonstrates the anatomical variations in ARM drainage. *1* Tradition teaching of the lymphatics from the arm running juxtaposed the axillary vein either above or below; *2* sling low in the axilla; *3* lateral apron; *4* medial apron, the latter two usual consisting of multiple *blue* nodes; *5* entwined cord of lymphatics

may translate into a lower incidence of lymphedema with SLNB and axillary lymph node dissection.

Since our original report in 2007 [19], there have been many other reports using variable methods for ARM. However, in the literature to date, there are only seven studies with >50 patients undergoing ARM (two ALND only and five SNB ± completion ALND) in 859 patients undergoing axillary surgery for breast cancer [45]. Overall, the lymphedema incidence ranged from 0 to 5.7 % during ARM assisted SNB and 4–14 % during ARM lymphatic preservation at ALND. Crossover (SLN=ARM) nodes were identified in between 0 and 9.6 % of patients. Metastases were identified in 0–35 % of these patients with crossover nodes excised. ARM nodes could not technically be preserved in between 11.1 and 17.5 % of patients with ARM nodes identified, and metastases were found in 0–18.5 % of ARM nodes from these patients. All patients where ARM nodes were found to be positive were inpatients with > N2 disease. Of note is that N2 and N3 patients would also receive radiation therapy, thus potentially negating chances of recurrence from leaving a positive ARM node(s) behind but also increasing LE. A randomized controlled trial with adequate follow-up is needed to formally evaluate these outcomes.

In a review of the literature, four studies of ARM were assessed at SNB, but between 10 and 31 % of patients went on to undergo a completion ALND [21, 24, 40, 46]. The ARM lymphatics or nodes were identifiable in between 38 and 100 % of patients. ARM crossover nodes were identified in patients undergoing SLNB between 0 and 10 % of patients, and metastases were present in between 0 and 20 % of these nodes as expected as the ARM is the SLN. ARM nodes or lymphatics were sacrificed during ALND in between 0 and 18 % of those identified, and of those excised the incidence of metastases was between 0 and 18.5 %. Low rates of 1.3 and 4 % in non-concordant nodes (ARM nodes that were not SLNs) were seen in the three studies that reported procedures using ARM as initially reported (split mapping, i.e., radioactivity in the breast and blue dye in the arm). Positive non-concordant blue nodes were only found in patients with heavily positive nodes (>N2) [21, 24, 39]. In nodes with N2 or higher metastatic disease, it is postulated that the lymphatic flow from the breast may back flow into the arm lymphatic drainage, and it is why split mapping is important to indicate when these nodes should be taken. The reported lymphedema rates were between 0 and 5.4 % for ALND. To date, long-term local recurrence rates were only reported in our study [24], which quoted figures of 1.2 and 0.4 % for breast and axillary recurrences, respectively; systemic recurrence was quoted as 6.4 % overall. The remaining study (Kuusk et al.) divided patients into SNB alone and ALND alone patients [47]. This study identified ARM nodes or lymphatics in 27 % of patients. Crossover nodes were present in 9.6 % (five patients) of patients; SLNs and metastases were present in one (20 %) of these which is what one would expect for an SLN positivity rate. Overall, 14.2 % of ARM lymphatics were sacrificed, with no involved nodes identified and an incidence of lymphedema of 5.7 % with no recurrences.

In the two studies, which performed ARM without breast injection in 203 consecutive breast cancer patients scheduled to undergo ALND alone [22, 36], ARM lymphatics or nodes were identified in 78.3 and 100 % of occasions. The preservation of ARM lymphatics was possible in 52.6 and 75 % of cases. The lymphedema rates ranged between 9 and 23 % in the ARM lymphatic preservation groups and between 33.3 and 40 % in the non-lymphatic preservation sacrifice group. There were no reported cases of local recurrence [48, 49].

In our unpublished follow-up data in our single institution trial, 642 patients have prospectively undergone 685 ARM procedures with an SLNB and/or ALND (presented at Society of Surgical Oncology, 2014). Objective lymphedema rates for SLNB and ALND were 0.8 % and 6.5 %, respectively, with 26-month median follow-up. Blue lymphatics were identified in 29.2 % (138/472) of SLNB and 71.8 % (153/213) of ALND. Crossover was seen in 3.8 % (18/472) of SLN and 5.6 % (12/213) of ALND. Blue node metastasis rate was 4.5 % (2/44). Axillary recurrence rate was 0.2 % and 1.4 % for SLNB and ALND, respectively. At 26-month median follow-up, objective LE is <1 % after SLNB and 6.5 % for ALND as measured by volume displacement.

5.6 Lymphatic Reanastomosis

A total of 81 blue ARM lymphatic transections occurred during our single institution study, 31 instances during SLNB and 50 during ALND. Crossover node resection was the necessary cause in 58 % (18/31) and 24 % (12/50) of the blue ARM transections during SLNB and ALND, respectively. Of the 31 patients where ARM lymphatic injury was identified at the time of SLNB, 15 (48.3 %) had a lymphatic reanastomosis/reapproximation performed. An additional 18 patients out of 50 (36 %) had similar reanastomosis of ARM lymphatics during ALND. Consistent reapproximation of lymphatics only occurred starting in 2011. In the subset of patients in which an identified blue lymphatic was transected, there was an overall lymphedema rate of 18.7 % (9/48) when not re-anastomosed and 0 % (0/33) when re-anastomosed ($p = 0.009$); this is over a median follow-up of 14 months (range 3–54 months).

5.7 Measurement of LE

Total limb volume measurement can be performed by water displacement [50], conic geometry (as used in this study) [51], perometry [52], or tissue changes by tonometry [53]. In the normal healthy person, the volume of the extracellular subcompartment is approximately 25 % of the total volume. Hence, these methods which measure total limb volume are thought to inherently suffer from a sensitivity four times less than any technique which measures extracellular volumes directly [54]. Lymphedema is not simply an increase in volume but also an alteration of the dermal and subcutaneous tissues accompanying the increase in protein concentration of the extracellular fluid. Such changes alter the resistance of the tissue to compression, and a measure of this resistance can be used to reflect the extent of the changes. Extracellular fluid volume measurement by magnetic resonance imaging (MRI) or computed tomography (CT) has also been used to determine the cross-sectional composition of the limb at small increments along the limb length [55, 56]. However, practical application of the procedure is severely limited due to both cost and availability (reviewed in [57]). Extracellular fluid volume measurement by bioelectrical impedance analysis (BIA), a method first used to assess body composition by nutritionists [58], has also been used successfully to quantify lymphedema [59, 60]. While this technique provides valuable information complementary to volume measurements, it is information about changes associated with lymphedema after the initial stages and as such may not be useful in the early diagnosis of the condition [54].

L-Dex® U400 is a noninvasive BIS tool to assess the extracellular fluid differences between the arms by measuring resistance to electrical current flow. At very low frequencies, the current travels predominantly through the extracellular fluid compartment of limbs. The L-Dex® U400 device uses an "impedance ratio" methodology to assess unilateral lymphedema of the arm. The resistance at 0 kHz (theoretical) in the affected/at-risk arm is compared to the resistance at 0 kHz (theoretical) in the unaffected arm as represented by the following ratio (unaffected to affected/at risk). By this method, the unaffected arm acts as an internal and subject-specific control with high sensitivity allowing for subclinical detection compared to traditional techniques. BIS uses standardized cutoffs and has been shown to have excellent interobserver variability. Measurements are made by attaching electrodes to the patient's skin. The current is imperceptible to patients and would be equivalent to that received by holding an AA battery. Once both arms are measured, the device calculates an L-Dex value. Abnormal L-Dex values include those outside the normal range (+/− 10 L-Dex units) and a change of >10 from baseline. Cornish et al. studied 102 female patients; 20 patients developed lymphedema in the 24 months after breast cancer surgery [59]. In each of these 20 cases using bioimpedance, predicted onset of lymphedema up to 10 months before the condition could be clinically diagnosed, thus allowing the early institution of preventative measures. This study will compare conical geometric LE assessment with that of BIA to determine comparative sensitivity and timing. This small study claimed a 100 % sensitivity of bioimpedance and demonstrated a vast improvement on the presently used circumferential technique which proved to have a sensitivity of only 5 % for the purposes of early detection.

5.8 Summary

Correction of any disability can come only with knowledge of the cause of that disability, and with that, a preventive strategy to at the very least decreases, if not prevents, the disability. Our preliminary data suggests that a significant number of patients are susceptible to arm lymphatic injury during an SLNB±ALND due to the ARM node anatomical location. Our data shows that injury to these arm lymphatic channels can be prevented by identification and preservation with the ARM procedure. Non-concordance (97.2 %) of arm and breast lymphatic drainage even in diseased axillae allows its use for SLNB as well as for ALND. Current preliminary data suggest that blue lymph nodes can be safely preserved. As many and varied procedures have failed to fix lymphedema, it is our estimation that prevention is the key to avoiding lymphedema. Axillary reverse mapping may help us further optimize the technique of axillary staging when performing SLNB. This study proposes an organized assessment of our newly developed intervention, ARM, to determine its effectiveness in reducing lymphedema after SLNB±ALND. Secondarily, this study will demonstrate the ability of ARM to identify arm-draining lymphatics for preservation during SLNB±ALND and assess the safety of its use for preserving arm-draining lymphatics (assess regional recurrence). The best way to assess the success of such interventions is yet to be determined.

References

1. Klimberg VS (2010) In: Klimberg VS, Bland K (eds) Master techniques in general surgery: breast surgery, 1st edn. LWW, New York
2. Ivens D, Hoe AL, Podd TJ, Hamilton CR, Taylor I, Royle GT (1997) Assessment of morbidity from complete axillary dissection. Br J Cancer 66:136
3. Somers RG, Jablon LK, Kaplan MJ, Sandler GL, Rosenblat NK (1992) The use of closed suction drainage after lumpectomy and axillary node dissection for breast cancer; a prospective randomized trial. Ann Surg 215:146
4. Petrek JA, Senie RT, Peters M et al (2001) Lymphedema in a cohort of breast carcinoma survivors 20 years after diagnosis. Cancer 92:1368–1377
5. Larson D, Weinstein M, Goldberg I et al (1986) Edema of the arm as a function of the extent of axillary surgery in patients with stage I-II carcinoma of the breast treated with primary radiotherapy. Int J Radiat Oncol Biol Phys 12:1575–1582
6. Nesvold IL, Dahl AA, Løkkevik E, Marit Mengshoel A, Fosså SD (2008) Arm and shoulder morbidity in breast cancer patients after breast-conserving therapy versus mastectomy. Acta Oncol 47(5):835–842
7. Passik SD, McDonald MV (1998) Psychosocial aspects of upper extremity lymphedema in women treated for breast carcinoma. Cancer 83:2817–2820
8. Tobin MB, Lacey HJ, Meyer L, Mortimer PS (1993) The psychosocial morbidity of breast cancer-related arm swelling. Psychological morbidity of lymphedema. Cancer 72:3248–3252
9. Schrenk P, Rieger R, Shamiyeh A et al (2000) Morbidity following sentinel lymph node biopsy versus axillary lymph node dissection for patients with breast carcinoma. Cancer 88:608–614
10. Haid A, Kuehn T, Konstantiniuk P, Köberle-Wührer R, Knauer M, Kreienberg R, Zimmermann G (2002) Shoulder-arm morbidity following axillary dissection and sentinel node only biopsy for breast cancer. Eur J Surg Oncol 28(7):705–710
11. Swenson KK, Nissen MJ, Ceronsky C, Swenson L, Lee MW, Tuttle TM (2002) Comparison of side effects between sentinel lymph node and axillary lymph node dissection for breast cancer. Ann Surg Oncol 9(8):745–753
12. Blanchard DK, Donohue JH, Reynolds C et al (2003) Relapse and morbidity in patients undergoing sentinel lymph node biopsy alone or with axillary dissection for breast cancer. Arch Surg 138:482–488

13. Schijven MP, Vingerhoets AJ, Rutten HJ et al (2003) Comparison of morbidity between axillary lymph node dissection and sentinel node biopsy. Eur J Surg Oncol 29:341–350
14. Ronka R, von Smitten K, Tasmuth et al (2005) One-year morbidity after sentinel node biopsy and breast surgery. Breast 14:28–36
15. Leidenius M, Leivonen M, Vironen J, von Smitten K (2005) The consequences of long-time arm morbidity in node-negative breast cancer patients with sentinel node biopsy or axillary clearance. J Surg Oncol 92:23–31
16. Mansel R, Fallowfield L, Kissin M et al (2006) Randomized multicenter trial of sentinel node biopsy versus standard axillary treatment in operable breast cancer: the ALMANAC trial. JNCI 98(9):599–609
17. McLaughlin SA, Wright MJ, Morris KT et al (2008) Prevalence of lymphedema in women with breast cancer 5 years after sentinel lymph node biopsy or axillary dissection: objective measurements. J Clin Oncol 26(32):5213–5219
18. Ashikaga T, Krag DN, Land SR et al (2010) Morbidity results from the NSABP B-32 trial comparing sentinel lymph node dissection versus axillary dissection. J Surg Oncol 102 (2):111–118
19. Thompson M, Korourian S, Henry-Tillman R et al (2007) Axillary Reverse Mapping (ARM): a new concept to identify and enhance lymphatic preservation. Ann Surg Oncol 14:1890–1895
20. Thompson M, Korourian S, Henry-Tillman RS, Adkins L, Mumford S, Westbrook K, Klimberg VS, Talley L, Korourian S (2007) ARM (Axillary Reverse Mapping): a new concept to identify and enhance lymphatic preservation. Ann Surg Oncol 14(2):84–85, Supplement
21. Boneti C, Korourian S, Bland K, Cox K, Adkins LL, Henry-Tillman RS, Klimberg VS (2008) Axillary reverse mapping: mapping and preserving arm lymphatics may be important in preventing lymphedema during sentinel lymph node biopsy. J Am Coll Surg 206 (5):1038–1042; discussion 1042–4
22. Klimberg VS (2008) A new concept toward the prevention of lymphedema: axillary reverse mapping. J Surg Oncol 97(7):563–564
23. Boneti C, Badgwell B, Robertson Y, Korourian S, Adkins L, Klimberg VS (2012) Axillary reverse mapping (ARM): initial results of phase II trial in preventing lymphedema after lymphadenectomy. Minerva Ginecol 64(5):421–430
24. Ochoa D, Korourian S, Boneti C, Adkins L, Badgwell B, Klimberg VS (2014) Axillary reverse mapping: five-year experience. Axillary reverse mapping: five-year experience. Surgery 156 (5):1261–1268. doi:10.1016/j.surg.2014.05.011. Epub 2014 Oct 17
25. Wilke LG, McCall LM, Posther KE, Whitworth PW, Reintgen DS, Leitch AM, Gabram SG, Lucci A, Cox CE, Hunt KK, Herndon JE 2nd, Giuliano AE (2006) Surgical complications associated with sentinel lymph node biopsy: results from a prospective international cooperative group trial. Ann Surg Oncol 13(4):491–500
26. Hayes SC, Janda M, Cornish B, Battistutta D, Newman B (2008) Lymphedema after breast cancer: incidence, risk factors and effect of upper body. J Clin Oncol 26:3536–3542
27. Albert US, Koller M, Kopp I, Lorenz W, Schulz KD, Wagner U (2006) Early self-reported impairments in arm functioning of primary breast cancer patients predict late side effects of axillary lymph node dissection: results from a population-based cohort study. Breast Cancer Res Treat 100(3):285–292
28. Shah C, Vicini FA (2011) Breast cancer-related arm lymphedema: incidence rates, diagnostic techniques, optimal management and risk reduction. Int J Radiat Oncol 81(4):907–914
29. Deutsch M, Land S, Begovic M, Sharif S (2008) The incidence of arm edema in women with breast cancer randomized on the National Surgical Adjuvant Breast and Bowel Project study B-04 to radical mastectomy versus total mastectomy and radiotherapy versus total mastectomy alone. Int J Radiat Oncol Biol Phys 70(4):1020–1024
30. Williams AF, Franks PJ, Moffatt CJ (2005) Lymphoedema: estimating the size of the problem. Palliat Med 19:300–313

31. Nielsen I, Gordon S, Selby A (2008) Breast cancer-related lymphoedema risk reduction advice: a challenge for health professionals. Cancer Treat Rev 34:621–628. [Epub ahead of print]
32. Foldi M (2004) Remarks concerning the consensus document (CD) of the International Society of Lymphology the diagnosis and treatment of peripheral lymphedema. Lymphology 37 (4):168–173
33. Kröger K (2008) Lymphoedema and lipoedema of the extremities. Vasa 37(1):39–51
34. Ponzone R, Mininanni P, Cassina E, Sismondi P (2008) Axillary reverse mapping in breast cancer: can we spare what we find? Ann Surg Oncol 15(1):390–391; author reply 392–3
35. Nos C, Kaufmann G, Clough KB, Collignon MA, Zerbib E, Cusumano P, Lecuru F (2008) Combined axillary reverse mapping (ARM) technique for breast cancer patients requiring axillary dissection. Ann Surg Oncol 15(9):2550–2555. Epub 2008 Jul 11
36. Ponzone R, Cont NT, Maggiorotto F, Cassina E, Mininanni P, Biglia N, Sismondi P (2009) Extensive nodal disease may impair axillary reverse mapping in patients with breast cancer. J Clin Oncol 27(33):5547–5551. Epub 2009 Oct 13
37. Bedrosian I, Babiera GV, Mittendorf EA, Kuerer HM, Pantoja L, Hunt KK, Krishnamurthy S, Meric-Bernstam F (2010) A phase I study to assess the feasibility and oncologic safety of axillary reverse mapping in breast cancer patients. Cancer 116(11):2543–2548
38. Casabona F, Bogliolo S, Ferrero S, Boccardo F, Campisi C (2008) Axillary reverse mapping in breast cancer: a new microsurgical lymphatic-venous procedure in the prevention of arm lymphedema. Ann Surg Oncol 15(11):3318–3319. Epub 2008 Aug 15
39. Kang SH, Choi JE, Jeon YS et al (2009) Preservation of lymphatic drainage from arm in breast cancer surgery: is it safe? Cancer Res 69(suppl 2):201
40. Casabona F, Bogliolo S, Valenzano Menada M, Sala P, Villa G, Ferrero S (2009) Feasibility of axillary reverse mapping during sentinel lymph node biopsy in breast cancer patients. Ann Surg Oncol 16(9):2459–2463. Epub 2009 Jun 9
41. Noguchi M, Yokoi M, Nakano Y (2010) Axillary reverse mapping with indocyanine fluorescence imaging in patients with breast cancer. J Surg Oncol 101(3):217–221
42. Shaitelman SF, Cromwell KD, Rasmussen JC, Stout NL, Armer JM, Lasinski BB, Cormier JN (2015) Recent progress in the treatment and prevention of cancer-related lymphedema. CA Cancer J Clin 65(1):55–81. doi:10.3322/caac.21253. Epub 2014 Nov 19. Review
43. Kim T, Giuliano A, Lyman G (2006) Lymphatic mapping and sentinel lymph node biopsy in early-stage breast carcinoma – a metaanalysis. Cancer 106:4–16
44. Klimberg VS, Rubio IT, Henry R, Cowan C, Colvert M, Korourian S (1999) Subareolar versus peritumoral injection for location of the sentinel lymph node. Ann Surg 229(6):860–864, discussion 864–5
45. Ahmed M, Rubio IT, Kovacs T, Klimberg VS, Douek M (2015) Systematic review of axillary reverse mapping in breast cancer. Br J Surg. doi:10.1002/Bjs.10041. [Epub ahead of print]
46. Han JW, Seo YJ, Choi JE, Kang SH, Bae YK, Lee SJ (2012) The efficacy of arm node preserving surgery using axillary reverse mapping for preventing lymphedema in patients with breast cancer. J Breast Cancer 15:91–97
47. Kuusk U, Seyednejad N, McKevitt EC, Dingee CK, Wiseman SM (2014) Axillary reverse mapping in breast cancer: a Canadian experience. J Surg Oncol 110:791–795
48. Gennaro M, Maccauro M, Sigari C et al (2013) Selective axillary dissection after axillary reverse mapping to prevent breast-cancer-related lymphedema. Eur J Surg Oncol J Eur Soc Surg Oncol Br Assoc Surg Oncol 39:1341–1345
49. Tausch C, Baege A, Dietrich D (2013) Can axillary reverse mapping avoid lymphedema in node positive breast cancer patients? Eur J Surg Oncol J Eur Soc Surg Oncol Br Assoc Surg Oncol 39:880–886
50. Geber LH (1998) A review of measures of lymphedema. Cancer 83:2803–2804
51. Kaulesar Sukul DMKS, den Hoed PT, Johannes EJ et al (1993) Direct and indirect methods for the quantification of leg volume: comparison between water displacement volumetry, the disk

model method and the frustum sign model method, using the correlation coefficient and the limits of agreement. J Biomed Eng 15:477–480
52. Stanton AW, Northfield JW, Holroyd B et al (1997) Validation of an optoelectronic limb volumeter (perometer). Lymphology 30:77–97
53. Bates DO, Levick JR, Mortimer PS (1994) Quantification of rate and depth of pitting in human edema using an electronic tonometer. Lymphology 27:159–172
54. Cornish BH, Chapman M, Hirst C, Mirolo B, Bunce LH, Ward LC, Thomas BJ (2001) Early diagnosis of lymphedema using multiple frequency bioimpedance. Lymphology 34:2–11
55. Werner GT, Scheck R, Kaiserling E (1998) Magnetic resonance imaging of peripheral lymphedema. Lymphology 31:34–36
56. Marotel M, Cluzan R, Ghabboun S et al (1998) Transaxial computer tomography of lower extremity lymphedema. Lymphology 31:180–185
57. Stanton AWB, Badger C, Sitzia J (2000) Non-invasive assessment of the lymphoedematous limb. Lymphology 33:122–135
58. Lukaski HC (1987) Methods for the assessment of human body composition: traditional and new. Am J Clin Nutr 46:537–556
59. Ward LC, Bunce IH, Cornish BH et al (1992) Multi-frequency bioelectrical impedance augments the diagnosis and management of lymphedema in post-mastectomy patients. Eur J Clin Invest 22:751–754
60. Cornish BH, Bunce IH, Ward LC (1996) Bioelectrical impedance for monitoring the efficacy of lymphedema treatment programmes. Breast Cancer Res Treat 38:169–176

Chapter 6
Ultrasound for Axillary Staging

Chiun-Sheng Huang

Abstract Ultrasound examination of the axillary lymph node has been demonstrated to be a useful tool in evaluating axilla lymph node status. Axillary ultrasound (AUS) was first used to identify positive lymph nodes preoperatively, so that patients could undergo axillary lymph node dissection (ALND) directly and be spared from sentinel lymph node biopsy (SLNB). Recent studies also focus on the application of AUS in surgical planning when AUS reveals negative nodal status. When AUS is negative, the chance of having more than three positive nodes is low. Therefore, when AUS is negative, one can plan immediate reconstruction after mastectomy, and there is no need of intraoperative SLN examination for breast-conserving surgery. If AUS reveals suspicious lymph node and ultrasound-guided biopsy proves the node to be metastatic, SLNB can be spared if mastectomy is planned. Axillary ultrasound is also helpful in guiding whether SLNB should be done before or after neoadjuvant chemotherapy. If AUS is negative, the chance of having positive SLN is relatively low, and it would be reasonable to proceed with SLNB. If AUS or ultrasound-guided biopsy is positive, one may consider SLNB after neoadjuvant chemotherapy. For node-positive patients undergoing neoadjuvant chemotherapy first, patients with negative AUS before SLNB can be considered to undergo SLNB alone after neoadjuvant chemotherapy.

Keywords Axillary staging • Sentinel lymph node biopsy • Axillary ultrasound • Neoadjuvant chemotherapy

6.1 Current Status of Sentinel Lymph Node Biopsy and Axillary Ultrasound in Axillary Staging

Sentinel lymph node biopsy (SLNB) is widely accepted by physicians and patients as an option of axillary staging due to its low incidence of morbidity. In its recent SLNB clinical practice guideline update, the American Society of Clinical Oncology made several recommendations, which include that clinicians should not

C.-S. Huang (✉)
National Taiwan University Hospital, National Taiwan University College of Medicine, No. 7, Chung Shan S. Rd., Taipei 10002, Taiwan
e-mail: huangcs@ntu.edu.tw

M. Toi et al. (eds.), *Personalized Treatment of Breast Cancer*,
DOI 10.1007/978-4-431-55552-0_6

recommend axillary lymph node dissection (ALND) for women with early-stage breast cancer who do not have nodal metastases and clinicians should not recommend ALND for women with early breast cancer who have one or two sentinel lymph node metastases and will receive breast-conserving surgery with conventionally fractionated whole-breast radiotherapy [1].

During the advent of SLNB, ultrasound examination of the axillary lymph node has also been demonstrated to be a useful tool in evaluating axilla lymph node status. Axillary ultrasound (AUS) was first used to identify positive lymph nodes preoperatively, so that patients could undergo ALND directly and be spared from SLNB. Recent studies also focus on the application of AUS in treatment decision-making when AUS reveals negative axillary lymph node status. The applications of ultrasound in axillary staging in conjunction with SLNB are reviewed in the following.

6.2 Axillary Ultrasound Can Identify Metastatic Lymph Node

Among different studies of different incidences of lymph node involvement in axillae, metastases were detected preoperatively by ultrasound-guided fine-needle aspiration cytology (US-FNAC), and 1.4–45 % of SLNB could be avoided [2–13]. In one large series of 726 patients (consisting of 732 axillae) with 67 % of T1 tumor, 30 % of T2 tumors, and 2.7 % of T3 or T4 tumors reported by van Rijk et al., about one-quarter of axillae were found to have suspicious lymph node by AUS, and about one-third of these axillae with suspicious ultrasound were proved by US-FNAC to have metastatic lymph node involvement by SLNB [9]. Those patients with normal AUS did not receive US-FNAC. The sensitivity and specificity were 35 % and 82 %, respectively, for AUS, and 21 % and 99.8 %, respectively, for US-FNAC. In this series, 58 of 732 (8 %) of axillae were diagnosed preoperatively to have lymph node metastasis. Therefore, 8 % of patients can be saved from SLNB and receive ALND directly.

Among the earlier studies, the percentage of metastatic lymph nodes diagnosed preoperatively by ultrasound-guided biopsy ranged from 5.7 to 80 %, and the percentage of SLNB avoided ranged from 1.4 to 45% [2–13]. In addition to the different incidences of metastatic lymph nodes among these studies, the explanation for the wide variation of rates could also be due to differences in the following factors: the percentage of lymph nodes visualized, the criteria of suspicious nodes detected by AUS, biopsied only the suspicious nodes or all nodes visualized, and the biopsy method (core needle biopsy (CNB) or FNAC).

The specificity of US-FNAC is higher than that of AUS, but the sensitivity of AUS is higher than that of US-FNAC, which implies that the false-negative rates of US-FNAC may be due to FNAC but not due to ultrasound. Two studies reported the use of CNB in biopsy of the lymph node [2, 3]. Complications associated with the

CNB procedure seem acceptable. Just like in the diagnosis of primary tumor, the false-negative rate is expected to be lower with CNB than with FNAC.

6.3 Ultrasound Evaluation Decreases False-Negative Rate of SLNB

Pre-SLNB evaluation of the axillary lymph node by AUS will help to decrease the false-negative rate of SLNB. As demonstrated in the study by Sato et al., the SLN identification rate for 262 total patients and 208 patients with negative AUS was 88.2 % and 98.6 %, respectively, while for 23 patients with T3 tumors and 6 patients with T3 tumors but negative AUS, the identification rate was 65.2 % and 100 %, respectively [14]. The false-negative rate of SLNB for all 262 patients and 208 patients with negative AUS was 10.8 % and 1.7 %, respectively, while for 23 patients with T3 tumors and 6 patients with T3 tumors but negative AUS, the false-negative rate was 35.7 % and 0 %, respectively.

6.4 Axillary Ultrasound Is Helpful in Large Tumor Staging

The incidence of lymph node metastasis demonstrated by ALND in breast cancer patients for different tumor sizes as reported by Silverstein et al. was 5 %, 16 %, 28 %, 47 %, 68 %, and 86 % in T1a, T1b, T1c, T2, T3, and T4 tumors, respectively [15]. Since the chance of lymph node involvement is low in small tumors, which makes the complications associated with ALND more undesirable, SLNB was first applied in small tumors to replace ALND [16–18]. In daily practice, SLNB generally has been applied to invasive breast cancers not larger than 3 cm and without clinical evidence of lymph node involvement [18–20]. Tumor size is limited to 3 cm or smaller for several reasons: first, nearly half of the T2 tumor may develop lymph node metastasis, which would necessitate a second procedure of ALND after SLNB and make SLND unnecessary; second is the incorrect perception that false-negative rate of SLNB could be high in a large tumor, due to a higher chance of the complete occupancy of cancer in the lymph node, which prevents the radiotracer entering the lymph node.

The recent ASCO SLNB guideline recommends that clinicians should not perform SNB for women who have large or locally advanced invasive breast cancers (tumor size T3/T4) [1]. Only one study of 64 patients with locally advanced breast cancers was found by the panels. The FNRs were 5.1 % for patients with locally advanced breast cancer and 5.8 % for those with early-stage breast cancer enrolled in different randomized trial comparing SLNB with ALND [21].

Actually, several studies, also non-randomized trials, have focused on the accuracy of SLNB in large breast cancer. In a prospective multi-institutional study of 2,085 breast cancer patients, the identification rate of SLN and false-negative rate were not significantly different in patients with T1, T2, and T3 tumors [22]. All patients received SLNB using dual tracer with radioactive colloid and blue dye, followed by ALND. The identification rate of SLN was 93.2 % and 97.8 % for T2 and T3 tumors, respectively, compared with that of 92.1 % for T1 tumors, and the false-negative rate was 6.8 % and 3.0 % for T2 and T3 tumors, respectively, compared with 9.2 % for T1 tumors. When the tumor size was categorized into a 1-cm difference, the SLN identification rate tended to be higher and false-negative rate lower in patients with larger tumors. Generally speaking, the identification rates of SLN (93–100 %) and false-negative rates of SLNB (3–6.8 %) were not worse in T2 and T3 tumors than those of T1 tumors [22–25]. In one study of 218 patients with T2 and T3 tumors and in the other study of 48 patients with tumor larger than 3 cm, both with negative SLN and not receiving ALND, none of the patients developed isolated axillary recurrence at a median follow-up of 31 months and 43 months, respectively [26, 27]. Based on the findings in these studies, it seems that SLNB is as accurate an axillary staging procedure in T2 and T3 breast cancers as in T1 cancers.

In addition, the sensitivity of AUS in detecting lymph node metastasis has been shown to increase as the tumor size increases. Koelliker et al. reported the sensitivity of ultrasound for T1, T2, T3, and T4 tumor was 56 %, 64–73 %, 82 %, and 100 %, respectively, and Somasundar et al. reported 35 % and 67 % for T1 and T2 tumors, respectively [11, 28]. This could be explained by larger metastasis depositing in lymph nodes of larger cancer, which make it easier to be detected by AUS [10, 13]. As mentioned previously, pre-SLNB evaluation of the axillary lymph node by ultrasound will help to decrease the false-negative rate of SLNB. The study by Sato et al. demonstrated that the false-negative rate of SLNB for all 262 patients and 208 patients with negative ultrasound was 10.8 % and 1.7 %, respectively, while for 23 patients with T3 tumors and 6 patients with T3 tumors but negative ultrasound, the false-negative rate was 35.7 % and 0 %, respectively [14]. Therefore, AUS is helpful for axillary staging in large tumor. Either the metastatic lymph node can be identified preoperatively, or accuracy of SLNB can be ensured by negative AUS.

6.5 Negative Ultrasound Indicates Fewer Nodal Metastases

Reports also suggest that when AUS or US-FNAC reveals negative axillary lymph node status, the chance of having more than three positive lymph nodes or tumor deposits in the lymph node >5 mm is low. The study by van Rijk et al. demonstrated that patients, whose axillary lymph node involvement was diagnosed by preoperative US-FNAC, had more positive nodes than patients whose axillary lymph node involvement could not be detected by US-FNAC (mean 4.3 vs. 2.2, median 3 vs.1.5; $p < 0.001$) [9]. The study by Bonnema et al. also demonstrated that the chance to detect metastatic lymph nodes by US-FNAC was higher when there were four or more positive nodes compared with when there was only one positive node [4]. In Swinson et al.'s series, none of 14 cases with micrometastasis (0.2–2 mm) of the lymph node were detected by US-FNAC, but 38 of 102 (37 %) cases with lymph node metastasis larger than or equal to 2 mm were detected by US-FNAC [13]. Fifty percent of cases with more than three positive nodes were detected preoperatively by US-FNAC, while only 15 % of cases with one positive node were diagnosed by US-FNAC. In this series, 278 of 369 (75 %) breast cancers were detected by screening. In a series of 286 patients having negative AUS before SLNB, 32 % of patients have positive SLNs of macrometastasis or micrometastasis and 9.2 % of 286 patients might have positive non-SLNs. The mean and median numbers of positive nodes (SLNs plus non-SLNs) were 1.7 and 1, respectively [29].

6.6 How to Find the Lymph Node in Axillary Ultrasound

To increase the percentage of metastatic lymph nodes diagnosed preoperatively, one needs to know how to visualize a lymph node. In the early reports, the percentage of the lymph node visualized in axillae was only 35–37 % [5, 8], while in more recent reports, it was 100 % [9]. A normal lymph node has a central fatty hilum and thin cortex, which sometimes is hard to detect from the surrounding fatty tissue of the axilla (Fig. 6.2). To find a lymph node, or even an SLN, in the axilla, one also needs to be aware of the frequent location of an SLN. In 98.4 % of our 974 patients, the hotspot detected on the axilla skin before SLNB was located in the area demarcated by the four landmarks of the hairline, a line tangential to and 2 cm below the center of the hairline, the lateral border of the pectoralis major muscle, and the midaxillary line (Fig. 6.1) [30].

6.7 Ultrasound Criteria of Metastatic Lymph Nodes

The diagnostic criteria of a metastatic lymph node by ultrasound vary among reports [2–4, 7–9, 11, 12, 31]. The following characteristics may suggest that a lymph node could be metastasized: the absence of or narrow fatty hilum, an eccentrically or concentrically increased thickness of cortex (more than 2 mm), an atypical cortex appearance (echo poor, inhomogeneous), and the ratio of longitudinal to transverse axis less than two (Fig. 6.2). In addition, if ultrasound examination is done after excisional biopsy, a benign axillary lymph node may look suspicious (with increased thickening of cortex) [7].

In one study using ultrasound alone without biopsy to evaluate axillary status, Sato et al. chose the absence of the hilum as the criteria of lymph node involvement

Fig. 6.1 Frequent locations of axillary sentinel lymph node

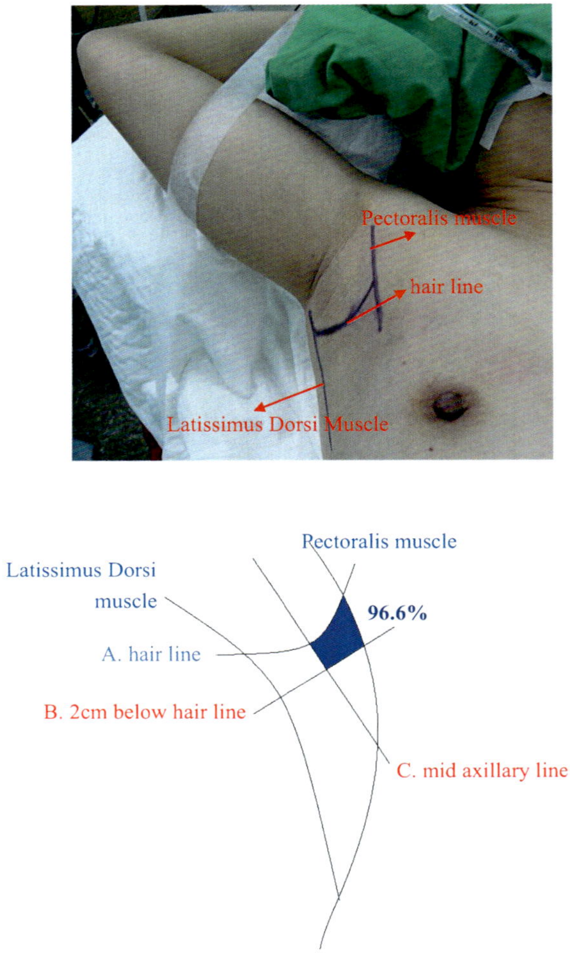

[14]. In 54 patients with abnormal ultrasound, 50 had lymph node metastasis and in 208 patients with normal ultrasound; only 62 had lymph node involvement. The PPV, sensitivity, and specificity calculated from these data were 93 %, 45 %, and 97 %, respectively. Maximum cortex thickness was the most significant feature in the study by Deurloo et al. to predict lymph node metastasis [8]. To obtain a high sensitivity at 95 %, and a low specificity at 44 %, a maximum cortex thickness of 2.3 mm was shown to be the most important criteria for biopsy. In a recent study by Koelliker et al., the PPV for the absence of the hilum, eccentric hilum, hypoechoic

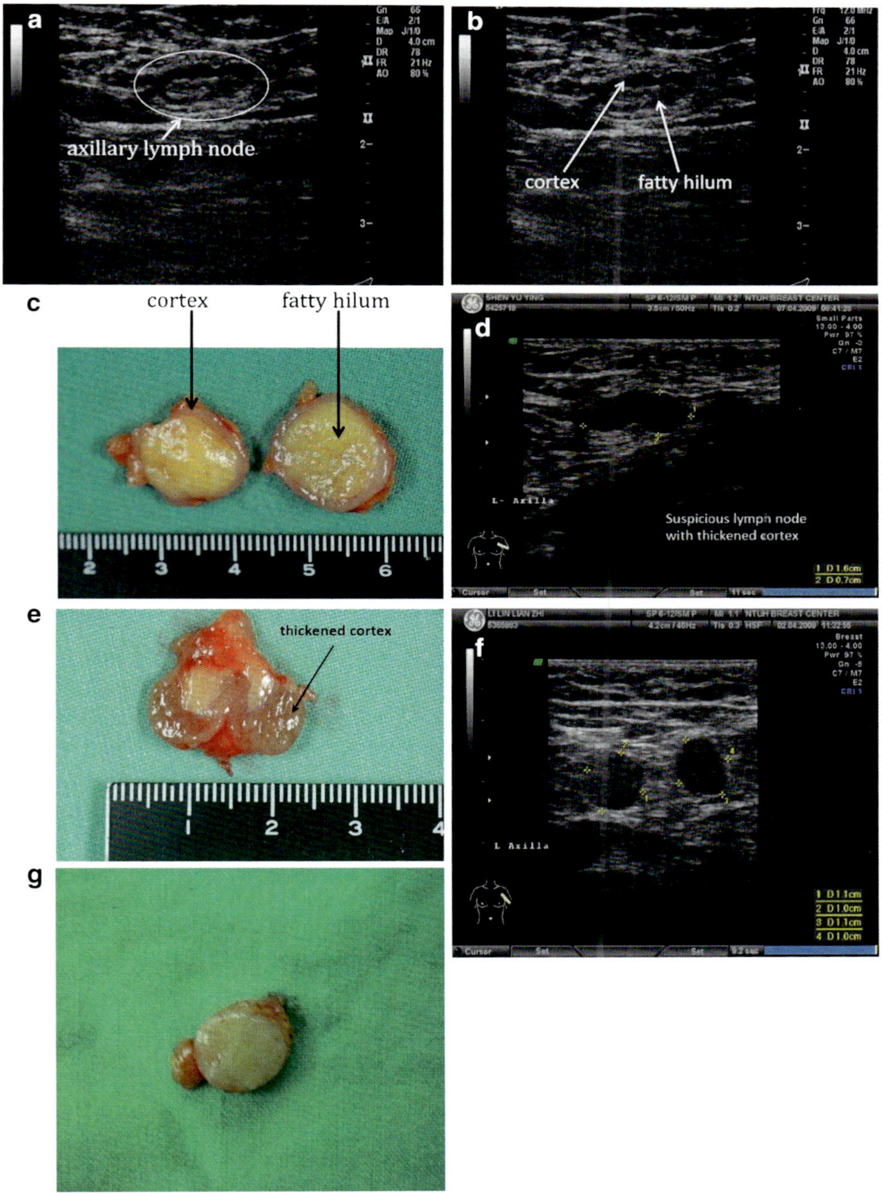

Fig. 6.2 Ultrasound images and photos of benign and suspicious axillary lymph nodes (**a**) A benign lymph node on AUS with thin cortex (**b**) Benign lymph node on AUS (**c**) Cut surface of a benign lymph node (**d**) A suspicious lymph node with thickened cortex (7 mm) (**e**) Cut surface of a lymph node with thickened cortex (**f**) A metastatic lymph node characterized by loss of the fatty hilum with rounding appearance (**g**) Cut surface of a metastatic lymph node

cortex, and thick or lobular cortex was 100 %, 94 %, 97 %, and 73 %, respectively [11].

In a study using ultrasound-guided CNB, the sensitivity of ultrasound to diagnose a metastatic lymph node based on the cortical thickening, the absence of the fatty hilum, and the nonhilar blood flow was 79 %, 33 %, and 65 %, respectively, and the PPV was 73 %, 93 %, and 78 %, respectively [3]. With the cortical thickness cutoff point set at 3 mm, the sensitivity and specificity of this parameter for the detection of metastatic nodes were 95 % (61 of 64 patients) and 6 % (2 of 36 patients), respectively. If 4 mm was used as the cutoff point, sensitivity decreased slightly to 88 % (56 of 64 patients) and specificity increased to 42 % (15 of 36 patients). Of the 191 needle-localized nodes, Cho et al. used a cutoff point of a cortical thickness of 2.5 mm and achieved a sensitivity of 85 % and specificity of 78 %. When AUS is negative, the chance of having positive node was about 11% [32].

6.8 Application of Axillary Ultrasound If Neoadjuvant Chemotherapy Is Not Planned

Based on the above studies, loss of the fatty hilum has the highest PPV in predicting positive lymph node. While different thickness of cortex will yield different values of sensitivity, specificity, NPV, and PPV, one may choose different criteria depending on how to apply AUS. For example, if a metastatic lymph node needs to be ruled out, a lymph node with loss of the fatty hilum or a cortical thickness more than 2 mm will receive US-FNAC. If the cytology is negative, SLNB will be done to confirm the status of axillary lymph node. With these criteria, the NPV will be the highest and the chance of having a metastatic lymph node will be the lowest. Hence, when AUS is negative and neoadjuvant chemotherapy is not planned, one can plan immediate reconstruction after mastectomy, and there is no need of intraoperative SLN examination (no unanticipated ALND, which is helpful for scheduling surgery) if breast-conserving treatment is planned and will be more comfortable to follow Z0011 conclusion to omit ALND when there are no more than two positive SLNs (Fig. 6.3a). If AUS reveals a suspicious lymph node and US-FNAC proves the node to be metastatic, SLNB can be spared if mastectomy is planned. If breast-conserving surgery is planned in a patient with suspicious AUS or positive US-FNAC but the lymph node is not palpable before US-FNAC, some people still think ALND can be spared if positive SLNs are not more than two, since only patients with palpable axillary nodes, but not patients with positive AUS, were excluded in Z0011 trial.

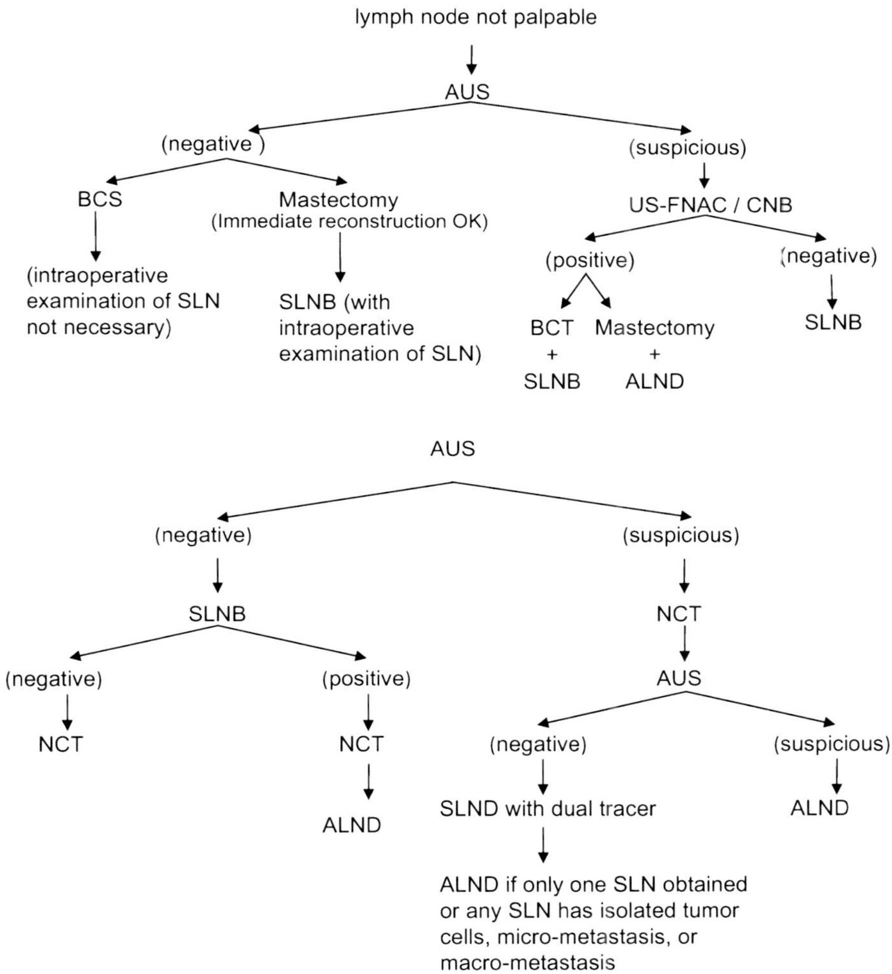

Fig. 6.3 Flowchart of proposed algorithm using ultrasound in conjunction with SLNB for axillary staging among patients receiving primary surgery or neoadjuvant chemotherapy (**a**) Neoadjuvant chemotherapy (NCT) not considered. *AUS* axillary ultrasound, *BCS* breast-conserving surgery, *US-FNAC* ultrasound-guided fine-needle aspiration cytology, *CNB* core needle biopsy, *SCNB* sentinel lymph node biopsy, *ALND* axillary lymph node dissection (**b**) Neoadjuvant chemotherapy (NCT) considered

6.9 Axillary Ultrasound for Guiding SLND Before or After Neoadjuvant Chemotherapy

The 2014 American Society of Clinical Oncology (ASCO) SLNB guideline recommends that SLNB may be offered before or after neoadjuvant systemic therapy but states that SLNB seems less accurate after neoadjuvant systemic therapy [1]. In general, when SLNB is done before neoadjuvant chemotherapy and SLN is negative, axillary staging is not necessary after neoadjuvant chemotherapy; while if SLN is positive, ALND is usually recommended after chemotherapy. The rationale of doing SLND after neoadjuvant chemotherapy is that about one-third of positive nodal status before chemotherapy will be converted to negative nodal status after chemotherapy. SLND done after neoadjuvant chemotherapy may save these patients from ALND.

Axillary ultrasound is helpful in guiding whether SLNB should be done before or after neoadjuvant chemotherapy. If AUS is negative, the chance of having positive SLNs is relatively low, and it would be reasonable to proceed with SLNB. Even there are positive SLNs, if the number of positive nodes is not more than two and breast-conserving treatment is planned after neoadjuvant chemotherapy, ALND may still be waived according to the conclusion of Z0011 study [33]. If AUS or ultrasound-guided biopsy is positive before neoadjuvant chemotherapy, one may consider SLNB after neoadjuvant chemotherapy.

The SENTINA study investigated the feasibility of SLNB before and after neoadjuvant chemotherapy [34]. It included 1,737 patients undergoing at least six cycles of an anthracycline-based chemotherapy. Among them, 76 % had T2 tumor, 6.4 % had T3 tumor, and 14.2 % had unknown tumor size; 1,022 patients were clinically node negative and 715 patients were clinically node positive. Clinical lymph node status was evaluated preoperatively by palpation and ultrasound. Palpable nodes were considered as negative nodal status if ultrasound showed benign-look lymph nodes. Basically, clinically node-negative status means negative AUS in SENTINA study. No uniformly standard for sonographic lymph node assessment is described in SENTINA. Lymph nodes were classified as suspicious if the hilum/cortex ratio >2:1 or total loss of the hilum.

Immunohistochemical staining of SLN was not required in SENTINA. Only 25 % of patients had FNA cytology or core needle biopsy confirmation for their positive nodal status. Of the 1,022 patients, who had negative AUS and underwent SLNB before neoadjuvant chemotherapy, 65 % had negative SLN. The IDR of second SLNB in patients who had positive sentinel nodes before neoadjuvant chemotherapy and had a second SLNB procedure after neoadjuvant chemotherapy was 76.2 % or 52.9 % with dual tracers (isotope and blue dye) or isotope only, respectively. Although 70.8 % had negative node revealed by second SLNB, the FNR of second SLNB was as high as 51.6 %.

Some previous studies support that SLNB alone seems feasible after neoadjuvant chemotherapy [35–40]. However, the identification rates and false-negative rates vary widely among different studies due to inclusion of patients of different stages and different nodal status before neoadjuvant chemotherapy. Three recent studies reported the application of AUS related to SLNB after neoadjuvant chemotherapy in patients presenting with positive axillary nodes.

Among the 715 patients presenting with initially suspicious nodes on AUS in SENTINA study, 17 % had persistent suspicious nodes after neoadjuvant chemotherapy and underwent ALND directly after neoadjuvant chemotherapy. AUS converted from positive to negative after neoadjuvant chemotherapy in 83 %

(592/715) of patients. The IDR of SLNB was 80 % (474/592) and FNR was 14.2 % (32/226) in these 474 patients who had successful SLNB. Of the 474 patients, 248 (52.3 %) had negative node and 226 (47.7 %) were node positive.

The FNR of SLND is significantly related to the number of resected sentinel lymph nodes in these patients who converted from node-positive to node-negative status on AUS after neoadjuvant chemotherapy and then underwent SLNB. The false-negative rate was 24.3 % for patients who had only one sentinel node removed, 18.5 % for patients who had two removed, and less than 10 % for patients who had three or more sentinel lymph nodes removed (9.6 % for patients who had at least two SLNs removed). The false-negative rate was also lower, although not significant in multivariate analysis, for 389 patients who underwent SLNB with dual tracers (isotope and blue dye) compared with 164 patients who received isotope alone (8.6 % vs. 16.0 %). But dual tracer was associated with a significant increase in the IDR (87.8 % vs. 77.4 %).

ACOSOG Z1071 trial included 701 eligible patients with cN1 (disease in movable axillary lymph nodes, 663 patients, T1 and T2 69 %, T3 and T4 30 %) or cN2 (disease in fixed or matted axillary lymph nodes, 38 patients) at presentation documented by fine-needle aspiration biopsy or core needle biopsy [41]. Seventy-four percent of patients received neoadjuvant chemotherapy with both anthracycline and taxane. The FNR of SLNB after neoadjuvant chemotherapy was 12.6 %. FNR significantly decreased when dual tracers (isotope and blue dye) were used for mapping ($P = 0.05$; FNR, 10.8 % dual tracer vs. 20.3 % single tracer) and when at least three SLNs were obtained ($P = 0.007$; FNR, 9.1 % for ≥ 3 SLNs vs. 21.1 % for 2). Multivariate analysis revealed that no other factors, such as chemotherapy duration, dual or single mapping agents, single or multiple injection sites, pre-chemotherapy tumor size, and lymph node status after chemotherapy, would affect the FNR of SLNB, once the number of SLNs harvested (2 vs. ≥ 3) was accounted for.

In Z1071 trial, 611 patients had an AUS examination before SLNB after neoadjuvant chemotherapy [42]. The AUS images were submitted for central review by a single radiologist. A lymph node was considered suspicious if the cortex was either focally or diffusely thickened (>3 mm thick) and the fatty hilum was deformed or absent, which is not quite different from the criteria of suspicious node in SENTINA. In the 470 cN1 patients with a post-chemotherapy AUS (negative or positive nodal status) and at least two SLNs removed, FNR of SLNB was 12.6 %. If only patients with post-chemotherapy normal AUS would have been selected for SLNB surgery with resection of at least two SLNs, the FNR would be 9.8 %.

There were no difference of clinical N stage at presentation, completion of all chemotherapy, the number of SLNs removed, and the number of additional axillary lymph nodes removed between patients with normal lymph nodes and those with suspicious nodes on AUS. Patients with post-chemotherapy suspicious nodal status on AUS were more likely to have positive nodes after neoadjuvant chemotherapy, two or more positive SLNs, additional positive nodes, greater number of involved nodes, and larger median SLN metastasis size, than patients with normal AUS findings. In patients with a normal AUS, 8.6 % had more than two positive SLNs. In patients with a normal AUS but positive SLNs, 62.6 % had no additional positive nodes in the ALND specimen.

SN FNAC study enrolled patients with T0-T3, N1-2, and M0-X breast cancer and biopsy-proven node-positive status receiving neoadjuvant chemotherapy [43]. Among them, 50 % were T2, 40 % were T3, 96 % received both anthracycline and taxane, and 57 % were ER or PR positive and Her2 negative. AUS before and after neoadjuvant chemotherapy was performed. Immunohistochemical staining of SLN was included in pathological examination of SLN, and SLN metastases of any size, including isolated tumor cells, were considered positive. The SLN identification rate was 87.6 %, and the FNR was 8.4 %. If isolated tumor cells in SLN had been considered negative nodal status, the FNR would have increased to 13.3 %. The average number of SLNs removed was 2.7. Although the size of SLN metastases did not correlate directly with the rate of positive non-SLNs, but the average number of residual positive nodes in the ALND after positive SLNs with isolated tumor cells, micrometastasis or macrometastasis after neoadjuvant chemotherapy was 0.7, 0.5, and 2.8, respectively. If only one SLN was obtained, the FNR increased to 18.2 %. In the presence of two or more than two SLNs, the FNR of SLNB decreased to 4.9 %. The FNR of SLNB mapping with dual tracers (isotope and blue dye) and single tracer (radiocolloid) was 5.2 % and 16.0 %, respectively, but the difference was not significant. AUS was also done before and after neoadjuvant chemotherapy. Its impact was not reported.

Based on the above three trials, harvesting only one SN is associated with a high FNR (SN FNAC, 18.2 %; ACOSOG Z1071, 31.5 %; SENTINA, 24.3 %) of SLNB done after neoadjuvant chemotherapy in patients with node-positive breast cancer. In the above three trials, 20–31 % of patients had only one SLN harvested [33, 41, 43]. As there is probably no way to increase the number of harvested SLNs, patients with only one SLN harvested after neoadjuvant chemotherapy better proceed to ALND. The FNR for patients with two or more than two SLNs and SN metastases >0.2 mm was 11.5 % in SN FNAC study, which is close to the FNR of 12.6 % reported in the ACOSOG Z1071 trial but much lower than the 18.5 % in SENTINA patients who had two removed (less than 10 % for patients who had three or more sentinel lymph nodes removed in SENTINA).

By applying immunohistochemical staining in the pathologic evaluation of the SLNs and considering SLN metastases of any size as positive, FNR becomes 8.4 % in SN FNAC trial. While immunohistochemical staining of SLN decreased the FNR in the SN FNAC study, it was not mandatory in both SENTINA and Z1071 trials.

The FNR of SLNB with resection of at least two SLNs in node-positive patients with negative AUS after neoadjuvant chemotherapy was 9.6 % in SENTINA trial and 9.8 % in Z1071 trial. In both trials, AUS was done after neoadjuvant chemotherapy but before SLNB. Patients with suspicious nodal status on AUS in SENTINA trial will undergo ALND directly without SLNB. The percentage of patients with positive nodes revealed by ALND was not reported in SENTINA trial. In this situation, one would use stricter criteria of AUS to select patients with positive nodal status for ALND. Although the AUS criteria of the suspicious node used in SENTINA trial (criteria of suspicious lymph node: hilum/cortex ratio >2:1 or total loss of the hilum) and Z1071 trial (criteria of suspicious node: the cortex was either focally or diffusely thickened (>3 mm thick) and the fatty hilum was deformed or absent) seem not very different, the central review by single radiologist would probably still use a stricter criteria, e.g., a thinner cortex, to define a negative nodal status [34, 42]. In SN FNAC study, AUS nodal status was also evaluated but not considered in the calculation of FNR of SLNB.

In summary, for patients with positive nodal status undergoing neoadjuvant chemotherapy, AUS should be performed before SLNB after neoadjuvant chemotherapy. Only patients with negative AUS can be considered to undergo SLNB alone after neoadjuvant chemotherapy. ALND should be considered not only for patients with micrometastatic or macrometastatic SLNs but also in patients with isolated tumor cells in SLN. Patients with only one SLN harvested after neoadjuvant chemotherapy better proceed to ALND. Dual tracer with isotope and blue dye should be used for SLNB mapping (Fig. 6.3b).

References

1. Lyman GH, Temin S, Stephen BE et al (2014) Sentinel lymph node biopsy for patients with early-stage breast cancer: American Society of Clinical Oncology clinical practice guideline update. J Clin Oncol 32(13):1365–1383
2. Damera A, Evans AJ, Cornford EJ et al (2003) Diagnosis of axillary nodal metastases by ultrasound-guided core biopsy in primary operable breast cancer. Br J Cancer 89:1310–1313
3. Abe H, Schmidt RA, Kulkarni K et al (2009) Axillary lymph nodes suspicious for breast cancer metastasis: Sampling with US-guided 14-gauge core-needle biopsy—Clinical experience in 100 patients. Radiology 25:41–49
4. Bonnema J, van Geel AN, van Ooijen B et al (1997) Ultrasound-guided aspiration biopsy for detection of nonpalpable axillary node metastases in breast cancer patients: new diagnostic method. World J Surg 21:270–274
5. de Kanter AY, van Eijck CHJ, van Geel et al (1999) Multicentre study of ultrasonographically guided axillary node biopsy in patients with breast cancer. Br J Surg 86:1459–1462
6. Kuenen-Boumeester V, Menke-Pluymers M, de Kanter AY et al (2003) Ultrasound-guided fine needle aspiration cytology of axillary lymph nodes in breast cancer patients. A preoperative staging procedure. Eur J Cancer 39:170–174
7. Bedrosian I, Bedi D, Kuerer HM et al (2003) Impact of clinicopathological factors on sensitivity of axillary ultrasonography in the detection of axillary nodal metastases in patients with breast cancer. Ann Surg Oncol 10(9):1025–1030
8. Deurloo EE, Tanis PJ, Gilhuijs KGA et al (2003) Reduction in the number of sentinel lymph node procedures by preoperative ultrasonography of the axilla in breast cancer. Eur J Cancer 39:1068–1073
9. van Rijk MC, Deurloo EE, Nieweg OE et al (2006) Ultrasonography and fine-needle aspiration cytology can spare breast cancer patients unnecessary sentinel lymph node biopsy. Ann Surg Oncol 13(1):31–35
10. Hinson JL, McGrath P, Moore A et al (2008) The critical role of axillary ultrasound and aspiration biopsy in the management of breast cancer patients with clinically negative axilla. Ann Surg Oncol 15(1):250–255

11. Koelliker SL, Chung MA, Mainiero MB et al (2008) Axillary lymph nodes: US-guided fine-needle aspiration for initial staging of breast cancer—Correlation with primary tumor size. Radiology 246(1):81–89
12. Gilissen F, Oostenbroek R, Storm R et al (2008) Prevention of futile sentinel node procedures in breast cancer: ultrasonography of the axilla and fine-needle aspiration cytology are obligatory. Eur J Surg Oncol 34(2008):497–500
13. Swinson C, Ravichandran D, Nayagam M et al (2009) Ultrasound and fine needle aspiration cytology of the axilla in the pre-operative Identification of axillary nodal involvement in breast cancer. Eur J Surg Oncol 35(2009):1152–1157
14. Sato K, Tamaki K, Tsuda H et al (2004) Utility of axillary ultrasound examination to select breast cancer patients suited for optimal sentinel node biopsy. Am J Surg 187(2004):679–683
15. Silverstein MJ, Skinner KA, Lomis TJ (2001) Predicting axillary nodal positivity in 2282 patients with breast carcinoma. World J Surg 25:767–772
16. Krag DN, Anderson SJ, Julian TB, Brown AM, Harlow SP, Ashikaga T, Weaver DL, Miller BJ, Jalovec LM, Frazier TG, Dirk Noyes R, Robidoux A, Scarth HMC, Mammolito DM, McCready DR, Mamounas EP, Costantino JP, Wolmark N, for the National Surgical Adjuvant Breast and Bowel Project (NSABP) (2007) Technical outcomes of sentinel-lymph-node resection and conventional axillary-lymph-node dissection in patients with clinically node-negative breast cancer: results from the NSABP B-32 randomised phase III trial. Lancet Oncol 7(10):881–888
17. Zavagno G, De Salvo GL, Scalco G et al (2008) A randomized clinical trial on sentinel lymph node biopsy versus axillary lymph node dissection in breast cancer results of the Sentinella/GIVOM Trial. Ann Surg 247(2):207–213
18. Veronesi U, Paganelli G, Viale G et al (2006) Sentinel-lymph-node biopsy as a staging procedure in breast cancer: update of a randomised controlled study. Lancet Oncol 7 (12):983–990
19. Bergkvist L, de Boniface J, Jo¨nsson P-E et al (2008) Axillary recurrence rate after negative sentinel node biopsy in breast cancer: three-year follow-up of the Swedish Multicenter Cohort Study. Ann Surg 247:150–156
20. Intra M, Rotmensz N, Mattar D et al (2007) Unnecessary axillary node dissections in the sentinel lymph node era. Eur J Cancer 43:2664–2668
21. Canavese G, Dozin B, Vecchio C et al (2011) Accuracy of sentinel lymph node biopsy after neo-adjuvant chemotherapy in patients with locally advanced breast cancer and clinically positive axillary nodes. Eur J Surg Oncol 37(8):688–694
22. Wong SL, Chao C, Edwards MJ et al (2001) Accuracy of sentinel lymph node biopsy for patients with T2 and T3 breast cancers. Am J Surg 67:522–528
23. Bedrosian I, Reynolds RC, Mick R et al (2000) Accuracy of sentinel lymph node biopsy in patients with large primary breast tumors. Cancer 88(11):2540–2545
24. Chung MH, Ye W, Giuliano AE (2001) Role for sentinel lymph node dissection in the management of large (=5 cm) invasive breast cancer. Ann Surg Oncol 8(9):688–692
25. Lelievre L, Houvenaeghel G, Buttarelli M et al (2007) Value of the sentinel lymph node procedure in patients with large size breast cancer. Ann Surg Oncol 14(2):621–626
26. Naik AM, Fey J, Gemignani M et al (2004) III. The risk of axillary relapse after sentinel lymph node biopsy for breast cancer is comparable with that of axillary lymph node dissection: a follow-up study of 4008 procedures. Ann Surg 240:462–471
27. Meretoja TJ, Leidenius MH, Heikkilä PS et al (2009) Sentinel node biopsy in breast cancer patients with large or multifocal tumors. Ann Surg Oncol 16:1148–1155
28. Somasundar P, Gass J, Steinhoff M et al (2006) Role of ultrasound-guided axillary fine-needle aspiration in the management of invasive breast cancer. Am J Surg 192(2006):458–461
29. Zgajnar J, Hocevar M, Podkrajsek M et al (2006) Patients with preoperatively ultrasonically uninvolved axillary lymph nodes: a distinct subgroup of early breast cancer patients. Breast Cancer Res Treat 97(3):293–299

30. Lo C, Lee P-C, Yen R-F et al (2014) Most frequent location of the sentinel lymph nodes. Asian J Surg 37(3):125–129
31. Krishnamurthy S, Snelge N, Bedi DG et al (2002) Role of ultrasound-guided fine–needle aspiration of indeterminate and suspicious axillary lymph nodes in the initial staging of breast carcinoma. Cancer 95(5):982–988
32. Cho N, Moon WK, Han W et al (2009) Preoperative sonographic classification of axillary lymph nodes in patients with breast cancer: node-to-node correlation with surgical histology and sentinel node biopsy results. Am J Roentgenol 193(6):1731–1737
33. Giuliano AE, Hunt KE, Ballman KV et al (2011) Axillary dissection vs no axillary dissection in women with invasive breast cancer and sentinel node metastasis: a randomized clinical trial. J Am Med Assoc 305(6):569–575
34. Kuehn T, Bauerfeind I, Fehm T et al (2013) Sentinel-lymph-node biopsy in patients with breast cancer before and after neoadjuvant chemotherapy (SENTINA): a prospective, multicentre cohort study. Lancet Oncol 14(7):609–618
35. Mamounas EP, Brown A, Anderson S et al (2005) Sentinel node biopsy after neoadjuvant chemotherapy in breast cancer: results from National Surgical Adjuvant Breast and Bowel Project Protocol B-27. J Clin Oncol 23:2694–2702
36. Classe J-M, Bordes V, Campion L et al (2009) Sentinel lymph node biopsy after neoadjuvant chemotherapy for advanced breast cancer: results of Ganglion Sentinelle et Chimiothérapie Neoadjuvante, a French prospective multicentric study. J Clin Oncol 27(5):726–732
37. Kelly AM, Dwamena B, Cronin P et al (2009) Breast cancer sentinel node identification and classification after neoadjuvant chemotherapy—systematic review and meta analysis. Acad Radiol 16(5):551–563
38. van Deurzen CHM, Vriens BEPJ, Tjan-Heijnen VCG et al (2009) Accuracy of sentinel node biopsy after neoadjuvant chemotherapy in breast cancer patients: a systematic review. Eur J Cancer 45:3124–3130
39. Gimbergues P, Abrial C, Durando S et al (2008) Sentinel lymph node biopsy after neoadjuvant chemotherapy is accurate in breast cancer patients with a clinically negative axillary nodal status at presentation. Ann Surg Oncol 15(5):1316–1321
40. Lee S, Kim EY, Kang SH et al (2007) Sentinel node identification rate, but not accuracy, is significantly decreased after pre-operative chemotherapy in axillary node-positive breast cancer patients. Breast Cancer Res Treat 102:283–288
41. Boughey JC, Suman VJ, Mittendorf EA et al (2013) Sentinel lymph node surgery after neoadjuvant chemotherapy in patients with node-positive breast cancer: the ACOSOG Z1071 (Alliance) clinical trial. J Am Med Assoc 310(14):1455–1461
42. Boughey JC, Ballman KV, Hunt KK et al (2015) Axillary ultrasound after neoadjuvant chemotherapy and its impact on sentinel lymph node surgery: results from the American College of Surgeons Oncology Group Z1071 Trial (Alliance). J Clin Oncol. doi:10.1200/JCO.2014.55.7827
43. Boileau J-F, Poirier B, Basik M et al (2015) Sentinel node biopsy after neoadjuvant chemotherapy in biopsy-proven node-positive breast cancer: the SN FNAC study. J Clin Oncol 33 (3):258–264

Chapter 7
One-Step Nucleic Acid Amplification (OSNA) Assay for Primary Breast Cancer

Seigo Nakamura and Katsutoshi Enokido

Abstract Recently, sentinel lymph node biopsy (SLNB) has become a standard procedure for N0 breast cancer. OSNA (one-step nucleic acid amplification, SYSMEX) is an automated assay system using cytokeratin 19 mRNA to detect lymph node metastasis of breast cancer in 30–40 min. OSNA has already been approved by health insurance in Japan since 2008.

For the next step, the feasibility of the OSNA assay in breast cancer patients treated by PST has been confirmed under multicenter trial; we compared the judgment of the OSNA assay and of pathological examination on lymph nodes dissected after receiving PST to evaluate the performance of the OSNA assay. The overall concordance rate between the OSNA assay and pathological examination was 91.1 % (275/302) with sensitivity of 88.3 % (53/60) and specificity of 91.7 % (222/242) (Osako et al. British Journal of Cancer (2013) 109, 1693–1698). These results are very similar to those of the Japanese clinical validation study in breast cancer patients without receiving PST which was conducted by the almost same protocol (Tamaki Y, et al. Clin Cancer Res, 2009, 15: 2879–2884). These results indicate the OSNA assay can be applicable for breast cancer patients after receiving PST as well as breast cancer patients without receiving PST.

The status of residual cancer burden in SLN after PST has been assumed as one of prognostic factors. Therefore, the accurate measurement of cancer burden using OSNA is a promising method especially in the setting of PST.

At the present, the prospective clinical trial has been conducted to assess local recurrence rate and disease-free survival (DFS) of patients with OSNA negative without ALND after PST. The study is also focusing on the inclusion criteria for SNB among the cases of positive to negative change in preoperative imaging.

Keywords One-step nucleic acid amplification • OSNA • Sentinel lymph node • SLN • CK19

S. Nakamura (✉) • K. Enokido
Department of Surgery, Division of Breast Surgical Oncology, Showa University School of Medicine, 1-5-8 Hatanodai, Shinagawa-ku, Tokyo 142-8666, Japan
e-mail: seigonak@med.showa-u.ac.jp

M. Toi et al. (eds.), *Personalized Treatment of Breast Cancer*,
DOI 10.1007/978-4-431-55552-0_7

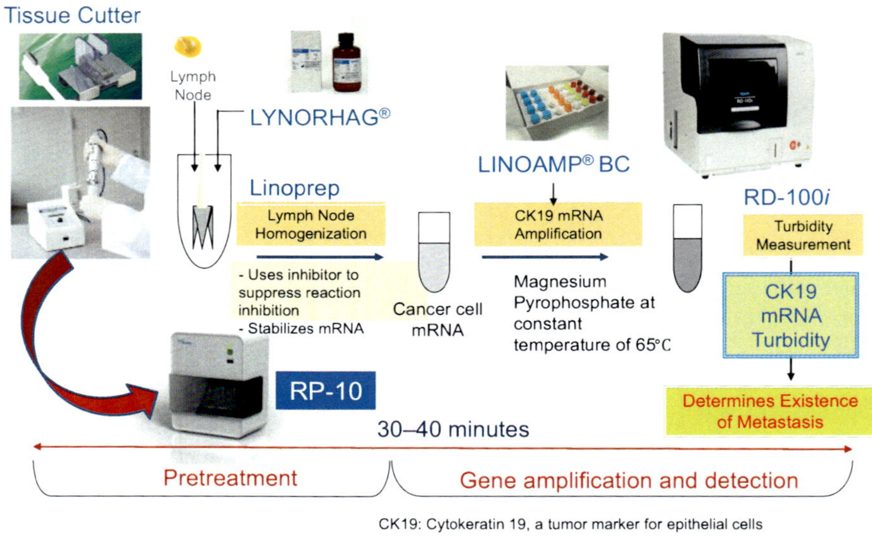

Fig. 7.1 Configuration of OSNA method for sentinel lymph node

7.1 Introduction

The one-step nucleic acid amplification (OSNA) method is an increasingly used procedure for intraoperative analysis of sentinel lymph node (SLN) status in breast cancer patients (Fig. 7.1) [1–5]. It measures cytokeratin 19 (CK19) mRNA copy numbers in homogenized samples of SLN; CK19 has been chosen for identifying node metastasis because most breast cancers express this molecule [6–9].

Pooled analysis of recent studies comparing OSNA with pathology indicated that OSNA is as accurate as pathology (96.3 % concordance rate) and is useful for making the decision to omit axillary dissection for OSNA-negative patients (97.4 % negative predictive value) [10, 11]. The advantage of OSNA over pathology is that the former allows the semiquantitative evaluation of total tumor volume in the node when a whole node is examined. OSNA is expected to be a powerful tool for the estimation of risk of non-sentinel lymph node metastasis and also patient prognosis [12].

7.2 Comparison Between OSNA Method and Conventional Sentinel Lymph Node Biopsy

Recently, sentinel lymph node biopsy has become a standard procedure for N0 breast cancer [12, 13]. Though accurate assessment of metastasis in sentinel lymph nodes (SLNs) of breast cancer is important, it causes a heavy workload for pathologists.

- OSNA stratifies metastasis into (++), (+) and (-) with specific cutoff values.

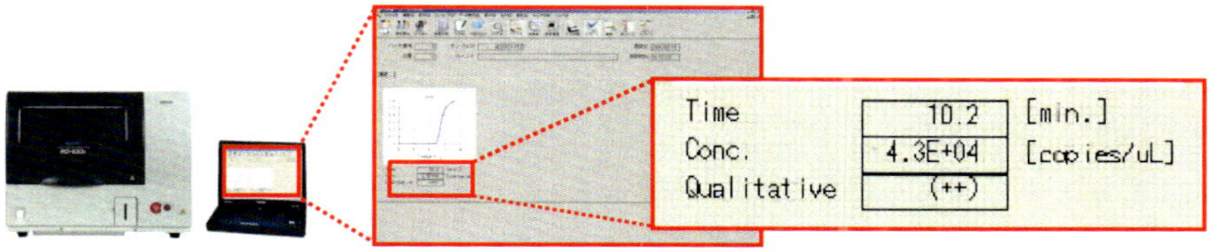

CK19 mRNA (copies/uL)	OSNA	Judgment
≥ 5,000	++	Positive
≥ 250, < 5,000	+	
< 250	-	Negative

Fig. 7.2 Semiquantitative judgment

OSNA (one-step nucleic acid amplification, SYSMEX) is a new automated assay system using cytokeratin 19 mRNA to detect lymph node metastasis of breast cancer in 30–40 min.

A multicenter clinical trial was conducted to evaluate the accuracy of the system in Japan, and OSNA has already been approved by health insurance since 2008.

In the first clinical trial, axillary lymph nodes obtained by axillary dissection were sectioned into four pieces, two of which were examined with the OSNA assay. The other two adjacent pieces were examined with H&E and immunohistochemical staining of cytokeratin 19. Serial sections at 0.2-mm intervals were used in the first trial (trial 1) to determine the specificity of the OSNA assay [10].

In the next trial (trial 2), three surfaces of the two blocks in 1.0–2.0-mm intervals from ordinal SLNs were used to compare the accuracy of the OSNA assay with that of a routine pathologic examination.

In trial 1, the sensitivity and specificity were 95.0 % (95 % confidence interval (95 % CI), 75.1–99.9 %) and 97.1 % (95 % CI, 91.8–99.4 %), respectively, for 124 axillary lymph nodes obtained from 34 patients.

In trial 2, the agreement between findings of the assay and of the concordance rate was 92.9 % (95 % CI, 90.1–95.1 %) in 450 axillary lymph nodes. Positive predictive value of macrometastasis by OSNA++ was 96.4 % in 164 patients [14].

Therefore, OSNA using CK19 mRNA is the appropriate method to examine SLN with enough rapidness to apply to intraoperative diagnosis.

Moreover, new findings are anticipated by estimating the volume of metastasis foci based on by OSNA. If CK19 mRNA copy numbers were fewer than 100 copies per μl of lysate, the result was designated as negative (pN0), whereas copy numbers between 100 and 250 copies per μl of lysate were designated as ITC. Copy numbers between 250 and 5000 copies per μl of lysate were designated as micrometastases, and more than 5,000 copies per μl of lysate were designated as macrometastases, per the manufacturer's recommendations (Fig. 7.2). In terms of equivalence to the results obtained by IHC, an OSNA-negative result is consistent with negative histology or with the presence of ITC, which were scored as pN0 and N0(i+), respectively [15–17].

7.3 OSNA Method in Several Clinical Guidelines

OSNA method in breast cancer has been approved by public health insurance in Japan since 2008. It is applicable in the field of gastric cancer and colon cancer [17–21]. Therefore, it has been covered by health insurance in gastric and colon cancer since 2013. In the clinical practice guideline by the Japanese Breast Cancer Society, OSNA method has been acquired recommendation grade of "A" as the same capability as pathological examination (H&E staining) [22]. It means few false negatives, high specificity compared with IHC. And the quantification of CK19 mRNA could have determined the cutoff values of macro- versus micrometastasis. The most important advantage of this method is the reduction of the burden on pathologists and laboratory operators.

UK NICE (National Institute for Health and Care Excellence) approved OSNA in Diagnostics Guidance 8 (published in August 2013). In their guidance, patients with early stage invasive breast cancer are recommended to use the OSNA method for measurement of the whole lymph node as a method for intraoperative analysis for sentinel lymph node metastasis.

7.4 TTL

There are several models to predict non-sentinel lymph node (NSLN) metastasis in the case of a positive sentinel lymph node (SLN) to avoid unnecessary dissection of axillary nodes. Although the American College of Surgeons Oncology Group Z0011 trial has defined a select cohort of patients in whom a completion axillary lymph node dissection (cALND) may be safely omitted, there are still a number of patients where prediction of non-SLN metastasis may be helpful for cALND decision-making. Multiple studies suggest that specific pathologic characteristics of the primary tumor and the SLN metastases are associated with an increased likelihood of additional positive non-SLN. Our study showed a whole-node analysis of non-sentinel lymph nodes (NSLNs) using the OSNA method in SLN metastasis-positive breast cancer patients. The rates of non-SLN metastasis positivity in those with SLN micrometastasis and macrometastasis were 44 % and 48 %, respectively, and this difference was not significant. When the study of non-SLN metastasis positivity was focused only on macrometastases, the rates of non-SLN metastasis positivity in patients with SLN micrometastasis and macrometastasis were 19 % and 22 %, respectively, and there was no significant difference [23]. Total tumoral load (TTL) in the SLNs assessed by OSNA is a predictive factor for additional non-SLN metastasis in the axillary lymph node dissection (ALND) [24, 25]. The objective was to develop a nomogram that predicts patient's risk of additional non-SLN metastasis incorporating TTL in the SLNs assessed by OSNA. Six hundred and ninety-seven consecutive patients with positive SLN evaluation by OSNA and a completion ALND were recruited. Pathologic features of the primary tumor and SLN metastases, including TTL, were collected. Multivariate logistic regression identified factors predictive of non-SLN metastasis. A nomogram was developed with these variables and validated in an external cohort. On multivariate logistic regression analysis, tumor size, number of affected SLN, Her2 overexpression, lymphovascular invasion, and TTL were each associated with the likelihood of additional NSLN metastasis ($p < 0.05$). The overall predictive accuracy of the nomogram, as measured by the AUC, was 0.7552 (95 % CI 0.7159–0.7945). When applied to the external cohort, the nomogram was accurate with an AUC = 0.678 (95 % CI 0.621–0.736). This novel nomogram that incorporates TTL assessed by OSNA performs well and may help clinicians to make decisions about ALND for individual patients. Moreover, the standardization of pathologic assessment by OSNA may help to achieve interinstitutional reproducibility among nomograms [26].

7.5 Significance of OSNA in Preoperative Systemic Therapy

The OSNA assay has been validated for breast cancer patients without receiving preoperative systemic therapy (PST) by several clinical studies and has currently become more popular as sentinel lymph node (SLN) examination method with the following two main advantages, (1) to allow examination of the whole portion of a node and (2) to allow intraoperative judgment of metastasis positive or negative [27, 28]. However, the feasibility of the OSNA assay in breast cancer patients treated by PST has never been confirmed. Therefore, multi-central clinical study was conducted in Japan [29].

In total, 302 lymph nodes from 80 breast cancer patients who underwent axillary dissection after chemotherapy were analyzed. Each node was cut into two or four slices. One piece or alternate pieces were evaluated by pathology, and the other (s) was examined using the OSNA assay. The results of the two methods were compared. The overall accuracy, sensitivity, and specificity of the OSNA assay compared with the reference pathology were 91.1 %, 88.3 %, and 91.7 %, respectively. Of the 302 lymph nodes, 66 (21.9 %) exhibited chemotherapy-induced histology. For these nodes, the accuracy, sensitivity, and specificity were 90.9 %,

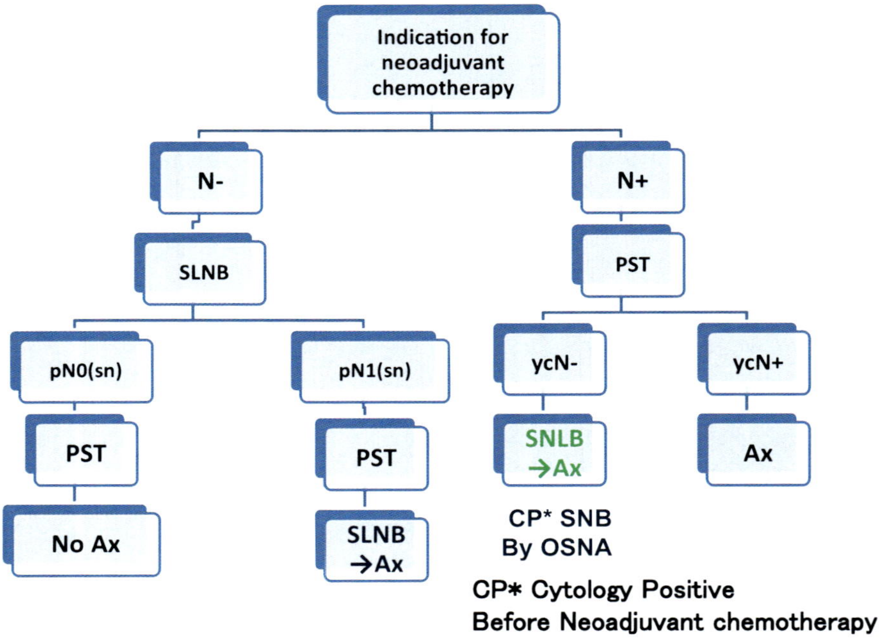

Fig. 7.3 SNB by OSNA trial in neoadjuvant setting

88.9 %, and 93.3 %, respectively. Therefore, the OSNA assay can detect the residual tumor burden as accurately as conventional pathology, although chemotherapy-induced histological changes are present. There was another multicenter prospective study performed in Japan from September 2011 to April 2013 in Japan. One hundred one breast cancer patients with positive axillary nodes, proven by ultrasound-guided fine needle aspiration, were entered (Fig. 7.3). After the confirmation of patients as clinically node negative by preoperative imaging following NAC, all patients underwent breast surgery, with SNB and complete axillary lymph node dissection. The sentinel lymph nodes were examined by hematoxylin-eosin staining, immunohistochemical analysis, or one-step nucleic acid amplification assay (OSNA). The false-negative rate and detection rate were analyzed, among the 101 patients analyzed. All cases presented with invasive ductal carcinoma, with a mean tumor size of 3.4 cm. Thirty-six cases were hormone receptor (HR) positive and HER2 negative (luminal subtype), 14 cases were HR positive and HER2 positive (triple-positive subtype), 27 cases were positive for HER2 (HER2-enriched subtype), and 24 cases were triple negative. After neoadjuvant chemotherapy, a complete clinical response in the primary tumor was seen in 24.8 %(25/101), a partial response in 66.3 %(67/101), and no response in 7.9 %(8/101). Pathological complete response of primary tumor was 39.6 %. The pathological complete nodal response rate was 42.2 %. The sentinel lymph node

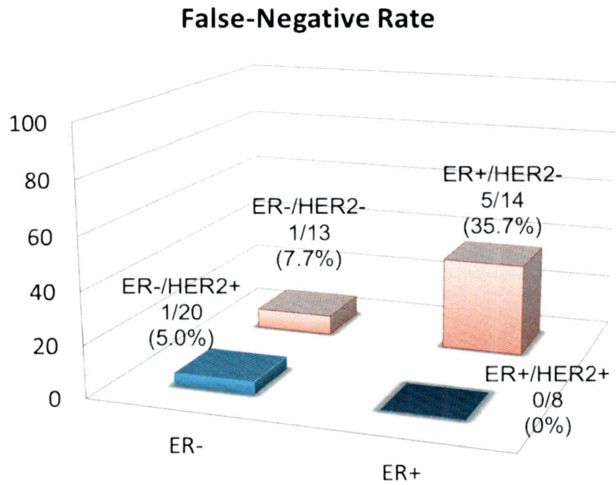

Fig. 7.4 False-negative rate in N+ tp N− after neoadjvant chemotherapy

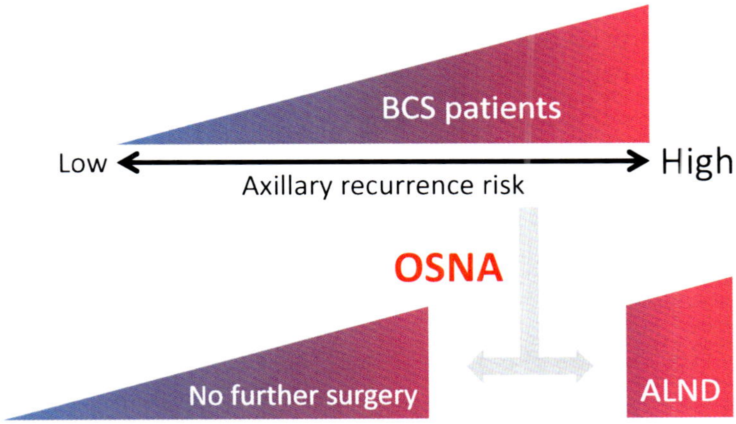

Fig. 7.5 Personalized axillary treatment by OSNA

could be identified in 91 of 101 cases (90.1 %). The identification rate according to the subtype was 88.9 % (32/36) of patients with luminal subtype, 100 %(14/14) of those with triple-positive subtype, 85.2 % (23/27) of those with HER2-enriched subtype, and 91.7 % (22/24)% of those with triple-negative breast cancer subtype. The false-negative rate was 35.7 % (5/14) for luminal subtype, 0 % (0/8) for triple-positive subtype, 5.0 % (1/20) for HER2-enriched subtype, and 7.7 % (1/13) for triple-negative subtype ($P = 0.03$) (Fig. 7.4). Therefore, SNB following NAC in patients with node-positive breast cancer was found to be technically feasible but is not recommended for the luminal subtype. However, it might be safely considered in selected patients, those with triple-positive subtype, HER2-enriched subtype, and triple-negative subtype breast cancers.

7.6 Future Perspectives

OSNA is an alternative method to diagnose metastasis in sentinel lymph node.

And it can assess the volume of metastatic cancer cells more accurately than conventional IHC examination. But it is still unknown whether the copy number is correlate DFS or OS. Therefore, registration trial for long-term follow-up will be warranted.

Even within 1 mm lymph node metastasis might be the same potential of recurrent risk especially after neoadjuvant chemotherapy [30]. Therefore, the prospective clinical trial has been conducted to assess local recurrence rate and disease-free survival (DFS) of patients with OSNA negative without ALND after PST. The study is also focusing on the inclusion criteria for SNB among the cases of positive to negative change in preoperative imaging.

References

1. Bernet L, Cano R, Martinez M, Duenas B, Matias-Guiu X, Morell L, Palacios J, Rezola R, Robles-Frias M, Ruiz I, Velasco A, Vieites B, Sevilla F, Torro J, Medrano J, Ballester B (2011) Diagnosis of the sentinel lymph node in breast cancer: a reproducible molecular method: a multicentric Spanish study. Histopathology 58(6):863–869
2. Le Frere-Belda MA, Bats AS, Gillaizeau F, Poulet B, Clough KB, Nos C, Peoc'h M, Seffert P, Bouteille C, Leroux A, Guillemin F, Blanc-Fournier C, Crouet H, Arnould L, Cuisenier J, Penault-Llorca F, Gimbergues P, Jacquemier J, Houvenaeghel G, Chatellier G, Lecuru F (2012) Diagnostic performance of one-step nucleic acid amplification for intraoperative sentinel node metastasis detection in breast cancer patients. Int J Cancer 130(10):2377–2386
3. Cserni G (2012) Intraoperative analysis of sentinel lymph nodes in breast cancer by one-step nucleic acid amplification. J Clin Pathol 65(3):193–199
4. Castellano I, Macri L, Deambrogio C, Balmativola D, Bussone R, Ala A, Coluccia C, Sapino A (2012) Reliability of whole sentinel lymph node analysis by one-step nucleic acid amplification for intraoperative diagnosis of breast cancer metastases. Ann Surg 255(2):334–342
5. Vilardell F, Novell A, Martin J, Santacana M, Velasco A, Diez-Castro MJ, Cuevas D, Panades MJ, Gonzalez S, Llombart A, Iglesias E, Matias-Guiu X (2012) Importance of assessing CK19 immunostaining in core biopsies in patients subjected to sentinel node study by OSNA. Virchows Arch 460(6):569–575
6. Chu PG, Weiss LM (2002) Keratin expression in human tissues and neoplasms. Histopathology 40(5):403–439
7. Tsujimoto M, Nakabayashi K, Yoshidome K, Kaneko T, Iwase T, Akiyama F, Kato Y, Tsuda H, Ueda S, Sato K, Tamaki Y, Noguchi S, Kataoka TR, Nakajima H, Komoike Y, Inaji H, Tsugawa K, Suzuki K, Nakamura S, Daitoh M, Otomo Y, Matsuura N (2007) One-step nucleic acid amplification for intraoperative detection of lymph node metastasis in breast cancer patients. Clin Cancer Res 13(16):4807–4816
8. Alvarenga CA, Paravidino PI, Alvarenga M, Dufloth R, Gomes M, Zeferino LC, Schmitt F (2011) Expression of CK19 in invasive breast carcinomas of special histological types: implications for the use of one-step nucleic acid amplification. J Clin Pathol 64(6):493–497
9. Parikh RR, Yang Q, Higgins SA, Haffty BG (2008) Outcomes in young women with breast cancer of triple-negative phenotype: the prognostic significance of CK19 expression. Int J Radiat Oncol Biol Phys 70(1):35–42

10. Tamaki Y, Akiyama F, Iwase T, Kaneko T, Tsuda H, Sato K, Ueda S, Mano M, Masuda N, Takeda M, Tsujimoto M, Yoshidome K, Inaji H, Nakajima H, Komoike Y, Kataoka TR, Nakamura S, Suzuki K, Tsugawa K, Wakasa K, Okino T, Kato Y, Noguchi S, Matsuura N (2009) Molecular detection of lymph node metastases in breast cancer patients: results of a multicenter trial using the one-step nucleic acid amplification assay. Clin Cancer Res 15 (8):2879–2884
11. Tamaki Y, Sato N, Homma K, Takabatake D, Nishimura R, Tsujimoto M, Yoshidome K, Tsuda H, Kinoshita T, Kato H, Taniyama K, Kamio T, Nakamura S, Akiyama F, Noguchi S, Japanese One-Step Nucleic Acid Amplification Study Group (2012) Routine clinical use of the one-step nucleic acid amplification assay for detection of sentinel lymph node metastases in breast cancer patients: results of a multicenter study in Japan. Cancer 118(14):3477–3483
12. Schem C, Maass N, Bauerschlag DO, Carstensen MH, Loning T, Roder C, Batic O, Jonat W, Tiemann K (2009) One-step nucleic acid amplification – a molecular method for the detection of lymph node metastases in breast cancer patients; results of the German study group. Virchows Arch 454(2):203–210
13. Visser M, Jiwa M, Horstman A, Brink AA, Pol RP, van Diest P, Snijders PJ, Meijer CJ (2008) Intra-operative rapid diagnostic method based on CK19 mRNA expression for the detection of lymph node metastases in breast cancer. Int J Cancer 122(11):2562–2567
14. Snook KL, Layer GT, Jackson PA, de Vries CS, Shousha S, Sinnett HD, Nigar E, Singhal H, Chia Y, Cunnick G, Kissin MW, Group OS (2011) Multicentre evaluation of intraoperative molecular analysis of sentinel lymph nodes in breast carcinoma. Br J Surg 98(4):527–535
15. Feldman S, Krishnamurthy S, Gillanders W, Gittleman M, Beitsch PD, Young PR, Streck CJ, Whitworth PW, Levine EA, Boolbol S, Han LK, Hermann R, Hoon DS, Giuliano AE, Meric-Bernstam F, Group USOSNAACS (2011) A novel automated assay for the rapid identification of metastatic breast carcinoma in sentinel lymph nodes. Cancer 117(12):2599–2607
16. Vegue LB, Rojo F, Hardisson D, Iturriagagoitia AC, Panades MJ, Velasco A, Bonet EL, Munoz RC, Polo L, Investigators BC-I (2012) Comparison of molecular analysis and histopathology for axillary lymph node staging in primary breast cancer: results of the B-CLOSER-I study. Diagn Mol Pathol 21(2):69–76
17. Vogelaar FJ, Reimers MS, van der Linden RL, van der Linden JC, Smit VT, Lipsm DJ, van de Velde CJ, Bosscha K (2014) The diagnostic value of one-step nucleic acid amplification (OSNA) for sentinel lymph nodes in colon cancer patients. Ann Surg Oncol 21(12):3924–3930
18. Güller U, Zettl A, Worni M, Langer I, Cabalzar-Wondberg D, Viehl CT, Demartines N, Zuber M (2012) Molecular investigation of lymph nodes in colon cancer patients using one-step nucleic acid amplification (OSNA): a new road to better staging? Cancer 118(24):6039–6045
19. Kumagai K, Yamamoto N, Miyashiro I, Tomita Y, Katai H, Kushima R, Tsuda H, Kitagawa Y, Takeuchi H, Mukai M, Mano M, Mochizuki H, Kato Y, Matsuura N, Sano T (2014) Multicenter study evaluating the clinical performance of the OSNA assay for the molecular detection of lymph node metastases in gastric cancer patients. Gastric Cancer 17(2):273–280
20. Yaguchi Y, Sugasawa H, Tsujimoto H, Takata H, Nakabayashi K, Ichikura T, Ono S, Hiraki S, Sakamoto N, Horio T, Kumano I, Otomo Y, Mochizuki H, Yamamoto J, Hase K (2011) One-step nucleic acid amplification (OSNA) for the application of sentinel node concept in gastric cancer. Ann Surg Oncol 18(8):2289–2296
21. Croner RS, Geppert CI, Bader FG, Nitsche U, Späth C, Rosenberg R, Zettl A, Matias-Guiu X, Tarragona J, Güller U, Stürzl M, Zuber M (2014) Molecular staging of lymph node-negative colon carcinomas by one-step nucleic acid amplification (OSNA) results in upstaging of a quarter of patients in a prospective, European, multicentre study. Br J Cancer 110 (10):2544–2550
22. Horii R, Honma N, Ogiya A, Kozuka Y, Fukuda T, Yoshida M, Ohsumi S, Mukai H (2015) The Japanese Breast Cancer Society Clinical Practice Guideline for pathological diagnosis of breast cancer. Breast Cancer 22(1):59–65

23. Ogiya A, Iwase T, Kitagawa D, Nakashima E, Sakai T, Miyagi Y, Iijima K, Morizono H, Makita M, Horii R, Akiyama F (2015) Non-sentinel lymph node analysis with one-step nucleic acid amplification in breast cancer patients. Breast 24(4):476–480
24. Espinosa-Bravo M, Sansano I, Pérez-Hoyos S, Ramos M, Sancho M, Xercavins J, Rubio IT, Peg V (2013) Prediction of non-sentinel lymph node metastasis in early breast cancer by assessing total tumoral load in the sentinel lymph node by molecular assay. Eur J Surg Oncol 39(7):766–773
25. Peg V, Espinosa-Bravo M, Vieites B, Vilardell F, Antúnez JR, de Salas MS, Delgado-Sánchez JJ, Pinto W, Gozalbo F, Petit A, Sansano I, Del Mar TM, Rubio IT (2013) Intraoperative molecular analysis of total tumor load in sentinel lymph node: a new predictor of axillary status in early breast cancer patients. Breast Cancer Res Treat 139(1):87–93
26. Rubio IT, Espinosa-Bravo M, Rodrigo M, Viguri A, Diaz M, Hardisson D, Sagasta A, Dueñas B, Peg V (2014) Nomogram including the total tumoral load in the sentinel nodes assessed by one-step nucleic acid amplification as a new factor for predicting nonsentinel lymph node metastasis in breast cancer patients. Breast Cancer Res Treat 147(2):371–380
27. Navarro-Cecilia J, Dueñas-Rodríguez B, Luque-López C, Ramírez-Expósito MJ, Martínez-Ferrol J, Ruíz-Mateas A, Ureña C, Carrera-González MP, Mayas MD, Martínez-Martos JM (2013) Intraoperative sentinel node biopsy by one-step nucleic acid amplification (OSNA) avoids axillary lymphadenectomy in women with breast cancer treated with neoadjuvant chemotherapy. Eur J Surg Oncol 39(8):873–879
28. Rebollo-Aguirre AC, Gallego-Peinado M, Sánchez-Sánchez R, Pastor-Pons E, García-García J, Chamorro-Santos CE, Menjón-Beltrán S (2013) Sentinel lymph node biopsy after neoadjuvant chemotherapy in patients with operable breast cancer and positive axillary nodes at initial diagnosis. Rev Esp Med Nucl Image Mol 32(4):240–245
29. Osako T, Tsuda H, Horii R, Iwase T, Yamauchi H, Yagata H, Tsugawa K, Suzuki K, Kinoshita T, Akiyama F, Nakamura S (2013) Molecular detection of lymph node metastasis in breast cancer patients treated with preoperative systemic chemotherapy: a prospective multicentre trial using the one-step nucleic acid amplification assay. Br J Cancer 109 (6):1693–1698
30. Fisher ER, Wang J, Bryant J, Fisher B, Mamounas E, Wolmark N (2002) Pathobiology of preoperative chemotherapy: findings from the National Surgical Adjuvant Breast and Bowel (NSABP) protocol B-18. Cancer 95(4):681–695

Chapter 8
Management of the Clinically Node-Negative Axilla in Primary Breast Cancer

Abdul Q. Alarhayem and Ismail Jatoi

Abstract Axillary lymph node status is an important prognostic factor in patients with primary breast cancer. Yet, management of the axilla in these patients has been controversial. Sentinel lymph node biopsy (SLNB) is a less morbid procedure with similar survival and recurrence when compared to axillary lymph node dissection (ALND) and has emerged as the standard of care for staging patients with clinically node-negative disease. The results of three randomized trials seem to suggest that completion ALND may not be necessary in all women with T1/T2 tumors that have sentinel node-positive tumors and a low burden of axillary disease. However, while patients with isolated tumor cells or micrometastatic disease in the sentinel node may forego further axillary treatment, we believe that those with macrometastatic disease on SLNB should undergo additional axillary treatment (either ALND or radiotherapy) until further evidence defining which patients may benefit from observation alone emerges.

Keywords Breast cancer • Axilla • Radiotherapy • Surgery

8.1 Background

Since antiquity, physicians have debated whether primary breast cancer is a local or systemic disease at inception. Galen viewed breast cancer as a systemic disease arising in the setting of excess "black bile" (*the humoral theory*), and this theory predominated until the end of the eighteenth century [1, 2]. At that time, French surgeons Jean-Louis Petit and Henri François Le Dran argued that breast cancer was a local disease, at the root of which were enlarged lymphatic glands. During the nineteenth century, German pathologist Rudolf Virchow's analysis of postmortem dissections led him to conclude that lymph nodes were indeed the nidus for the distant spread of epithelial cancers and suggested lymph node dissection be incorporated into the surgical management of all patients with breast cancer [3].

A.Q. Alarhayem • I. Jatoi (✉)
Division of Surgical Oncology and Endocrine Surgery, University of Texas Health Science Center at San Antonio, 7703 Floyd Curl Drive, San Antonio, TX 78229, USA
e-mail: Jatoi@uthscsa.edu

M. Toi et al. (eds.), *Personalized Treatment of Breast Cancer*,
DOI 10.1007/978-4-431-55552-0_8

In the late nineteenth century, William Halsted incorporated the tenets of Virchow's hypothesis and proposed the radical mastectomy as the operation of choice for the treatment of primary breast cancer [4]. In this operation, the tumor-containing breast, underlying pectoral muscles, and ipsilateral axillary contents were removed en bloc. The radical mastectomy remained the standard surgical treatment of primary breast cancer from the late nineteenth century until about the second half of the twentieth century and was very effective in achieving local control. If, in keeping with Virchow's hypothesis, breast cancer progressed in an orderly fashion from the breast to the axillary lymph nodes and then to distant sites, then resection of a node-negative cancer should have been curative. Yet, long-term follow-up of patients treated with the radical mastectomy revealed that 30 % of node-negative breast cancer patients died of metastatic disease [5].

In the early 1960s, Bernard Fisher argued that breast cancer was systemic at inception. Fisher disputed the impact of the radical mastectomy on overall survival, attributing the apparent survival advantage to the fact that patients in the latter half of the twentieth century were seeking medical attention sooner than women a century prior, and harbored smaller tumors. He subsequently developed randomized trials comparing less aggressive, breast-conserving surgical treatments to mastectomy [6, 7].

8.2 Significance of Lymph Node Metastasis

There has been considerable controversy as to whether nodal metastasis is a marker of tumor chronology or tumor biology. Mittra et al. have argued that nodal metastasis is simply an indicator of tumor chronology. These authors have concluded that the worse outcome in patients with node-positive versus node-negative tumors is simply due to lead-time bias (e.g., detecting the cancer at a later point in time) [8].

Other authors argued that nodal involvement was a marker of an aggressive phenotype and might be secondary to the accumulation of genomic aberrancies in cancer cells [9, 10]. Jatoi et al. found nodal status to be a good predictor of outcome after recurrence. In women with early stage breast cancer, nodal metastasis present at the time of initial breast cancer diagnosis was associated with a shorter interval from the time of recurrence to the time of death, when compared to patients without nodal metastasis. Moreover, as the extent of nodal involvement at the time of initial diagnosis increased, the interval of time from recurrence to death decreased [11]. Younger age, higher tumor grade, larger tumor size, and lymphovascular invasion are each predictors of lymph node metastases, and these are also indicators of aggressive tumor phenotype [3].

However, a recent review of 2957 cases found patients with triple-negative breast cancer, an aggressive cancer subtype, found that these patients do not have a higher risk for nodal metastases [12].

Taken together, these studies suggest that nodal metastasis is perhaps an indicator of both tumor chronology and biology. There is a correlation between tumor size and nodal metastasis (larger tumors are more likely to harbor nodal metastasis than smaller tumors), which suggests that nodal metastasis is an indicator of tumor chronology. However, nodal metastasis may occur earlier in the natural history of the more aggressive tumors, suggesting that nodal metastasis is perhaps also a marker of tumor phenotype [13].

8.3 Evaluation of Axillary Nodal Status

As mentioned above, nodal status remains a key determinant of overall prognosis in patients with primary breast cancer. Yet clinical examination of the axilla is notoriously unreliable for correct preoperative staging of the lymph nodes, with false-positive rates approaching 30 %, even with experienced clinicians [14]. Also, up to 30 % of clinically node-negative patients are found to have nodal involvement following ALND (Axillary Lymph Node Dissection) [15]. Axillary staging with surgery thus remains an important component of the care of these patients.

In developed nations, the vast majority of breast cancer patients are clinically node negative at the time of initial diagnosis [16]. Indiscriminate total axillary dissection therefore seems unjustified. However, inadequate axillary management at the time of initial diagnosis may place these patients at unacceptable high risks for axillary recurrence [14, 17].

Attempts have been made to enhance the accuracy of axillary assessment through supplementation with ultrasound (US), combined with FNAC (Fine Needle Aspiration Cytology) or core needle biopsy of suspicious lesions. While this practice allows for improved preoperative assessment of lymph node status [18], the sensitivity of US remains low when lymph nodes are non-palpable [19, 20]. Even with the use of PET/CT, the reported mean sensitivity is 63 % and a mean specificity of 94 %. Similar to US, in patients with non-palpable lymph nodes, sensitivity of PET/CT is low [21]. In a meta-analysis of nine studies, MRI was found to have a mean sensitivity of 90 % and specificity of 90 % in assessing axillary lymph nodes [22].

8.4 Axillary Lymph Node Dissection (ALND)

The lymph nodes in the axilla are divided into three compartments based on their anatomic relationship to the pectoralis minor muscle. Lymph nodes lateral to the pectoralis minor muscle are classified as level I nodes, those posterior to its lateral and medial borders are classified as level II nodes, and those medial to the muscle are classified as level III nodes. Level III nodal dissection generally requires dividing the pectoralis minor muscle; this is usually not done unless lymph nodes are palpable at this level. Until recently, axillary lymph node dissection (ALND) was standard practice for all patients with breast cancer. Not only did ALND impact local control (recurrence), but it was crucial to staging patients with potential therapeutic ramifications.

A randomized study in 514 patients with T1/T2/T3 and N0/1a/1b breast cancer undergoing mastectomy found longer operative times and greater blood loss associated with level III dissections compared to level I nodal dissection with no differences in OS and DFS at 10 years (level III, 89.6 % and 76.6 % vs. level I, 87.8 % and 74.1 %, respectively) [23]. Another trial randomized 1209 women with stage II breast cancer who had undergone mastectomy to level II versus level III axillary node dissection. Similarly, there was no difference in DFS or OS at 10 years (level II 86.6 % vs. level III 85.7 %, HR = 1.02; $P = 0.931$) [24].

Current practice guidelines recommend level I and II ALND with removal of ten or more nodes. This avoids misclassification of node-positive patients as node-negative tumors, and the number of lymph nodes removed correlates with a reduction in the rate of subsequent axillary recurrence [25, 26].

The impact of ALND on survival and local control in patients with primary breast cancer was assessed in two large, randomized prospective trials, the National Surgical Adjuvant Breast and Bowel Project (NSABP)-04 and King's/Cambridge.

In the NSABP-04 trial, 1,665 clinically node-negative patients with primary breast cancer were randomized to no axillary treatment versus axillary radiotherapy versus ALND. In this study, 18 % of the patients who received no initial axillary treatment went on to develop axillary adenopathy within 5 years, subsequently requiring an ALND. In contrast, axillary adenopathy developed in only 2 % of patients whose axilla had initially been treated with either surgery (ALND) or radiotherapy (RT). However, there were no significant differences in mortality in clinically node-negative patients who received mastectomy + axillary dissection versus mastectomy + axillary radiotherapy versus mastectomy alone.

The King's/Cambridge trial randomized 2,243 clinically node-negative patients to receive total mastectomy and immediate postoperative radiotherapy to the axilla versus total mastectomy and observation of the axilla. The observation group did not receive RT unless there was progression or recurrence of the disease in the axilla. At 10 years of follow-up, there was no significant difference in survival between the two groups, but there was a highly significant increased risk of local recurrence in patients not receiving immediate postoperative RT [27].

Even after 25 years of follow-up, the B-04 trial continues to demonstrate no significant differences in long-term mortality in clinically node-negative patients who received mastectomy + ALND versus those who received mastectomy + axillary radiotherapy versus mastectomy + observation of the axilla [28].

Both the NSABP-04 and King's/Cambridge trials indicate that treatment of the axilla (with either ALND or RT) in patients with clinically node-negative breast cancer substantially reduced the risk of axillary relapse at 5 years (by approximately 90 %). However, permutations in the management of the axilla (delayed axillary management versus RT versus surgery) had no effect on mortality.

Another important finding was that RT and surgical extirpation were equally effective in achieving local control of the axilla [29].

It may be argued that breast cancer patients enrolled in the trials discussed above had larger cancers with greater nodal disease burden compared to patients seen today. Approximately 15–25 % of patients today have nodal involvement at the time of breast cancer diagnosis compared to approximately 50 % three decades ago [30–33]. Also the majority of patients today (even those with small T1N0 tumors) are treated with adjuvant systemic therapy, which has been shown to improve local control [29, 34, 35].

8.5 Sentinel Lymph Node Biopsy (SLNB)

In patients with primary breast cancer who are clinically node positive (palpable axillary nodes or histological confirmation of metastasis to the axillary nodes), ALND is essential for local control.

However, the vast majority of patients are clinically node negative at the time of presentation. The sentinel lymph node biopsy (SLNB) technology was introduced as a means of assessing nodal status in these patients, while avoiding the morbidity associated with unnecessary ALND.

Sentinel lymph node biopsy (SLNB) is based on the hypothesis that if the first lymph node in the basin to receive lymphatic drainage from a tumor (the sentinel lymph node) is free of metastatic tumor, then all other nodes in the basin should be free of tumor as well, obviating the need for an ALND [36].

The first published use of SLNB was by Krag and colleagues in 1993, with an intraparenchymal injection of radionucleotide-labeled sulfur colloid and a gamma probe [37]. They were able to identify the SLN in 82 % of patients.

When periareolar injection of blue dye was first employed in lymphatic mapping of the breast, it was only successful in identifying the sentinel node in two-thirds of patients. Giuliano and colleagues found blue dye mapping SLNB could accurately predict axillary nodal status in 95.6 % of patients [38].

A randomized prospective trial by Morrow and colleagues compared both blue dye and radioactive colloid in combination versus the use of blue dye alone and found sentinel node identification rates were >95 % in both groups [39].

There is consensus that dual localization methods are associated with a short learning curve and maximize identification rates while maintaining low false-negative rates [40–44].

SLNB has also consistently been found to be a much less morbid procedure than the standard ALND (see Table 8.1).

Extensive axillary dissection has been associated with arm swelling and reduced mobility. While the risk of major motor nerve injury following an ALND is <1 % in most reports, reduced arm mobility, numbness and paresthesias, can be as high as 40 % at 1 year [45].

The Milan trial by Veronesi and colleagues randomized 512 patients to ALND versus SLNB (with ALND only in patients with positive SLNs). Patients undergoing SLNB reported significantly less axillary pain (8 % vs. 39 %), numbness (1 %

Table 8.1 A summary of three non-inferiority prospective randomized trials evaluating survival and locoregional recurrence in early stage breast cancer with low-burden axillary disease

Trial	Pathology	Axillary Rx	5-year survival		5-year axillary recurrence	
			No ALND	ALND	No ALND (%)	ALND (%)
IBCSG 23	Tumor ≤5 cm, N0, and micrometastatic disease on SLNB	SLNB vs. ALND	OS 97.5 %	97.6 %	<1	<1
			DFS 87.8 %	84.4 %		
			OS, $p=0.73$; DFS, $p=0.16$			
ACOSOG Z0011	T1/T2 N0, <3 +ve SLN	SLNB vs. ALND	OS 92.5 %	91.8 %	<1	<1
			DFS 83.9 %	82.2 %		
			OS, $p=0.25$; DFS, $p=0.14$			
AMAROS	T1/T2 N0, <3 +ve SLN	Axillary RT vs. ALND	OS 92.5 %	93.3 %	1.19	0.43
			DFS 82.7 %	86.9 %		
			OS, $p=0.34$; DFS, $p=0.18$			

AMAROS trial: The 5-year lymphedema rate was 28 % in the ALND group versus 14 % in the AR group, $p<0.001$

vs. 68 %), and better overall arm mobility (0 % vs. 21 % mobility restriction) than those randomized to the ALND arm of the trial [46].

In the NSABP B-32, SLNB was associated with significantly fewer shoulder abduction deficits (75 % vs. 41 %; $P<0.001$), lymphedema (7–9 % vs. 13–14 %), arm numbness (31.0 % vs. 8.1 %; $P<0.001$), and tingling (13.5 % vs. 7.5 %; $P<0.001$) compared to ALND [47]. In a meta-analysis of 98 prospective or retrospective cohort studies and randomized control trials, patients undergoing ALND were significantly more likely to develop lymphedema compared with patients undergoing a sentinel lymph node dissection (RR = 3.07, 2.20–4.29) [48].

Similarly, at 12 months, the axillary lymphatic mapping against nodal axillary clearance (ALMANAC) trial found SLNB to be associated with significantly less lymphedema (relative risk [RR], 0.37) and sensory loss (RR, 0.37) compared to ALND. SLNB alone was also associated with shorter time to resumption of normal daily activities ($P<0.001$), as well as improved patient-recorded quality of life and arm functioning scores ($P\leq 0.003$) [49].

The sentinel node versus axillary clearance (SNAC) trial randomized 1,083 patients to routine axillary clearance or SLNB (followed by axillary clearance if the SLN was positive or not detected). At 1 year, compared to routine ALND, the

SLNB group had a significant decrease in arm swelling, wound infection, impaired shoulder motion, and numbness/paresthesia [50].

A meta-analysis of seven randomized controlled trials with a total of 9608 patients found SLNB (with completion ALND if SLNB was positive) was associated with lower rates of infection (OR = 0.58, $P = 0.0011$), seroma (OR = 0.40, $P = 0.0071$), arm swelling (OR = 0.30, $P = 0.0028$), and numbness (OR = 0.25, $P = 0.0018$) compared to standard ALND [51].

Based on these results, consensus statements from the American Society of Clinical Oncology and the National Comprehensive Cancer Network recommend initial axillary evaluation with SLND rather than ALND in patients with early stage breast cancer who are clinically node negative. In patients with a negative SLNB, ALND may be omitted without an adverse impact on recurrence or survival. When metastases are identified on SLND, a completion ALND (cALND) has, until recently, been generally recommended [52].

Numerous trials have found that patients with clinically node-negative breast cancer who undergo SLNB have similar survival and local recurrence rates compared to those who undergo standard ALND.

Veronesi et al. randomized 341 women with clinical T1N0 breast cancer and a negative sentinel lymph node (SLN) to SLNB alone or SLNB followed by ALND. The false-negative rate of SLNB was 5 % (8/174) when compared to ALND. At 7-year follow-up, there was no difference in local or distant recurrence between the groups. More importantly, disease-free and overall survival was equivalent between the two groups [46].

The NSABP B-32 trial randomized patients with clinically N0 invasive breast cancer to either SLNB plus ALND or SLNB alone (followed by ALND only if SLNB were positive). At 8 years, there was no significant difference in overall survival (OS 92 %, ALND vs. 90 %, SLNB), disease-free survival (DFS 82 %, ALND vs. 82 %, SLNB), local recurrence ($P = 0.55$), or regional recurrence ($P = 0.22$).

In a subsequent meta-analysis of 48 studies that included almost 15,000 node-negative breast cancer patients with a tumor-negative SLNB and no subsequent ALND, the overall axillary recurrence rate was found to be 0.3 % at a median follow-up of 34 months [53].

Another systematic review, performed by the ASCO expert guideline panel, that included 69 eligible trials of SLND in early stage breast cancer representing 8059 patients, was successful in identifying the SLN in 95 % of patients with a median false-negative rate of 7.3 % [54, 55].

Taken together, these studies suggest that SLNB is less morbid than ALND and can predict spread of tumor to regional nodes in $\geq$95 % of cases, with no adverse effect on OS, DFS, or locoregional recurrence.

Importantly, despite SLNB being associated with a 5–10 % false-negative rate (i.e., patients with negative SLNB who undergo ALND and subsequently found to have disease on ALND), the rates of regional recurrence reported in the studies mentioned above are consistently $<$1 % [47, 56, 57].

While the widespread use of SLNB for initial axillary evaluation in clinically node-negative breast cancers has reduced morbidity, Ronka et al. cited an increase in cost associated with the procedure compared to ALND due to the need of preoperative lymphoscintigraphy, intraoperative γ-probe use, and prolonged operative time while waiting for frozen section results [58].

Also, with up to 20 % false negatives on frozen section (*see next section*), a second surgical procedure for axillary node dissection may be required [59].

Several studies however found length of hospital stay to be the primary driver of cost and that SLNB, while involving more expensive techniques, was overall less expensive than ALND [60].

8.6 Management of Sentinel Node-Positive Breast Cancer

Increased use of SLNB technology during the past 15 years has led to improved techniques of histopathological analysis. The sentinel node is often subjected to a more detailed histological examination than nodes that are harvested with ALND. Thus, pathologists are more likely to uncover a metastatic deposit in a sentinel node than in other nodes in the axillary basin. Although this has the potential to improve staging accuracy, it has also given rise to a new dilemma; the detection of occult disease in the sentinel node, namely *micrometastases and isolated tumor cells*. The seventh edition of the American Joint Committee on Cancer (AJCC) defines *macrometastases* as foci of tumor greater than 2.0 mm, *micrometastases* as tumor deposits greater than 0.2 mm and/or more than 200 cells but less than 2.0 mm, and *isolated tumor cells* (*ITCs*) as clusters of cells not greater than 0.2 mm or fewer than 200 cells [61].

Compared to standard ALND, SLNB using H&E staining combined with IHC is associated with an increased detection of both macro- (42 % vs. 29 %; $P < 0.03$) and micrometastatic disease (16 % vs. 3 %; $P < 0.0005$) [62]. In recent years, the results of three large randomized trials have provided further insights into the optimal management of patients with low-volume axillary disease detected on SLNB: the IBCSG 23, the ACOSOG Z0011, and the AMAROS trials (see Table 8.1).

8.7 IBCSG 23-01

Between 2001 and 2010, the International Breast Cancer Study Group (IBCSG) randomized 934 patients with primary breast tumors ≤5 cm and with one or more sentinel lymph nodes with micrometastases (≤2 mm) and no extracapsular extension, to undergo SLNB alone versus completion ALND. Two-thirds of patients had tumors <2 cm, more than 80 % were estrogen receptor positive, and almost all patients (90 %) underwent lumpectomy and radiotherapy. Following serial sectioning, evaluation consisted of either H&E staining or IHC.

In patients undergoing ALND following SLNB, the 5-year overall and disease-free survival rates were equivalent in patients undergoing completion ALND versus SLNB alone. Axillary recurrence was <1 % in both arms of the trial.

Patients who underwent ALND were more likely to report lymphedema, sensory neuropathy, and wound infection when compared to patients treated with SLNB alone.

This trial was a non-inferiority trial and criticized for lower-than-projected event rates and low accrual that resulted in early closure (target accrual, 1960; actual accrual, 934) [63]. Nonetheless, the results of this trial are interpreted to mean that ALND can be safely avoided in patients with SLNB showing micrometastases in the sentinel node.

The development of newer SLN evaluation techniques such as immunohistochemistry (IHC), molecular marking, and reverse transcriptase-polymerase chain reaction (RT-PCR) has resulted in a dramatic increase in the detection of micrometastatic disease in lymph nodes [64].

The clinical significance of H&E-negative IHC-positive SLN metastasis was examined in the American College of Surgeons Oncology Group (ACOSOG) Z0010, a prospective observational study. Of 3326 breast cancer patients with H&E-negative SLNs, 10 % were found to have occult metastases with IHC. At a median of 6.3-year follow-up, there was no increased risk of recurrence or death in patients with IHC micrometastatic disease versus those without (DFS 90 % vs. 92 %, $P = 0.82$) [65].

Similarly, in the NSABP B-32, of 3887 patients with H&E-negative SLNs, 15.9 % had IHC detectable metastases. Through 10 years of follow-up, there was a 4 % difference in DFS ($P = 0.02$) between patients with IHC-positive and IHC-negative SLNs, yet there was no statistically significant difference in OS [66]. Current consensus guidelines thus advise against routine IHC testing, recommending multilevel nodal sectioning with H&E staining alone [67, 68].

In view of these results, for patients with micrometastases on SLNB, ALND can be safely avoided with no adverse impact on locoregional recurrence or survival.

While the IBCSG only enrolled women with micrometastatic disease on SLNB, the ACOSOG Z0011 and the AMAROS trials were primarily dedicated to patients with macrometastatic disease on SLNB.

8.8 ACOSOG Z0011

The Z0011 trial randomized 891 patients with early stage breast cancer (T1/T2) and one to two positive SLNs (detected by H&E only) to completion ALND versus no axillary treatment. All patients were treated with lumpectomy, tangential field radiation therapy, and, when indicated, adjuvant systemic therapy.

At a median follow-up of 6.3 years, there was no difference in local or regional recurrence between the two groups (SLNB 0.5 % and 1.6 % vs. ALND 0.9 % and 3.1 %, respectively, $P = 0.45$). Also, there was no statistically significant difference in DFS (SLNB 83.9 % vs. ALND 82.2 %, $P = 0.14$) or OS [69].

The following considerations are important in interpreting the findings of the Z0011:

1. All patients received whole-breast irradiation (WBI) with opposing standard tangential fields. Although designed to treat the breast, it's well known that WBI also includes a significant portion of the lower axilla in the treatment field. Based on published data, 51 % of level I and 26 % of level II axillary nodes received 95 % of the prescribed dose [70–73]. Thus, the results of this trial can only be applied to patients who receive lumpectomy with radiotherapy.
2. Women enrolled were low risk with favorable breast cancers (69 % T1 tumors, 83 % ER positive tumors).
3. It was a non-inferiority trial, and it was underpowered. It failed to meet its accrual target and had lower-than-expected event rates, and almost 20 % of patients were lost to follow-up. This is attributable to low recurrence rates in the patient population.
4. The follow-up duration was also relatively short. ER-positive tumors are notorious for metastatic "dormancy," whereby regional recurrence does not occur for many years after resection of the primary tumor [74].

The extent of tangential axillary radiation in the Z0011 trial was a subject of considerable criticism. Radiation oncologists were not blinded to patients' treatment assignments and, given the lack of uniform field design, may have preferentially treated patients on the SLN-only arm with high tangents to include a component of axillary level I/level II more often than those in the ALND arm. Detailed radiation treatment records for 228 patients were submitted for post hoc central review, and it was determined that high tangents were used in up to 50 % of patients and that 19 % received directed regional nodal RT using >3 fields [72, 75].

8.9 AMAROS Trial

The AMAROS (After mapping of the axilla: Radiotherapy or surgery?) trial set out to determine if axillary radiotherapy (ART) could serve as an alternative to surgery in patients with early stage breast cancer (T1/T2, N0) and low-volume axillary disease. In this trial, 1,425 women with a positive SLNB were randomized to either completion ALND or ART. About 60 % of patients had macrometastases, 29 % had micrometastases, and 12 % had ITCs on SLNB.

In patients undergoing ALND, additional nodal disease was detected in 33 % of patients (similar rates are expected in those undergoing ART). Median follow-up was 6.1 years.

Axillary recurrence at 5 years was 0.43 % in the ALND group and 1.19 % in the axillary RT group. Also, there were no significant differences in DFS (ALND, 86.9 % vs. ART, 82.7 %; $p = 0.18$) and OS (ALND, 93.3 % vs. ART, 92.5 %; $p = 0.34$) between the two groups. At 5 years, the authors also found the rate of lymphedema in the surgery group to be twice that of the radiotherapy group.

The AMAROS trial was not blinded, and this may have contributed to a systematic bias whereby investigators may have been more inclined to note lymphedema in those undergoing ALND. Nonetheless, this difference in lymphedema rates did not translate into improved patient quality of life; and no differences in shoulder mobility were found between the two groups.

As in the Z0011 trial, the AMAROS trial was underpowered, and there were fewer axillary recurrences than predicted. Patient and tumor characteristics were also both quite favorable, as 74 % of patients had T1 tumors, 77 % had only one positive SLN, and 40 % had only micrometastatic disease or ITCs. The authors concluded SLNB plus axillary RT could serve as an alternative to ALND.

AMAROS also raised the question about whether omission of ALND in patients with positive SLNB would impact adjuvant therapy decisions due the loss of information derived from histopathological analysis of axillary contents. This was addressed in a multivariate analysis of the factors associated with the administration of adjuvant chemotherapy in the first 2000 women enrolled in the AMAROS trial. Age, tumor grade, multifocality, and the size of the SLN metastasis were all associated with the use of adjuvant systemic therapy. The extent of nodal involvement was not a factor, suggesting that this decision could be based on the primary tumor and sentinel node, not axillary contents [76].

8.10 Conclusion

In summary, the IBCSG 23-01, ACOSOG Z0011, and AMAROS trials seem to suggest that a completion ALND may not be necessary in all women with T1/T2 tumors that are clinically node negative and have low axillary tumor burden (see Table 8.1).

Patients with micrometastatic disease may forego axillary treatment with no increased risk of recurrence or adverse survival effects. However, patients with macrometastatic disease on SLNB should undergo some form of axillary treatment (ALND vs. ART) until further evidence defining which patients may benefit from observation alone emerges.

References

1. Sakorafas GH, Safioleas M (2009) Breast cancer surgery: an historical narrative. Part I. From prehistoric times to Renaissance. Eur J Cancer Care 18(6):530–544
2. Sakorafas G, Safioleas M (2010) Breast cancer surgery: an historical narrative. Part II. 18th and 19th centuries. Eur J Cancer Care 19(1):6–29
3. Virchow R (1863) Cellular pathology (transl. Chance F). Philadelphia, JB Lippincott
4. Halsted WS (1894) I. The results of operations for the cure of cancer of the breast performed at the Johns Hopkins Hospital from June, 1889, to January, 1894. Ann Surg 20(5):497
5. Bonadonna G, Valagussa P (1988) The contribution of medicine to the primary treatment of breast cancer. Cancer Res 48(9):2314–2324

6. Jatoi I, Kaufmann M (2010) Management of breast diseases. Springer, Heidelberg. xvii, 671 p. p
7. Travis K (2005) Bernard Fisher reflects on a half-century's worth of breast cancer research. J Natl Cancer Inst 97(22):1636–1637
8. Mittra I (1993) Axillary lymph node metastasis in breast cancer: prognostic indicator or lead-time bias? Eur J Cancer 29(3):300–302
9. Patani N, Dwek M, Douek M (2007) Predictors of axillary lymph node metastasis in breast cancer: a systematic review. Eur J Surg Oncol (EJSO) 33(4):409–419
10. Yoshihara E, Smeets A, Laenen A, Reynders A, Soens J, Van Ongeval C et al (2013) Predictors of axillary lymph node metastases in early breast cancer and their applicability in clinical practice. Breast 22(3):357–361
11. Jatoi I, Hilsenbeck SG, Clark GM, Osborne CK (1999) Significance of axillary lymph node metastasis in primary breast cancer. J Clin Oncol 17(8):2334
12. Gangi A, Mirocha J, Leong T, Giuliano AE (2014) Triple-negative breast cancer is not associated with increased likelihood of nodal metastases. Ann Surg Oncol 21(13):4098–4103
13. Smeets A, Ryckx A, Belmans A, Wildiers H, Neven P, Floris G et al (2013) Impact of tumor chronology and tumor biology on lymph node metastasis in breast cancer. SpringerPlus 2 (1):1–7
14. Specht MC, Fey JV, Borgen PI, Cody HS 3rd (2005) Is the clinically positive axilla in breast cancer really a contraindication to sentinel lymph node biopsy? J Am Coll Surg 200(1):10–14
15. Sacks N, Baum M (1993) Primary management of carcinoma of the breast. Lancet 342 (8884):1402–1408
16. Harbeck N, Thomssen C (2011) A new look at node-negative breast cancer. Oncologist 16 (Suppl 1):51–60
17. Voogd A, Coebergh J-W, Driel OR, Roumen RH, Beek MPM, Vreugdenhil A et al (2000) The risk of nodal metastases in breast cancer patients with clinically negative lymph nodes: a population-based analysis. Breast Cancer Res Treat 62(1):63–69
18. Nori J, Vanzi E, Bazzocchi M, Bufalini FN, Distante V, Branconi F et al (2007) Role of axillary ultrasound examination in the selection of breast cancer patients for sentinel node biopsy. Am J Surg 193(1):16–20
19. Rajesh Y, Ellenbogen S, Banerjee B (2002) Preoperative axillary ultrasound scan: its accuracy in assessing the axillary nodal status in carcinoma breast. Breast 11(1):49–52
20. Sapino A, Cassoni P, Zanon E, Fraire F, Croce S, Coluccia C et al (2003) Ultrasonographically-guided fine-needle aspiration of axillary lymph nodes: role in breast cancer management. Br J Cancer 88(5):702–706
21. Cooper KL et al (2011) Positron emission tomography (PET) for assessment of axillary lymph node status in early breast cancer: a systematic review and meta-analysis. Eur J Surg Oncol 37 (3):187–198
22. Harnan SE, Cooper KL, Meng Y, Ward SE, Fitzgerald P, Papaioannou D et al (2011) Magnetic resonance for assessment of axillary lymph node status in early breast cancer: a systematic review and meta-analysis. Eur J Surg Oncol: J Eur Soc Surg Oncol Br Assoc Surg Oncol 37 (11):928–936
23. Kodama H, Nio Y, Iguchi C, Kan N (2006) Ten-year follow-up results of a randomised controlled study comparing level-I vs level-III axillary lymph node dissection for primary breast cancer. Br J Cancer 95(7):811–816
24. Tominaga T, Takashima S, Danno M (2004) Randomized clinical trial comparing level II and level III axillary node dissection in addition to mastectomy for breast cancer. Br J Surg 91 (1):38–43
25. Axelsson CK, During M, Christiansen PM, Wamberg PA, Soe KL, Moller S (2009) Impact on regional recurrence and survival of axillary surgery in women with node-negative primary breast cancer. Br J Surg 96(1):40–46
26. Axelsson CK, Mouridsen HT, Zedeler K (1992) Axillary dissection of level I and II lymph nodes is important in breast cancer classification. Eur J Cancer 28(8–9):1415–1418

27. Party CRCW (1980) Cancer research campaign (King's/Cambridge) trial for early breast cancer: a detailed update at the tenth year. Lancet 316(8185):55–60
28. Fisher B, Jeong J-H, Anderson S, Bryant J, Fisher ER, Wolmark N (2002) Twenty-five-year follow-up of a randomized trial comparing radical mastectomy, total mastectomy, and total mastectomy followed by irradiation. N Engl J Med 347(8):567–575
29. Buchholz TA, Tucker SL, Erwin J, Mathur D, Strom EA, McNeese MD et al (2001) Impact of systemic treatment on local control for patients with lymph node-negative breast cancer treated with breast-conservation therapy. J Clin Oncol: Off J Am Soc Clin Oncol 19(8):2240–2246
30. Weaver DL, Rosenberg RD, Barlow WE, Ichikawa L, Carney PA, Kerlikowske K et al (2006) Pathologic findings from the breast cancer surveillance consortium. Cancer 106(4):732–742
31. Rivadeneira DE, Simmons RM, Christos PJ, Hanna K, Daly JM, Osborne MP (2000) Predictive factors associated with axillary lymph node metastases in T1a and T1b breast carcinomas: analysis in more than 900 patients. J Am Coll Surg 191(1):1–6; discussion -8
32. Bleyer A, Welch HG (2012) Effect of three decades of screening mammography on breast-cancer incidence. N Engl J Med 367(21):1998–2005
33. Carter CL, Allen C, Henson DE (1989) Relation of tumor size, lymph node status, and survival in 24,740 breast cancer cases. Cancer 63(1):181–187
34. Group EBCTC (2005) Effects of chemotherapy and hormonal therapy for early breast cancer on recurrence and 15-year survival: an overview of the randomised trials. Lancet 365 (9472):1687–1717
35. Kaplan HG, Malmgren JA, Atwood M (2009) T1N0 triple negative breast cancer: risk of recurrence and adjuvant chemotherapy. Breast J 15(5):454–460
36. Nagashima T, Sakakibara M, Nakano S, Tanabe N, Nakamura R, Nakatani Y et al (2006) Sentinel node micrometastasis and distant failure in breast cancer patients. Breast Cancer 13 (2):186–191
37. Krag DN, Weaver DL, Alex JC, Fairbank JT (1993) Surgical resection and radiolocalization of the sentinel lymph node in breast cancer using a gamma probe. Surg Oncol 2(6):335–339; discussion 40
38. Giuliano AE, Kirgan DM, Guenther JM, Morton DL (1994) Lymphatic mapping and sentinel lymphadenectomy for breast cancer. Ann Surg 220(3):391–398; discussion 8-401
39. Morrow M, Rademaker AW, Bethke KP, Talamonti MS, Dawes LG, Clauson J et al (1999) Learning sentinel node biopsy: results of a prospective randomized trial of two techniques. Surgery 126(4):714–720; discussion 20-2
40. Derossis AM, Fey J, Yeung H, Yeh SDJ, Heerdt AS, Petrek J et al (2001) A trend analysis of the relative value of blue dye and isotope localization in 2,000 consecutive cases of sentinel node biopsy for breast cancer1. J Am Coll Surg 193(5):473–478
41. Cody HS III, Fey J, Akhurst T, Fazzari M, Mazumdar M, Yeung H et al (2001) Complementarity of blue dye and isotope in sentinel node localization for breast cancer: univariate and multivariate analysis of 966 procedures. Ann Surg Oncol 8(1):13–19
42. Linehan DC, Hill AD, Akhurst T, Yeung H, Yeh SD, Tran KN et al (1999) Intradermal radiocolloid and intraparenchymal blue dye injection optimize sentinel node identification in breast cancer patients. Ann Surg Oncol 6(5):450–454
43. Hung W, Chan C, Ying M, Chong S, Mak K, Yip A (2005) Randomized clinical trial comparing blue dye with combined dye and isotope for sentinel lymph node biopsy in breast cancer. Br J Surg 92(12):1494–1497
44. McMasters KM, Tuttle TM, Carlson DJ, Brown CM, Noyes RD, Glaser RL et al (2000) Sentinel lymph node biopsy for breast cancer: a suitable alternative to routine axillary dissection in multi-institutional practice when optimal technique is used. J Clin Oncol 18 (13):2560–2566
45. Hladiuk M, Huchcroft S, Temple W, Schnurr BE (1992) Arm function after axillary dissection for breast cancer: a pilot study to provide parameter estimates. J Surg Oncol 50(1):47–52

46. Veronesi U, Paganelli G, Viale G, Luini A, Zurrida S, Galimberti V et al (2003) A randomized comparison of sentinel-node biopsy with routine axillary dissection in breast cancer. N Engl J Med 349(6):546–553
47. Krag DN, Anderson SJ, Julian TB, Brown AM, Harlow SP, Ashikaga T et al (2007) Technical outcomes of sentinel-lymph-node resection and conventional axillary-lymph-node dissection in patients with clinically node-negative breast cancer: results from the NSABP B-32 randomised phase III trial. Lancet Oncol 8(10):881–888
48. Tsai RJ, Dennis LK, Lynch CF, Snetselaar LG, Zamba GK, Scott-Conner C (2009) The risk of developing arm lymphedema among breast cancer survivors: a meta-analysis of treatment factors. Ann Surg Oncol 16(7):1959–1972
49. Mansel RE, Fallowfield L, Kissin M, Goyal A, Newcombe RG, Dixon JM et al (2006) Randomized multicenter trial of sentinel node biopsy versus standard axillary treatment in operable breast cancer: the ALMANAC Trial. J Natl Cancer Inst 98(9):599–609
50. Gill G (2009) Sentinel-lymph-node-based management or routine axillary clearance? One-year outcomes of Sentinel Node Biopsy Versus Axillary Clearance (SNAC): a randomized controlled surgical trial. Ann Surg Oncol 16(2):266–275
51. Kell MR, Burke JP, Barry M, Morrow M (2010) Outcome of axillary staging in early breast cancer: a meta-analysis. Breast Cancer Res Treat 120(2):441–447
52. Lyman GH, Temin S, Edge SB, Newman LA, Turner RR, Weaver DL et al (2014) Sentinel lymph node biopsy for patients with early-stage breast cancer: American Society of Clinical Oncology clinical practice guideline update. J Clin Oncol 32(13):1365–1383
53. van der Ploeg IMC, Nieweg OE, van Rijk MC, Valdés Olmos RA, Kroon BBR (2008) Axillary recurrence after a tumour-negative sentinel node biopsy in breast cancer patients: a systematic review and meta-analysis of the literature. Eur J Surg Oncol 34(12):1277–1284
54. Kim T, Giuliano AE, Lyman GH (2006) Lymphatic mapping and sentinel lymph node biopsy in early-stage breast carcinoma: a metaanalysis. Cancer 106(1):4–16
55. Lyman GH, Giuliano AE, Somerfield MR, Benson AB 3rd, Bodurka DC, Burstein HJ et al (2005) American Society of Clinical Oncology guideline recommendations for sentinel lymph node biopsy in early-stage breast cancer. J Clin Oncol: Off J Am Soc Clin Oncol 23 (30):7703–7720
56. Krag DN, Julian TB, Harlow SP, Weaver DL, Ashikaga T, Bryant J et al (2004) NSABP-32: Phase III, randomized trial comparing axillary resection with sentinal lymph node dissection: a description of the trial. Ann Surg Oncol 11(3):208S–210S
57. van der Ploeg IM, Nieweg OE, van Rijk MC, Valdes Olmos RA, Kroon BB (2008) Axillary recurrence after a tumour-negative sentinel node biopsy in breast cancer patients: a systematic review and meta-analysis of the literature. Eur J Surg Oncol: J Eur Soc Surg Oncol Br Assoc Surg Oncol 34(12):1277–1284
58. Rönkä R, Smitten K, Sintonen H, Kotomäki T, Krogerus L, Leppänen E et al (2004) The impact of sentinel node biopsy and axillary staging strategy on hospital costs. Ann Oncol 15 (1):88–94
59. Holck S, Galatius H, Engel U, Wagner F, Hoffmann J (2004) False-negative frozen section of sentinel lymph node biopsy for breast cancer. Breast (Edinb, Scotl) 13(1):42–48
60. Classe J, Baffert S, Sigal-Zafrani B, Fall M, Rousseau C, Alran S et al (2012) Cost comparison of axillary sentinel lymph node detection and axillary lymphadenectomy in early breast cancer. A national study based on a prospective multi-institutional series of 985 patients 'on behalf of the Group of Surgeons from the French Unicancer Federation'. Ann Oncol 23(5):1170–1177
61. Edge SB, Compton CC (2010) The American Joint Committee on Cancer: the 7th edition of the AJCC cancer staging manual and the future of TNM. Ann Surg Oncol 17(6):1471–1474
62. Giuliano AE, Dale PS, Turner RR, Morton DL, Evans SW, Krasne DL (1995) Improved axillary staging of breast cancer with sentinel lymphadenectomy. Ann Surg 222(3):394–401
63. Galimberti V, Cole BF, Zurrida S, Viale G, Luini A, Veronesi P et al (2013) Axillary dissection versus no axillary dissection in patients with sentinel-node micrometastases (IBCSG 23-01): a phase 3 randomised controlled trial. Lancet Oncol 14(4):297–305

64. Viale G, Maiorano E, Mazzarol G, Zurrida S, Galimberti V, Luini A et al (2001) Histologic detection and clinical implications of micrometastases in axillary sentinel lymph nodes for patients with breast carcinoma. Cancer 92(6):1378–1384
65. Giuliano AE, Hawes D, Ballman KV, Whitworth PW, Blumencranz PW, Reintgen DS et al (2011) Association of occult metastases in sentinel lymph nodes and bone marrow with survival among women with early-stage invasive breast cancer. JAMA 306(4):385–393
66. Julian T, Anderson S, Krag D, (eds) (2013) 10-year follow-up results of occult detected sentinel node disease: NSABP B-32, a randomized phase III clinical trial to compare sentinel node resection to conventional axillary dissection in clinically node-negative breast cancer patients [Z]. 2013 San Antonio Breast Cancer Symposium, Texas, USA
67. Network NCC (2014) NCCN Clinical Practice Guidelines in Oncology (NCCN Guidelines): breast cancer. Version 3.2014. 1 Apr 2014
68. Pilewskie ML, Morrow M (2014) Management of the clinically node-negative axilla: what have we learned from the clinical trials? Oncology (Williston Park, NY) 28(5):371–378
69. Giuliano AE, Hunt KK, Ballman KV, Beitsch PD, Whitworth PW, Blumencranz PW et al (2011) Axillary dissection vs no axillary dissection in women with invasive breast cancer and sentinel node metastasis: a randomized clinical trial. JAMA 305(6):569–575
70. Shah-Khan M, Boughey JC (2012) Evolution of axillary nodal staging in breast cancer: clinical implications of the ACOSOG Z0011 trial. Cancer Control: J Moffitt Cancer Cent 19 (4):267–276
71. Caudle AS, Hunt KK, Kuerer HM, Meric-Bernstam F, Lucci A, Bedrosian I et al (2011) Multidisciplinary considerations in the implementation of the findings from the American College of Surgeons Oncology Group (ACOSOG) Z0011 study: a practice-changing trial. Ann Surg Oncol 18(9):2407–2412
72. Jagsi R, Chadha M, Moni J, Ballman K, Laurie F, Buchholz TA et al (2014) Radiation field design in the ACOSOG Z0011 (Alliance) trial. J Clin Oncol 56:5838
73. Giuliano AE, McCall L, Beitsch P, Whitworth PW, Blumencranz P, Leitch AM et al (2010) Locoregional recurrence after sentinel lymph node dissection with or without axillary dissection in patients with sentinel lymph node metastases: the American College of Surgeons Oncology Group Z0011 randomized trial. Ann Surg 252(3):426–433
74. Zhang XH-F, Giuliano M, Trivedi MV, Schiff R, Osborne CK (2013) Metastasis dormancy in estrogen receptor-positive breast cancer. Clin Cancer Res 19(23):6389–6397
75. Haffty BG, Hunt KK, Harris JR, Buchholz TA (2011) Positive sentinel nodes without axillary dissection: implications for the radiation oncologist. J Clin Oncol 29(34):4479–4481
76. Straver ME, Meijnen P, van Tienhoven G, van de Velde CJ, Mansel RE, Bogaerts J et al (2010) Role of axillary clearance after a tumor-positive sentinel node in the administration of adjuvant therapy in early breast cancer. J Clin Oncol: Off J Am Soc Clin Oncol 28(5):731–737

Chapter 9
Lymphatic Mapping and Optimization of Sentinel Lymph Node Dissection

Tomoharu Sugie and Takashi Inamoto

Abstract Sentinel lymph node (SLN) biopsy is a standard of care for axillary staging in breast cancer. The modalities involving radioisotope (RI) and blue dye are the most widely used for SLN mapping. Near-infrared fluorescence imaging using indocyanine green (ICG) visualizes superficial lymphatic flow from tumor to SLN transcutaneously and directs the surgeon to the tumor-draining SLN in the axillary basin. This novel method achieves a high detection of SLN comparable with the RI method, and the additional use of ICG fluorescence maximizes the detection impact of RI. The ICG fluorescence method is reliable and safe and would be an acceptable alternative to SLN mapping using radioactive tracers in early breast cancer.

Keywords Lymphatic mapping • Near-infrared fluorescence • Indocyanine green • Sentinel lymph node

9.1 Introduction

The theory of the radical mastectomy with axillary lymph node dissection (ALND) was that removal of breast cancer cells as far as they extended might have benefit of not only local control of breast cancer but also survival. The alternative theory that breast cancer was a systemic disease at inception induced total mastectomy to partial mastectomy in early breast cancer treatment based upon results of randomized control trials. However, data from meta-analyses suggest that inadequate local therapy can increase risk of local recurrence [1]. ALND has been used for the past century as a means of preventing lymph node metastasis of breast cancer. Because ALND confers a high probability of complications such as arm edema (lymphedema) and neuropathy (locomotors disorder, pain, etc.), reduction in patient QOL is a major problem of ALND. In the 1990s, the concept of sentinel lymph nodes

T. Sugie (✉)
Department Surgery, Kansai Medical University, 2-3-1 Shinmachi, Hirakata, Osaka 573-1191, Japan
e-mail: sugiet@hirakata.kmu.ac.jp

T. Inamoto
Faculty of Health Care, Tenri Health Care University, Nara, Japan

M. Toi et al. (eds.), *Personalized Treatment of Breast Cancer*,
DOI 10.1007/978-4-431-55552-0_9

(SLNs) directly receiving lymphatic drainage from the tumor was proposed. As SLNs represent metastatic status of regional lymph nodes, removal of SLNs can be alternative to completion of ALND for diagnosis of axillary status.

Since this concept was first applied in 1992 to melanoma patients by Morton et al. [2], its application to various fields has been attempted. In the field of breast cancer, the validity of the SLN biopsy was evaluated in 1993 by Krag et al. [3] using a radioisotope (RI) and during approximately the same period by Giuliana et al. [4] using blue dye. Thereafter, many reports supporting the validity of the SLN biopsy using RI, blue dye, or the combination of both have been published. On the basis of large multicenter clinical studies, the mapping involving RI and/or blue dye becomes currently a standard method used worldwide.

9.2 SLN Mapping Using Near-infrared (NIR) Fluorescence Imaging Technique

At present, the standard methods achieve a high detection rate of SLN with a low false negative rate. In a meta-analysis by Kim et al., the median detection rate by the standard methods was 96 %, with a false negative rate of 7.3 % [5]. The RI method is advantageous with respect to a high SLN detection rate, but its applicability is restricted in high-volume hospitals that have nuclear medicine departments and radiation protection areas. The blue dye method is advantageous with respect to cost-effectiveness but has some drawbacks, such as a low SLN detection rate and the necessity of trained surgical skill [6].

To overcome the issues of the standard methods, Kitani et al. [7] reported in 2005 the application of indocyanine green (ICG) instead of RI and NIR fluorescence imaging system in breast cancer. The ICG fluorescence method utilizes the optic fluorescent characteristics of ICG within the NIR optic window (700–900 nm). The advantages of the NIR light include high tissue penetration due to less absorbance by water and hemoglobin and low autofluorescence. The ICG fluorescence method is currently adopted at the discretion of the physicians in view of the following advantages: (1) no risk for exposure to radiation, (2) applicable outside of large hospitals because this method does not requires nuclear medicine or a radiation protection area, (3) optimal for intraoperative SLN localization because it enables real-time imaging of lymphatic flow over the skin, and (4) requiring little skill. The technical aspects of SLN mapping using each modality are summarized in Table 9.1.

Table 9.1 Technical aspects of SLN mapping using each modality

Tracers	Advantage	Disadvantages
RI	High detection rate	Expensive
		No real-time guidance
		Requirement of permitted facilities
Dye	Cost-effective	Low detection rate
		Cannot be seen over the skin
		Requires training
ICG fluorescence	High detection rate	More LNs removed
	Real-time guidance	Unable to detect SLNs over the skin
	Visualizing lymphatic ducts	The limit of detection is 1–2 cm

9.3 Current Perspective of ICG Fluorescence Method

9.3.1 Current Devices for ICG Fluorescence Method

For the detection device, the NIR fluorescence imager, photodynamic eye (PDE, Hamamatsu Photonics, Hamamatsu Co., Japan) device, is widely used in the majority of clinical studies. This handheld device is composed of a light-emitting diode (LED) and a charge couple device (CCD) camera (Fig. 9.1a). The LED produces light at a wavelength of 760 nm to activate ICG, the CCD converts fluorescence light at a wavelength of 830 nm to digital imaging, and the filter of the camera cuts off the region of light at a wavelength below 820 nm. This ICG fluorescence method visualizes subcutaneous lymphatic flow in real-time (Fig. 9.1b) and directs orderly and sequential dissection to harvest SLNs (Fig. 9.1c, d). Another commercially available device is the Hyper Eye Medical System (HEMSTM, Mizuho Co. Toyo Japan). The HEMES can acquire both ICG fluorescence and color video imaging simultaneously, and this real-time imaging can direct the surgeon to the SLNs in the axilla without switching on or off the surgical light [8]. The FLARE and MIN-FLARE systems, which are not commercially available, have two light sources for the visible (400–650 nm) and NIR (760 nm) optic range and it can overlay the NIR signal on the color video image of the operation field [9]. There is no report of a direct comparison among these three devices. Each study, however, has reported highly successful detection rates, demonstrating that the diagnostic performance of ICG fluorescence is reliable and reproducible independent of the device.

9.3.2 Optimization of the ICG Fluorescence Signal

ICG is an amphiphilic molecule and quickly binds to plasma proteins in the vascular compartment. The protein-bound ICG fluorescence exhibits increased

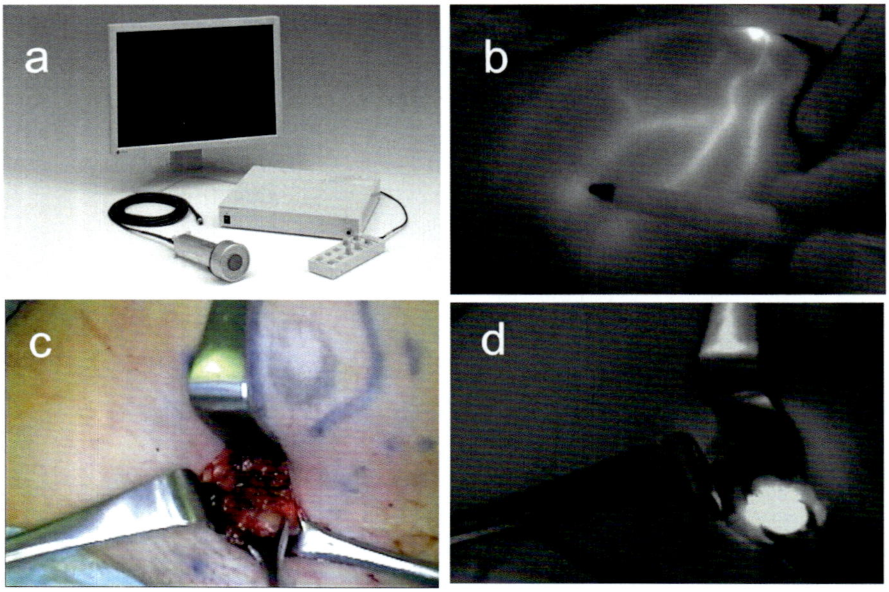

Fig. 9.1 (**a**) Photodynamic Eye (PDE) system (Hamamatsu Photonics, Japan). (**b**) Subcutaneous lymphatic mapping using ICG fluorescence. (**c**) ICG fluorescence navigation to the sentinel lymph nodes. (**d**) Removal of the SLN with a high ICG florescence signal

hydrostatic diameter, and this hydrostatic diameter is important for retention in the SLN. In general, there is a nonlinear association between ICG concentration and the intensity of an ICG fluorescence signal, and a high ICG concentration leads to decreased fluorescence intensity by fluorescence quenching. An optimal concentration of ICG absorbed to human serum albumin (ICG: HSA) was investigated for SLN biopsy in breast cancer patients. An ICG: HSA injection of 400–800 μM achieved the highest signal-to-background ratio (SBR) for SLNs compared with higher concentrations [10]. In melanoma, a dose of 600 μM ICG: HAS was optimal to obtain high SBR [11]. An ICG concentration of 0.5 % (5 mg/ml; 6.4 mM) was widely used following the original report in 2005 [7]. Although this dose is approximately tenfold higher than the optimal dose reported, a high detection rate was obtained in subsequent studies. For studies of lymphatic function or intracellular optical imaging, several compounds containing ICG, such as liposomal formulation of ICG or bovine serum albumin-coated polymeric nanocapsules loaded with ICG, have been developed [12, 13]. These new technologies could develop NIR fluorescence imaging for cancer detection and treatment.

9.3.3 Technical Aspects of SLN Mapping Using ICG Fluorescence

Several technical issues should be addressed to optimize lymphatic mapping for axillary staging. For the site of ICG injection, the subareolar site is acceptable in the case of intradermal or subcutaneous injection because these superficial injections yield a favorable visualization of lymphatic drainage and high fluorescence signals in the axillary basin compared with deep injection in the peritumoral site. It is still unknown whether ICG should be injected in the subareolar and the peritumoral site together or the subareolar site alone. Indeed, injection in the peritumoral site directs ICG to deep lymphatic flow and sometimes reveals extra-axillary drainage in the breast (i.e., inframammary chain). However, the main purpose of SLN biopsy is axillary staging, and we believe that subareolar injection alone is acceptable for the routine SLN mapping irrepective of tumor location [14].

After the induction of general or local anesthesia, 1 ml of ICG at a concentrate of 0.05–0.5 % is injected into the periareolar area, and a brief massage promotes the movement of ICG toward the axilla. As it takes 1–5 min for ICG to reach the axilla, NIR fluorescence imaging must be performed shortly after ICG administration. Fluorescence streaming can be detected on the skin surface by directing PDE onto the breast. During this process, blood vessels are sometimes visualized. The distinction between blood vessels and lymph ducts is easy because the flow rate of ICG through blood vessels is higher than through lymph ducts. ICG fluorescence in blood stream is quickly washed out, whereas it persists in lymphatic stream and visualizes lymphatic ducts longer.

As the fluorescence signal is attenuated by adipose tissue and cannot penetrate more than 2 cm in depth, fluorescent afferent lymphatic channels are interrupted at the site where they enter the axillary space. To press the skin over SLN using a plastic hemisphere decreases the distance between the skin and SLNs and helps to visualize fluorescent SLNs [15]. When SLNs cannot be identified over the skin, the skin incision made 2 cm distal to the site where the fluorescence signal disappears is recommended. While taking care to avoid injury of lymph ducts otherwise spoiling the operation field with spilled ICG, the anatomical and didactic dissection can be achieved in the axillary basin, and the fluorescence-emitting SLNs are exposed below the fascia [16].

Of the fluorescence-emitting lymph nodes, the lymph node to which the lymph ducts enter first is removed as the first SLN. The next fluorescence-emitting lymph nodes, if any, are removed as the second and subsequent SLNs. Furthermore, lymph nodes palpable in the operative field are also resected as SLNs. The ICG fluorescence method leads to this sequential and orderly SLN removal.

9.3.4 Definition of SLN Using ICG Fluorescence

SLN is defined as the first lymph node(s) to which cancer cells are most likely to spread from a primary tumor. In clinical practice, however, tracer positivity is commonly used as a surrogate for lymphatic drainage, and the identification of SLNs depends heavily on the specificity of the agent(s) used for the mapping. Using NIR fluorescence imaging system, SLNs can be categorized based on both the positivity of the fluorescent signal and the anatomical site in conjunction with lymphatic flow. For the RI method, the hottest SLN represents the definitive SLN, whereas the brightest SLN for fluorescence is only a good candidate for the definitive SLN; however, the quantification of the fluorescence signal has not yet been established. For the ICG fluorescence method, the removed SLN can be classified as follows:

1. Definitive SLN: This single node is the most proximal lymph node along the subcutaneous lymphatic flow and uptakes ICG fluorescence. This node is usually harvested first during the dissection procedure and sometimes exhibits the green color when 0.5 % ICG is used. This first lymph node represents actual lymph node status in the axilla.
2. Probable SLNs: These lymph nodes usually appeared adjacent to the first lymph node with fluorescence signals. One to two nodes are often harvested in the second and/or further tier.
3. Less probable SLNs: Palpable lymph nodes without any fluorescence signal may be included in this category

9.3.5 Comparison Between ICG Fluorescence and Blue Dye

The cumulative results for the ICG fluorescence method demonstrate that the ICG fluorescence method achieved a higher SLN detection rate (99–100 %) compared with the use of blue dye [17–22]. A large prospective study [23] comparing the ICG fluorescence method and the blue dye method in detection of SLNs reported that the ICG fluorescence method detected a significantly larger number of SLNs than did the blue dye method, and the median difference in the number of SLNs identified between the two methods was one (range 0–6, $p < 0.001$). The overall detection rate and the false negative rates for the ICG fluorescence and the blue dye method was 99 % and 78 % ($p < 0.001$) and 0 % and 30 %, respectively. A recent meta-analysis [24] also confirmed that the ICG fluorescence method is significantly superior to the blue dye method for SLN detection (OR 18.37, 95 % CI 8.63–39.10). When ICG is used under visible light, the SLN detection rate is only 73.8 %, whereas ICG can achieve a high detection rate using NIR imaging system. Van den Vorst and colleagues [25] reported that blue dye did not have any impact on SLN detection when ICG fluorescence is used in combination with radioactivity. On the basis of these results, blue dye can be spared when NIR imaging system is used.

9.3.6 Comparison Between ICG Fluorescence and RI

Several clinical trials have already demonstrated that the ICG fluorescence method is safe and can achieve a high SLN detection rate comparable with or superior to the RI method. Murawa et al. [26] analyzed the accuracy of SLN biopsy with the RI method and the ICG fluorescence method in 20 patients with breast cancer. In that study, the SLN detection rate for RI and ICG was 85 % and 100 %, the sensitivity in 13 lymph node metastasis-positive cases was 77 % and 92 %, and the false negative rate was 23 % and 8 %, respectively. The prospective direct comparison between the ICG fluorescence method and the RI method revealed that the SLN detection rate with the ICG fluorescence method was higher than that with the RI method (100 % v 91.3 %, $p < 0.001$) [27]. Other clinical trials [28, 29] also showed clinical utility of the ICG fluorescence method compared with the RI method, although these analyses do not have enough statistical power because of small cohort studies. As summarized in Table 9.2, the recent prospective study [30], which recruited 821 early breast cancer patients with clinically node-negative disease, demonstrated that there was no difference between the ICG fluorescence and the RI method for overall SLN detection rate (97.2 % v 97.0 %, $p = 0.88$) and for tumor-positive SLN detection rate (93.3 % v 90 %, $p = 0.18$). However, the additional use of ICG fluorescence with RI significantly improved the detection rate for overall and tumor-positive SLN compared with RI alone (99.8 % v 97.0 %, $p < 0.001$, 97.2 % v 90 %, $p < 0.001$, respectively). On the basis of these results, the ICG fluorescence method could be considered an alternative and additional method to SLN detection using RI in breast cancer.

9.3.7 SLN Biopsy After Preoperative/Neoadjuvant Systemic Therapy

SLN biopsy after preoperative/neoadjuvant systemic therapy (NACT) was previously not recommended because of a high false positive rate. However, several clinical studies have revealed that the sensitivity of SLN biopsy after NACT is not

Table 9.2 Detection rate for SLN

SLN detection	% (n/N)	p
Overall ($N = 821$)		
RI	97.0 (796/821)	
ICG fluorescence	97.2 (798/821)	0.88
RI+ICG fluorescence	99.8 (819/821)	<0.001
Positive node ($N = 180$)		
RI	90.0 (162/180)	
ICG fluorescence	93.3 (168/180)	0.18
RI+ICG fluorescence	97.2 (175/180)	<0.001

inferior to that before systemic therapy. Recent meta-analyses reported that the conventional RI method provided a detection rate of 90–90.5 % and a false negative rate of 10–12 % [31, 32] and that there is no significant difference in SLN detection between the groups before and after NACT. Based on these findings, the 2014 ASCO guidelines reported that SLN biopsy may be offered after NACT [33]. Chemotherapeutic agents, however, might cause fibrosis and obstruction of lymphatic channels, which leads to a less accurate procedure using the conventional RI method. As the hydrodynamic diameter of ICG (<1 nm) is smaller than that of RI (>50 mm), ICG may potentially reach the first SLN or the further tier more easily than RI. In the SENTIA trial [34], the false negative rate for SLN mapping was 14.2 % for patients who converted from clinically node-positive to node-negative disease after NACT. For the detection technique, the additional use of blue dye tended to improve the false negative rate. This false negative rate was also associated with the number of SLNs harvested, and the accuracy of SLN biopsy was apparently improved when more than two SLNs were harvested. ICG fluorescence yields the mean number of 2.3 SLNs removed [30] and has the potential to localize SLNs even in narrow lymphatic channels after NACT. As ICG would be a suitable method for SLN mapping after NACT, a large-scale clinical trial is required to confirm the clinical utility of ICG after NACT in patients with axillary involvement.

9.4 Conclusions

The cumulative results clearly demonstrate the advantage of NIR fluorescence imaging using ICG for SLN mapping in breast cancer. The ICG fluorescence method could be considered as an alternative and an accebtable additional method to SLN mapping using RI in breast cancer. This nonradioactive imaging system has the potential to be widely adopted in accordance with efforts to reduce radiation exposure.

References

1. Halsted CP, Benson JR, Jatoi I (2014) A historical account of breast cancer surgery: beware of local recurrence but be not radical. Future Oncol 10(9):1649–1657
2. Morton DL, Wen DR, Wong JH et al (1992) Technical details of intraoperative lymphatic mapping for early stage melanoma. Arch Surg 127:392–399
3. Krag DN, Weaver DL, Alex JC, Fairbank JT (1993) Surgical resection and radiolocalization of the sentinel node in breast cancer using a gamma probe. Surg Oncol 2:335–339
4. Giuliano AE, Kirgan DM, Kuenther JM, Morton DL (1994) Lymphatic mapping and sentinel lymphadenectomy for breast cancer. Ann Surg 220:398–401
5. Kim T, Giuliano AE, Lyman GH (2006) Lymphatic mapping and sentinel lymph node biopsy in early-stage breast carcinoma. Cancer 106:4–16

6. Morrow M, Rademaker AW, Bethke KP et al (1999) Learning sentinel node biopsy: results of a prospective randomized trial of two techniques. Surgery 126:714–720
7. Kitai T, Inomoto T, Miwa M, Shikayama T (2005) Fluorescence navigation with indocyanine green for detecting sentinel lymph nodes in breast cancer. Breast Cancer 12:211–215
8. Yamauchi K, Nagafuji H, Nakamura T et al (2011) Feasibility of ICG fluorescence-guided sentinel node biopsy in animal models using the HyperEye Medical System. Ann Surg Oncol 18:2042–2047
9. Troyan SL, Kinzard V, Gibbs-Strauss SL et al (2009) The FLARE intraoperative near-infrared fluorescence imaging system: a first-in-human clinical trial in breast cancer sentinel lymph node mapping. Ann Surg Oncol 16:2943–2952
10. Mieog JS, Troyan SL, Hutteman M et al (2011) Towards optimization of imaging system and lymphatic tracer for near-infrared fluorescent sentinel lymph node mapping in breast cancer. Ann Surg Oncol 18:2483–2491
11. van der Vorst JR, Schaafsma BE, Verbeek FP et al (2013) Dose optimization for near-infrared fluorescence sentinel lymph node mapping in patients with melanoma. Br J Dermatol 168:93–98
12. Proulx ST, Luciani P, Derzsi S et al (2010) Quantitative imaging of lymphatic function with liposomal indocyanine green. Cancer Res 70:7053–7062
13. Bahmani B, Gupta S, Upadhyayula S et al (2011) Effect of polyethylene glycol coatings on uptake of indocyanine green loaded nanocapsules by human spleen macrophages in vitro. J Biomed Opt 16:051303
14. Sugie T (2010) Controversy of axillary diagnosis and treatment. In: Toi M, Winer EP (eds) Local and systemic management of primary breast cancers. Kyoto University Press, Kyoto, pp 61–71
15. Kitai T, Kawashima M (2012) Transcutaneous detection and direct approach to the sentinel node using axillary compression technique in ICG fluorescence-navigated sentinel node biopsy for breast cancer. Breast Cancer 19:343–348
16. Sugie T, Kassim KA, Takeuchi M et al (2010) A novel method for sentinel lymph node biopsy by indocyanine green fluorescence technique in breast cancer. Cancers 2:713–720
17. Abe H, Mori T, Umeda T et al (2011) Indocyanine green fluorescence imaging system for sentinel lymph node biopsies in early breast cancer patients. Surg Today 41:197–202
18. Tagaya N, Yamazaki R, Nakagawa A et al (2008) Intraoperative identification of sentinel lymph node by near-infrared fluorescence imaging in patients with breast cancer. Am J Surg 195:850–853
19. Takeuchi M, Sugie T, Abdelazeem K et al (2012) Lymphatic mapping with fluorescence navigation using indocyanine green and axillary surgery in patients with primary breast cancer. Breast J 18:535–541
20. Aoyama K, Kamio T, Ohchi T et al (2011) Sentinel lymph node biopsy for breast cancer patients using fluorescence navigation with indocyanine green. World J Surg Oncol 9:157
21. Hirano A, Kamimura M, Ogura K et al (2012) A comparison of indocyanine green fluorescence imaging plus blue dye and blue dye alone for sentinel node navigation surgery in breast cancer patients. Ann Surg Oncol 19:4112–4116
22. Inoue T, Nishi T, Nakano Y et al (2014) Axillary lymph node recurrence after sentinel lymph node biopsy performed using a combination of indocyanine green fluorescence and the blue dye method in early breast cancer. Breast Cancer. doi:10.1007/s12282-014-0573-8
23. Sugie T, Sawada T, Tagaya N et al (2013) Comparison of the indocyanine green fluorescence and blue dye methods in detection of sentinel lymph nodes in early-stage breast cancer. Ann Surg Oncol 20:2213–2218
24. Ahmed M, Purushotham AD, Douek M (2014) Novel techniques for sentinel lymph node biopsy in breast cancer: a systematic review. Lancet Oncol 15:e351–e362
25. van der Vorst JR, Schaafsma BE, Verbeek FP et al (2012) Randomized comparison of near-infrared fluorescence imaging using indocyanine green and 99(m)technetium with or without

patent blue for the sentinel lymph node procedure in breast cancer patients. Ann Surg Oncol 19:4104–4111
26. Murawa D, Hirche C, Dresel S, Hünerbein M (2009) Sentinel lymph node biopsy in breast cancer guided by indocyanine green fluorescence. Br J Surg 96:1289–1294
27. Wishart GC, Loh SW, Jones L, Benson JR (2012) A feasibility study (ICG-10) of indocyanine green (ICG) fluorescence mapping for sentinel lymph node detection in early breast cancer. Eur J Surg Oncol 38:651–656
28. Schaafsma BE, Verbeek FP, Riebergen DD et al (2013) Clinical trial of combined radio-and fluorescence-guided sentinel lymph node biopsy in breast cancer. Br J Surg 100:137–144
29. Verbeek FP, Troyan SL, Mieog JS et al (2014) Near-infrared fluorescence sentinel lymph node mapping in breast cancer: a multicenter experience. Breast Cancer Res Treat 143:333–342
30. Sugie T, Kinoshita T, Masuda N et al (2016) Evaluation of the clinical utility of the ICG fluorescence method compared with the radioisotope method for sentinel lymph node biopsy in breast cancer. Ann Surg Oncol 23:44–50
31. Kelly AM, Dwamena B, Cronin P, Carios RC (2009) Breast cancer sentinel node identification and classification after neoadjuvant chemotherapy-systematic review and meta analysis. Acad Radiol 16:551–563
32. van Deurzen CH, Vriens BE, Tjan-Heijnen VC et al (2009) Accuracy of sentinel node biopsy after neoadjuvant chemotherapy in breast cancer patients: a systematic review. Eur J Cancer 45:3124–3130
33. Lyman GH, Temin S, Edge SB et al (2014) Practice. Sentinel lymph node biopsy for patients with early-stage breast cancer: American Society of Clinical Oncology clinical practice guideline update. J Clin Oncol 32:1365–1383
34. Kuehn T, Bauerfeind I, Fehm T et al (2014) Sentinel-lymph node biopsy in patients with breast cancer before and after neoadjuvant chemotherapy (SENTINA): a prospective, multicenter cohort study. Lancet Oncol 14:609–618

Part III
Radiation Therapy

Chapter 10
Personalisation of Radiotherapy for Breast Cancer

Ian H. Kunkler, Carol Ward, Corey Speers, Lori Pierce, Felix Feng, James Meehan, and Simon P. Langdon

Abstract The role of radiotherapy is well established in the multidisciplinary management of breast cancer. However, its use could be customised further with the intent of enhancing tumour cell radiosensitisation and reducing normal cell toxicity. The importance of tumour heterogeneity and the microenvironment in the response to radiotherapy is under intense scrutiny, and the value of molecular profiling is being increasingly recognised. Genome-wide association studies are likely to play an important role in elucidating the molecular pathogenesis of radiotoxicity in the emerging area of radiogenomics. Biomarkers of tumour radiosensitivity should help indicate potentially responsive and unresponsive cancers. Further understanding of the tumour microenvironment and better preclinical models will help identify targets to enhance radiosensitivity or reverse radioresistance.

Keywords Radiotherapy • Partial breast irradiation • Radiosensitivity • Tumour heterogeneity • Tumour microenvironment

10.1 Introduction

Adjuvant radiotherapy continues to play a key role in the multidisciplinary management of breast cancer. Its objective is to eradicate residual tumour after surgery. Adjuvant radiotherapy has traditionally been restricted to the postoperative setting after breast-conserving surgery and selectively after mastectomy. It has an established role in locally advanced disease either following systemic therapy

I.H. Kunkler (✉)
Edinburgh Cancer Research Centre, Western General Hospital, Crewe Road South, Edinburgh EH4 2XU, UK
e-mail: iankunkler@yahoo.com

C. Ward • J. Meehan • S.P. Langdon
Division of Pathology, Institute of Genetics and Molecular Medicine, University of Edinburgh, Western General Hospital, Edinburgh, UK

C. Speers • L. Pierce • F. Feng
Department of Radiation Oncology, University of Michigan, Ann Arbor, MI, USA

M. Toi et al. (eds.), *Personalized Treatment of Breast Cancer*,
DOI 10.1007/978-4-431-55552-0_10

where inflammatory changes or peau d'orange preclude mastectomy or postmastectomy. Recently, it has been investigated in the preoperative setting in an early phase clinical trial in combination with neoadjuvant chemotherapy [1].

The Oxford overview shows that, after mastectomy and breast-conserving therapy, radiotherapy reduces significantly both local recurrence and breast cancer mortality. At 15 years of follow-up, for every four recurrences prevented in the first 5 years, one breast cancer death can be avoided [2]. As the incidence of breast cancer rises globally, as a consequence of early detection from breast-screening programmes and rising life expectancy, demands for adjuvant irradiation are likely to rise. Using models of evidence-based recommendations, 83 % of patients with breast cancer will require external beam irradiation [3]. Increasing pressures on limited radiotherapy resources pose challenges for better selection of patients predicted to benefit from irradiation. The rationale for personalisation of radiotherapy is therefore strong. There are two possible areas of individual modulation: tumour and normal tissue radiosensitivity. Scope for modulation of the former seems a more realistic prospect than the latter, given how little we understand about the genetic basis of normal tissue radiosensitivity. With the rising population of older patients in whom comorbidities may preclude surgery and chemotherapy, the understanding of normal tissue radiosensitivity and the interaction with comorbidities will become increasingly important [4].

Traditionally, the treatment of breast cancer has been based on evidence from patients in clinical trials with a limited range of clinicopathological characteristics (typically TNM staging, grade, ER status, etc.). Where data show clinically significant benefit from intervention (surgery/drug/radiation), which reached a predefined threshold (e.g. 3 % in overall survival benefit at 5 years), the results are applied to all patients meeting the eligibility criteria for that trial. In the case of adjuvant radiotherapy for breast cancer, the application of a boost of irradiation to the site of excision after breast-conserving surgery (with clear margins) and whole breast irradiation is predominantly applied to women under the age of 50 where most benefit in reducing local recurrence is obtained [5].

10.2 The Rationale for Treatment Personalisation

The development of high-throughput sequencing and improvements in our understanding of the molecular mechanisms underlying malignant transformation and progress have facilitated a move away from a 'one size fits all' approach to efforts to personalise treatment for breast cancer [6]. One of the major limitations of the 'one size fits all' approach has been the underrepresentation of older patients in clinical trials of adjuvant radiotherapy, in part due to the historical exclusion of such patients due to arbitrary age eligibility caps at around 70 years. Advances in the therapeutic ratio for adjuvant radiotherapy either have to achieve a higher level of local control for the same or lower levels of acute and late radiation-induced toxicity or the same level of local control for lower levels of radiotoxicity.

Much of the current focus on the personalisation of the treatment of breast cancer has been driven by two developments. The first has been risk assessment in early stage breast cancer to avoid overtreatment, in particular in node-negative disease with the application of molecular profiling [7]. The second is the availability of targeted therapies, particularly for HER2-positive disease. Much less attention and research has been devoted to customising radiotherapy to the biology of the cancer and to the sensitivity of normal tissues to irradiation. This field is still in its infancy. Progress has been hampered in part because radiotherapy is not accepted as a targeted therapy and therefore personalization is not viewed in the same way as targeted therapies such as trastuzumab for HER2-positive cancers.

10.3 Advances in Radiation Planning and Delivery

Already, there has been significant progress in personalising radiotherapy through the application of 3D treatment planning with radiation portals customised to maximise target coverage whilst minimising irradiation of critical structures such as the heart and the lungs. More recent developments have been the application of intensity-modulated (IMRT) and image-guided radiation therapy (IGRT) to optimise dose distribution [8]. Much less progress has been made in understanding the biological factors which underlie differences in radiosensitivity between patients. We are therefore some way from an assay which would predict clinical radiation response for individual patients [9]. Gilbert Fletcher, a pioneer in the development of radiotherapy, compared the successful development of a radiotherapy predict assay to the quest for the Holy Grail [9, 10].

10.4 Importance of Tumour Heterogeneity

The heterogeneity within tumours is an acknowledged component in resistance to both radiation and systemic therapy. Studies in renal cancer have demonstrated that each area of a tumour displays specific genomic arrangements [11]; these findings are now being replicated in breast cancer [12, 13]. Such heterogeneity has a significant influence on radio and chemotherapy [14]. Differences in radiation sensitivity are apparent amongst patients with similar types of breast cancer, which may reflect disparities in the mutational burden of these tumours [15]. Variation in response can also be caused by the presence of radioresistant breast cancer stem cells [16–18], and further by the induction of 'stemness' by radiation treatment itself [19, 20].

10.5 Enhancing the Efficacy of Adjuvant Radiation Therapy

Adjuvant radiotherapy is a potent agent in the multidisciplinary armamentarium of anticancer therapy in breast cancer both in terms of locoregional therapy and survival. The 2005 Early Breast Cancer meta-analysis of adjuvant radiotherapy after breast-conserving surgery and mastectomy showed a direct relationship between the absolute reduction in locoregional recurrence at 5 years and an improvement in long-term survival at 15 years [2]. This equated to a 4:1 ratio with one breast cancer death being avoided for every four locoregional recurrences prevented by radiotherapy. This was the first evidence of a systemic effect of radiation in breast cancer. However, this equation proved to be erroneous because of the competing risks of local and distant disease, the lack of definition of time to locoregional recurrence and the systemic effect of RT [21]. As a result, the EBCTCG decided to report the effects of RT on first recurrence whether locoregional or distant. The Oxford overviews of adjuvant postoperative radiotherapy for breast cancer after breast-conserving surgery and mastectomy show that it has a higher effect to locoregional control and overall survival [22, 23]. It halves approximately the risk of first recurrence at 10 years after breast-conserving surgery [22] and improves long-term survival. For patients treated by mastectomy and axillary clearance (at least level II), the overview shows that radiotherapy reduced mortality from breast cancer by 20 % in women with one to three positive lymph nodes (rate ratio [RR], irradiated vs. not, 0 · 80, 95 % CI 0 · 67–0 · 95; 2p = 0 · 01) and by 13 % in women with at least four positive axillary nodes (RR 0 · 87, 95 % CI 0 · 77–0 · 99; 2p = 0 · 04) [23].

It is important to recognise that the benefits of radiotherapy as a local therapy in terms of survival need to be seen in the context of systemic therapy. Systemic therapy reduces the risks of both local and distant recurrence. With the ability of systemic therapy to control micrometastatic disease, locoregional control assumes even greater importance. However whilst these meta-analyses provide important insights to the effectiveness of locoregional radiotherapy, they do not predict individual patient benefit. Indeed, the magnitude of benefit might be larger amongst the radiosensitive population of patients since the benefits in the overview may be diluted by patients with radioresistant tumours. Hence, the dividends of being able to predict radiotherapy benefit by biomarkers may be substantial if they are more accurate than conventional clinicopathological factors. This is an area of active investigation. Personalisation of breast cancer radiotherapy can be considered in a number of ways: (1) selection for treatment based on clinicopathological factors and molecular features, (2) optimising dose distribution within the irradiated volumes and (3) minimising locoregional morbidity by minimising dose to critical structures, particularly the lung and heart.

10.6 Theories of Breast Cancer Spread

Personalisation of radiotherapy must consider the heterogeneity of breast cancer. In the first half of the twentieth century, breast cancer was believed to be a disease that spread from the primary site to the regional nodes (the Halstedian hypothesis), giving a rationale for aggressive locoregional treatment. This was succeeded by the view of breast cancer as a systemic disease (the Fisher hypothesis), based on the observation that patients developed distant metastases despite the primary site being controlled. Fisher argued that patients could be divided into two categories; those tumours with the ability to spread to distant sites and those that lacked that ability [24]. Neither view was valid for all breast cancers [25]. The current 'spectrum' theory advanced by Samuel Hellman is that breast cancer is a 'heterogeneous disease...[with] a spectrum of proclivities extending from a disease that remains local throughout its course to one that is systemic when first detectable' [26, 27]. Although some tumours have not metastasised from the primary site at the time of diagnosis, there is no current reliable method to detect micrometastatic disease. Failure to achieve local control may facilitate metastatic spread and reduce survival. Hellman's theory acknowledges that the higher the chance that systemic disease is present at the time of diagnosis, the lower the impact of local therapy. This may explain why the survival advantage of locoregional postmastectomy radiotherapy in the Danish Cooperative Breast Group trials is seen in the subgroup of good prognosis ER or PgR-positive, HER2-negative patients and not in ER or PgR-negative or HER2-positive patients where the latter have probably developed distant metastases [28]. With the recognition that breast cancer is a heterogeneous range of diseases with distinct molecular subtypes (luminal A, luminal B, HER2/neu), optimal strategies for different subsets of patients may be necessary [29].

Molecular profiling might assist in identifying patients (a) at sufficiently low risk of relapse that radiation might be avoided, (b) at sufficiently high risk of locoregional recurrence who might benefit from additional radiation dose or combination with systemic therapy, (c) with early breast cancer who would benefit from postmastectomy radiotherapy and (d) suitable for partial breast irradiation [29]. In addition, molecular targets that may be related to radiation resistance might be found.

10.7 Personalisation of Radiotherapy, Heterogeneity and Tumour/Normal Tissue Radiosensitivity

Improving the therapeutic gain of radiation (i.e. improving local control for the same level of normal tissue toxicity) for individual breast cancer patients is an enormous challenge because of tumour heterogeneity and the limited understanding of the genetic basis of tumour and normal tissue radiosensitivity. Breast cancer is a spectrum of diseases with heterogeneity at molecular, histopathological and clinical levels [30]. This heterogeneity includes the tumour microenvironment and its different cellular components involving many different biological processes including angiogenesis, tumour metabolism and the immune response. New approaches on combining drugs targeting the pH regulatory mechanisms of breast cancer in preclinical models in combination with radiation are discussed later in this chapter.

10.8 Selection of Patients on Clinicopathological Factors

Already, we have some degree of personalisation of adjuvant radiotherapy based on clinicopathological factors. For example, patients under the age of 50 benefit from an additional boost dose to the site of excision following breast-conserving surgery and postoperative whole breast irradiation [5]. The biological mechanism underlying the impact of young age still remains poorly understood.

10.9 Biomarkers of Tumour Radiosensitivity

It is a common clinical experience that local control rates following adjuvant systemic therapy and radiotherapy based on traditional clinicopathological factors (tumour size, grade, nodal status and clinical stage) do not reliably predict clinical outcome. One of the holy grails of radiation oncology in general and breast cancer in particular has been to identify reliable and clinically applicable biomarkers of tumour radiosensitivity which could select patients likely to benefit and those that would either derive no or minimal benefit. Patients with no evidence of radiosensitivity might be spared the toxicity of radiation therapy and offered alternative systemic approaches. Those with low or moderate radiosensitivity might be subject to combinatorial approaches with drugs increasing radiosensitivity. There is, however, a limited number of studies, all retrospective showing promise for molecular markers of breast cancer radiosensitivity. Prospective studies and randomised trials will be needed to evaluate their clinical utility.

The variables which determine radiosensitivity can be categorised into three groups: (i) intrinsic radiosensitivity, (ii) tumour oxygenation status and (iii) tumour proliferative potential (Tpot). Clonogenic cell survival assays have been the cornerstone for measuring intrinsic radiosensitivity. However, they are difficult to do as the ex vivo plating efficiency is around 1 % and none of these assays is applicable in the clinic. The Eppendorf probe has been the main method of measuring intratumoural oxygenation status but is impractical to apply in breast cancer and other solid deep-seated tumours. Tpot is a measure of tumour-doubling time based on flow cytometry from a tumour biopsy stained with bromodeoxyuridine. However, it is a weak predictor of outcome [9].

10.10 Gene Expression Classifiers

Genomic profiling technologies have allowed the stratification of human breast tumours into clinically useful groups and have further aided in the personalization of the treatment of breast cancer. The genomic era has produced an exponential increase in our understanding of cancer biology and has greatly accelerated cancer drug development. With the advent and implementation of microarray expression profiling, it is now possible to evaluate gene expression in tumours on a genome-wide basis. These advances have led to the utilisation of gene expression profiling to not only subtype cancers, but to predict prognosis and disease-free survival and determine optimal treatment.

Emerging gene expression data suggests that breast cancer is a clinically heterogeneous disease. This clinical heterogeneity is driven to a large extent by abnormal gene expression within tumours. Investigators now have the ability to identify the gene expression fingerprint of an individual's tumour. This information may be used to rationally design treatment regimens for patients in the future and also to predict the clinical course of an individual's disease, including response to a radiation treatment. Genetic profiles of tumours are now being correlated with clinical outcome, and several prognostic and predictive indicators have emerged based on this research. Additionally, transcriptional and proteomic profiling is advancing our understanding of the RNA and protein alterations in human cancers. Despite early limitations, genomic classifiers are now being used clinically to better risk stratify patients and guide rational therapy decisions by clinicians.

Multiple gene sets have been developed in an attempt to stratify patients based on the gene expression signature of their tumours. One of the first of these was the Rotterdam gene set. It was developed to predict the prognosis of patients with lymph node-negative (LNN) breast cancer [31]. Markers were selected separately from ER-negative and ER-positive tumours and were combined into a single 76-gene prognostic signature that was able to predict distant metastatic recurrence with a sensitivity of 93 % and a specificity of 48 % [31]. This prognostic indicator performed better than standard, clinical variables in a multivariate analysis (hazard ratio [HR], 5.55; 95 % confidence interval [CI], 2.46–12.5). Subsequently, this test was also validated using two other sets of patients with early stage breast cancer that were not included in the original study. This test is now FDA-approved and is clinically used to identify patients who should receive chemotherapy. The success of this gene expression profiling approach to address clinically relevant uncertainties underscores the utility of such profiling in the management of breast cancer.

Subsequent gene expression profiles have been developed and are now being used clinically to help identify individual tumours that will respond to chemotherapy. One such example is OncotypeDx®. This 21-gene assay was derived from 250 candidate genes chosen from gene expression profiling experiments, published literature and genomic databases and then correlated with breast cancer recurrence in 447 patients [32, 33]. Sixteen cancer-related genes and five reference genes were selected from the candidate genes. The 16 cancer-related genes were then used to develop an algorithm based on the expression levels of these genes, thus allowing a Recurrence Score™ (RS) to be computed for each specimen. This RS correlated with the rate of distant recurrence at 10 years. The OncotypeDx® assay was externally validated in the National Surgical Adjuvant Breast and Bowel Project (NSABP) clinical trial B-14, which examined the effect of adjuvant tamoxifen in patients with hormone receptor-positive LNN breast cancer [32, 33]. The results of this analysis showed that 7 % of low-risk patients (RS <18) relapsed, whereas 31 % of high-risk patients (RS >31) relapsed. Subsequent studies have shown that the RS is independently associated with sensitivity to chemotherapy and mortality [33, 34]. The OncotypeDx® assay is now FDA-approved for use in profiling the risk and need for chemotherapy responsiveness in breast cancers. It is now in wide clinical use by oncologists to determine which patients would benefit from chemotherapy.

OncotypeDx® is not the only prognostic gene profiling test being used clinically. Other tests currently approved include Mammaprint [35], Mammostrat [36], Prosigna [37–39] and CellSearch [40]. These tests, which also mainly rely on the use of gene expression technologies and molecular signatures, underscore the power and utility of such approaches at identifying expression derangements and the potential for treatment personalisation for individual patients.

In addition to defining molecular subtypes of cancers and predicting prognosis and disease-free survival, gene expression classifiers have been used to determine optimal treatment [7, 41–44]. Several groups have already used expression profiling to identify gene signatures of chemotherapeutic resistance [41, 42, 45]. These studies have identified tumour gene expression profiles associated with response to chemotherapy including docetaxel [41, 42], adriamycin/cyclophosphamide [46], paclitaxel, fluorouracil, doxorubicin, cyclophosphamide [47] and epirubicin, cyclophosphamide and paclitaxel [48] in the neoadjuvant setting. Together, these studies indicate the potential to not only determine the likelihood of response to a particular therapy, but may be incorporated into ways to personalise radiation therapy.

As mentioned previously, gene expression assays have been developed to predict clinical outcomes in breast cancer. The main focus of these has been to predict systemic rather than local recurrence. The 70-gene signature was the first to identify patients who are at higher risk of systemic relapse. This signature was developed using a cohort of 78 patients with axillary node-negative, ER-positive or ER-negative early stage breast cancer all under the age of 55 years with tumours up to 5 cm in size [46]. This approach identified 70 genes that were able to identify women with a significantly increased risk of distant metastasis and death from breast cancer. Not surprisingly, genes associated with cell cycle regulation, invasion, metastasis and angiogenesis predominantly comprised the 70-gene signature. Interestingly, this signature also was able to identify *BRCA1* mutation carriers based on the expression level of these genes. This was one of the first successful applications of the gene expression analysis to guide clinical care. Prior to the development of genomic tools, a number of prognostic approaches to assess tumour radiosensitivity were developed including hypoxic fraction, DNA strand break and repair, intrinsic radiosensitivity and proliferation cell fraction [49].

Despite the development of numerous gene expression signatures to predict survival, distant metastasis and response to chemotherapy in patients with breast cancer (i.e. OncotypeDX®, Mammaprint®, Prosigna®) there has, until recently, been no attempt to develop signatures predictive of radiation response. One of the first attempts to identify such a radiation response came from a group out of the University of Chicago [45]. This group derived an IFN-related DNA damage resistance signature and then applied it to 34 cancer cell lines from the NCI60 panel. The genes in this signature that correlated most robustly with radiation resistance (SF-2Gy) were retained within the signature and then applied to patient datasets. The authors found that the IFN-related DNA damage resistance signature was able to predict response to both chemo- and radiotherapy. Though not further developed into a clinically translatable test, it was the first proof-of-principle attempt to develop a molecular signature predictive of radiation response.

One test recently proposed for clinical practise is borrowed heavily from the existing OncotypeDx® test, a test that was developed to predict response of patients with ER-positive, lymph node-negative breast cancer to adjuvant chemotherapy. This spin-off of the OncotypeDx® test was recently reported to estimate local recurrence risk in the absence of radiotherapy in women with DCIS after breast-conserving surgery [50]. Whilst not yet validated in a prospectively run clinical trial, it does suggest the potential power of molecular signatures to personalise treatment decisions regarding the need for adjuvant radiation treatment.

More recently, a ten-gene expression signature (AR, cJun, STAT1, PKC, RelA, cABL, SUMO1, CDK1, HDAC1 and IRF1) has been described by Eschrich et al. [51]; this signature was developed initially in studies using a panel of 48 cancer cell lines before being validated in three independent datasets (rectal, esophageal and head and neck cancers) [51]. In these initial validation studies, the signature was able to accurately predict which patients were at increased risk of recurrence based on the expression of these ten genes. Furthermore, when applied to two independent breast cancer datasets (totalling 503 patients), it indicated that the radiosensitivity signature may also act as a predictive biomarker for breast cancer, though these studies looked at distant metastasis and not local recurrence [51].

A final and most recent signature has been developed by investigators at the University of Michigan [52]. Previous attempts to identify signatures predictive of response to radiation using gene expression data have relied on expression data from patient tumour samples for signature development and have repeatedly failed external validation. The University of Michigan group instead assessed the intrinsic radiation sensitivity of 21 breast cancer cell lines and identified a panel of 147 genes whose expression was significantly correlated with radiation sensitivity. This 147-gene signature was then trained, locked and validated on cohorts of patients with early stage breast cancer treated with radiation therapy after breast-conserving surgery for whom local recurrence data was available. This radiation sensitivity signature (RSS) was shown to effectively and accurately identify patients with high rates of local recurrence based on predicted radiation resistance as reflected by the RSS score. This was the first signature to specifically identify patients with increased rates of local recurrence, not systemic progression, after radiation treatment. Like the signature developed by Eschrich et al., this signature awaits external validation before it can be effectively translated into clinical care.

10.11 Personalising Approaches to Minimise Radiation-Induced Toxicity

In the clinic, we see wide variations in the intensity of acute and late radiation reactions (e.g. skin erythema and breast fibrosis). It is estimated, based on studies of internal mammary irradiation, that patient-specific factors account for 49–90 % of these differences [53], but the exact reasons for these variations or how they might be modified based on genetic profiles of radiosensitivity are little understood. In older patients, radiotoxicity might also interact with comorbidities such as heart disease and diabetes. Currently, no clinically applicable assays predict normal tissue radiosensitivity. Preclinical tests using lymphocyte and fibroblast radiosensitivity proved too complex and non-replicable to be used clinically [54].

In vitro tests of radiosensitivity in humans demonstrate a nearly normal distribution, implying that normal tissue sensitivity is a polygenic trait; therefore, most of the clinically observed variation in radiosensitivity is likely to be due to low-penetrance genetic variants [55]. The radiosensitivity phenotype is possibly influenced by multiple loci ranging from rare variants with large effects to common variants with minor effects [56]. The scope for modulating the response of individual patients by any form of drug therapy in the foreseeable future is therefore likely to be limited.

One promising new approach to understanding the genetic basis of normal tissue radiosensitivity is the emerging field of radiogenomics which investigates the influence of genetic variation on radiation response [57]. The long-term goal of this research is to develop SNP-based risk models to stratify patients for individualised radiotherapy protocols [58]. Genetic association studies initially focussed on candidate genes involved in known radioresponse pathways and sought to identify functional SNPs (single nucleotide polymorphisms) that influence normal tissue radiotoxicity [57]. SNPs within the XRCC family of genes, ATM and TGFB1 genes have all been suggested to be involved in radiotoxicity in breast cancer patients [59]. Transforming growth factor Beta 1 (TGFB1) is one of the candidate genes considered to be involved in the genesis of radiation-induced breast/chest wall fibrosis [60]. However, data analysis of SNPs in predicting radiation toxicity shows conflicting results. For example, the independent validation of SNPs in 46 genes previously published to be associated with radiosensitivity was not confirmed in the UK RAPPER study [60]. The more recently introduced genome-wide association studies (GWAS) could play an important role in elucidating the molecular pathogenesis of radiotoxicity [60]. An important finding in many of the GWAS studies is that the identified SNPs are not in known genes or pathways already considered to be key candidates [57]. Furthermore, many of the SNPs are found in noncoding regions without any known or obvious function.

The principal challenge for emerging radiogenomics consortia is the availability of accurately reported toxicity data [61]. Risk models incorporating genetic assays as well as comorbidities, radiation dose and the volume irradiated require development [62, 63].

What is presently achievable on an individual basis is maximising the homogeneity of dose distribution in the breast and reducing where possible exposure of critical structures such as the lungs and the heart to radiation. Acute toxicities have been defined as those occurring within 90 days of treatment, affecting tissues such as the skin which have a rapid renewal rate. Late toxicities occur more than 90 days after radiotherapy [56]. The changing shape of the breast in the transverse and sagittal planes makes it difficult to irradiate homogeneously. There is level I evidence that the application of intensity-modulated radiotherapy (IMRT) reduces acute skin toxicity [64] and improves cosmesis [65] compared to standard RT.

10.12 Minimising Radiation-Induced Cardiac Toxicity

Before the advent of 3D planning, it was difficult to assess how much of the heart was being irradiated by postoperative radiotherapy after breast-conserving surgery or mastectomy. The Oxford overview showed that an approximately 2 % 20-year reduction in breast cancer mortality from adjuvant radiation therapy was counterbalanced by a similar percentage of non-breast-cancer mortality (mainly cardiac) [66]. Much of the cardiac morbidity and mortality may have been accounted for by older radiation techniques where the doses delivered to the heart were higher. However, minimising cardiac exposure has been a contemporary priority in adjuvant radiotherapy for breast cancer. A study of two cohorts of women from Denmark and Sweden shows that there is a linear relation between mean heart dose and the rate of major coronary events with an increase of 7.4 % per Gy [67]. A prospective trial has shown that active breathing control can reduce mean heart dose by =/> 20 % of patients in 88 % of cases [68].

10.13 Personalisation of Radiotherapy: Preclinical Models

Most preclinical research in oncology begins with the use of panels of cell lines that reflect the relevant cancer and its diverse subtypes. This is an oversimplistic model that neither replicates the in vivo tumour microenvironment nor the heterogeneity found in breast and other tumours (see above). Single-cell sequencing illustrates that tumours are made up from many distinct clones with varied mutations [69]. Therefore, even in cancers of the same subtype, different clones and mutations will be present that will determine the outcome of both systemic and radiation treatment. Cell line-derived xenograft models are extremely useful to monitor tumour growth, drug pharmacokinetics, efficacy and toxicity and have the added benefit of modelling the oxygen and pH gradients found in the tumour microenvironment, but the models are still dependent on available cell lines. Genetically engineered mouse models allow investigation of specific mutations, but although they can closely replicate clinical trial results, they are not personalised tumours.

One method that can examine a specific patient's tumour directly is tumour grafting or patient-derived xenografts (PDXs) [70]. In this model, cells from digested patient tumour tissue are transferred to immunodeficient mice, and then passaged from host to host. PDXs of human breast cancer accurately duplicate receptor expression, growth, metastatic capability and pathology of the actual tumour [71, 72]. However, these models have substantial costs, because PDXs must be sustained in mice, and like other xenografts, tumour growth can take time to establish [73]. Although these and other animal models are extremely useful, all have limitations and none are suitable for fast, high-throughput methodology [74, 75].

However, primary tumour material (explants) from a specific breast cancer patient can be investigated ex vivo, using pretreatment biopsy material [76, 77]. This method can be a useful adjunct in the thrust for personalised treatment, allowing analysis of a heterogeneous tumour, with an intact microenvironment and stromal tissue [78]. In our laboratory, pieces of tissue from all breast cancer subtypes are placed in a collagen matrix and cultured with or without drug or radiation treatment. Changes can be perceived within 5 days in most cases. Therefore, this system could be used to investigate tumour responses to a specific therapy. Our studies indicate that these cultures can be maintained with minimum management for at least 30 days [77]. Such cultures can be continuously observed and examined when necessary and lysed or fixed for analysis when required.

Using the explant model, we are currently investigating the radioresponsiveness of individual breast cancer patient tumours to radiotherapy (Fig. 10.1). This figure illustrates the use of tumour tissue obtained from pretreatment breast cancer patient biopsies. In Fig. 10.1a, the invasive growth of an untreated single explant is monitored for 10 days. This control explant could be treated with drug or radiation and the effects on further growth or invasion monitored. Figure 10.1b shows a radiosensitive explant in which no further growth or invasion has occurred in tissue treated with 5GY radiation, compared with control explants, where invasive growth has increased by approximately 500 %. Contrast this with Fig. 10.1c, where 5GY radiation treatment has had no effect on explant growth in comparison to untreated control explants, showing that tumour material from this patient is radiation resistant. Use of this experimental system could (a) allow personalisation of radiation treatment and (b) permit therapeutic strategies for radiation sensitisation to be assessed in a more physiological model using actual breast cancer tissue.

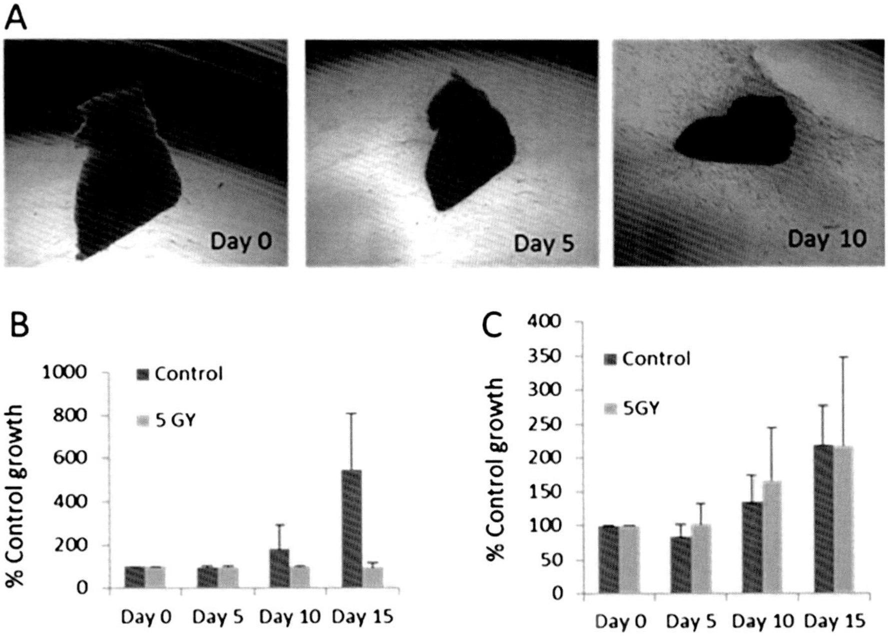

Fig. 10.1 Personalised assessment of radiosensitivity using pretreatment breast cancer patient biopsy material. (**a**) Tumour biopsy material was trimmed to remove fat. 1 mm^3 pieces were cultured in a collagen matrix and growth monitored over 10 days. (**b**) Illustration of a radiosensitive tumour treated with 5GY radiation and monitored for 15 days. Data shown indicates changes in growth normalised to Day 0 area ($n = 4 \pm$ SD). (**c**) Illustration of a radioresistant tumour treated with 5GY radiation and monitored for 15 days. Data shown indicates changes in growth normalised to Day 0 area ($n = 4 \pm$ SD)

10.14 The Radioresistant Tumour Microenvironment: Novel Therapeutic Targets

Hypoxia causes significant resistance to both radio- and chemotherapy and is found in approximately 40 % of all breast cancers and 50 % of advanced breast cancers demonstrating oxygen concentrations under 0.3 % [79]. Tumour cells use aerobic glycolysis to provide fuel and components for growth, even in the presence of sufficient oxygen [80, 81]. This leads to the excess production of CO_2, lactate and protons, which lowers the intracellular pH (pHi). However, several ion pumps, enzymes and transporters preserve pHi between 7.0 and 7.4 [80]. These include carbonic anhydrase (CA) IX, a hypoxia-inducible factor-1 (HIF-1)-induced enzyme that catalyses the conversion of CO_2 and H_2O to hydrogen ions and $HCO3^-$; the hypoxia-activated Na+/H+ exchanger 1 (NHE1), which extrudes hydrogen for sodium ions; monocarboxylate transporters (MCTs), which are H+/lactate transporters; and finally, V-ATPases, which act as H^+-transporters [80]. However, these proteins, whilst contributing to the alkaline pHi found in hypoxic cancer cells, lead to acidosis in the tumour microenvironment, facilitating invasion and metastasis and also increasing resistance to both systemic and radiation treatment [82]. Radiation resistance increases because hypoxia decreases cell proliferation and DNA damage is augmented in proliferative cell populations; lactate, via its antioxidant properties, has also been linked to resistance mechanisms in several tumours [82–84]. Therefore, targeting the adaptation mechanisms induced by the changing microenvironment may offer new targeted therapies. Currently, preclinical strategies are exploring novel compounds that disrupt pH regulation in concert with radiation and systemic drug therapies [85–87].

Preclinical research in our laboratory suggested that NHE1 inhibitors could sensitise breast cancer cells to radiation (unpublished data); however, phase III clinical trials of these drugs reported increased levels of stroke [88]. Several xenograft models have shown enhanced sensitivity to radiation in colorectal and small cell lung cancer using MCT1 inhibitors [89, 90]. MCT1 and MCT4 require an accessory molecule, CD147, for correct situation in the plasma membrane. Silencing of CD147 in breast cancer cells caused robust inhibition of lactate production and glycolysis [91]. Strategies that reduce lactate concentration in the tumour microenvironment should reduce radiation resistance [83, 92, 93]. Invasion and metastasis of breast cancer cells can be inhibited by blocking V-ATPase activation [94, 95]. Some inhibitors are too toxic to be used clinically, but several proton pump inhibitors (PPIs) are used therapeutically, with negligible contraindications, and these compounds also act as V-ATPase inhibitors [96]. Radiation resistance may be partly influenced by the induction of autophagy, which is V-ATPase-dependent [97]; therefore, PPIs may increase sensitivity to radiation.

Currently, CAIX inhibition is a promising therapeutic objective. This enzyme is often overexpressed in breast cancer, where it correlates with poor prognosis [98], but it is infrequently found in normal breast tissue. CAIX knockdown in murine models show that the consequences are limited to gastric hyperplasia, implying limited toxicity issues [99, 100]. Knockdown of CAIX has been linked to radiation sensitisation [101], and a novel class of sulfamate CAIX inhibitors enhanced the effects of radiation in a colorectal cancer model, both in vitro and in vivo [86, 87]. Preclinical research in our laboratory suggests that these novel inhibitors may sensitise breast cancer to radiation using several models.

10.15 Personalisation of Treatment Through Monitoring Strategies

Because of the erratic tumour vasculature, tumour hypoxia is discontinuous. If tumour oxygenation could be monitored in real time, radiation treatment could be given when oxygen concentrations in the tumour were at their highest to achieve maximal efficiency. Alternatively, hypoxic areas could be treated with larger radiation doses to increase efficacy. Oxygen and metabolic indicators can be observed in real time using microphysiometry equipment in in vitro research [64], and currently, biosensors are being developed that would permit personalised monitoring of tumour hypoxia in real time [http://www.see.ed.ac.uk/drupal/impact] and allow optimal radiation treatment strategies to be scheduled with the greatest clinical benefit for each patient.

Acknowledgements We gratefully acknowledge support from the EU-financed FP7 (HEALTH-F2-2009-222741) METOXIA collaborative programme, the EPSRC-financed IMPACT project, ECMC, the Aitken Breast Cancer Research Fund and the Breast Cancer Institute.

References

1. Bondiau PY, Courdi A, Bahadoran P et al (2013) Phase 1 clinical trial of stereotactic body radiation therapy concomitant with neoadjuvant chemotherapy for breast cancer. Int J Radiat Oncol Biol Phys 85:1193–1199
2. Clarke M, Collins R, Darby S et al (2005) Effects of radiotherapy and of differences in the extent of surgery for early breast cancer on local recurrence and 15-year survival. An overview of the randomised trials. Lancet 366:2087–2106
3. Barton MB, Jacob S, Shafiq J et al (2014) Estimating the demand for radiotherapy from the evidence: a review of changes from 2003 to 2012. Radiother Oncol 112:40–144
4. Overgaard J (2015) Gazing at the crystal ball of European radiotherapy. Nat Rev Clin Oncol 12:5–6
5. Bartelink H, Maingon P, Poortmans P et al (2015) Whole-breast irradiation with or without a boost for patients treated with breast-conserving surgery for early breast cancer: 20-year follow-up of a randomised phase 3 trial. Lancet Oncol 16:47–56
6. Arnedos M, Soria JC, Andre F et al (2015) Personalized treatment of cancer patients: a reality in daily practice, a costly dream or a shared vision of the future from the oncology community? Cancer Treat Rev 10:1192–1198
7. Van't Veer LJ, Dai H, van der Vijver MJ et al (2002) Gene expression profiling predicts clinical outcome of breast cancer. Nature 415:530–536
8. Bucci M, Bevan A, Roach M III (2005) Advances in radiation therapy: conventional to 3D, to IMRT to 4D and Beyond. CA Cancer J Clin 55:117–154
9. Torres-Roca JF, Stevens CW (2008) Predicting response to clinical radiotherapy: past, present and future directions. Cancer Control 15:151–156
10. Peters LJ (1990) The ESTRO Regaud lecture. Inherent radiosensitivity of tumor and normal tissue cells as a predictor of human tumor response. Radiother Oncol 17:177–190
11. Gerlinger M, Rowan AJ, Horswell S et al (2012) Intratumor heterogeneity and branched evolution revealed by multiregion sequencing. N Engl J Med 366:883–892
12. Russnes HG, Navin N, Hicks J, Borresen-Dale A-L (2011) Insight into the heterogeneity of breast cancer through next-generation sequencing. J Clin Invest 121:3810–3818
13. Desmedt C, Voet T, Sotiriou C et al (2012) Next generation sequencing in breast cancer: first take home messages. Curr Opin Oncol 24:597–604
14. Suit H, Skates S, Taghian A et al (1992) Clinical implications of heterogeneity of tumour response to radiation therapy. Radiother Oncol 25:251–260
15. Jiang H (2009) The combined status of ATM and p53 link tumour development with therapeutic response. Genes Dev 59:1895–1909
16. Baumann M, Krause M, Hill R (2008) Exploring the role of cancer stem cells in radioresistance. Nat Rev Cancer 8:545–554

17. Duru N, Fan M, Candas D et al (2012) HER-2-associated radioresistance of breast cancer stem cells isolated from HER-2 negative breast cancer cells. Clin Cancer Res 18:6634–6647
18. Philips TM, McBride WH, Pajonk F (2006) The response of CD24 (-/low) /CD44+ breast cancer – initiating cells to radiation. J Natl Cancer Inst 98:1772–1785
19. Lagadec C, Vlashi E, Della Donna I et al (2012) Radiation-induced reprogramming of breast cancer cells. Stem Cells 30:33–844
20. Lagadec C, Vlashi E, Della Donna I et al (2010) Survival and self-renewing capacity of breast cancer initiating cells during fractionated radiation treatment. Breast Cancer Res 12:R3
21. Harris JR (2014) Fifty years of progress in radiation therapy for breast cancer. ASCO Educational Book. Am Soc Clin Oncol 21–25
22. EBCTCG (Early Breast Cancer Trialists' Collaborative Group) (2011) Effect of radiotherapy after breast-conserving surgery on 10-year recurrence and 15-year breast cancer death: meta-analysis of individual patient data for 10 801 women in 17 randomised trials. Lancet 378:1707–1716
23. EBCTCG (Early Breast Cancer Trialists' Collaborative Group) (2014) Effect of radiotherapy after mastectomy and axillary surgery on 10-year recurrence and 20-year breast cancer mortality: meta-analysis of individual patient data for 8135 women in 22 randomised trials. Lancet 383:2127–2135
24. Fisher B (1980) Laboratory and clinical research in breast cancer – a personal adventure: the David A. Karnofsky Memorial Lecture. Cancer Res 40:3863–3874
25. Punglia RS, Morrow M, Winer EP et al (2007) Local therapy and survival in breast cancer. N Engl J Med 356:2399–2405
26. Hellman S (1994) Karnofsky memorial lecture: natural history of small breast cancers. J Clin Oncol 12:22229–22234
27. Hellman S, Harris JR (1987) The appropriate breast cancer paradigm. Cancer Res 47:339–342
28. Kyndi M, Sørensen FB, Knudsen H et al (2008) Danish Breast Cancer Cooperative Group Estrogen receptor, progesterone receptor, HER-2, and response to postmastectomy radiotherapy in high-risk breast cancer: the Danish Breast Cancer Cooperative Group. J Clin Oncol 26:1419–1426
29. Haffty B, Buccholz T (2010) Molecular predictors of loco-regional recurrence in breast cancer: ready for prime time? J Clin Oncol 28:1627–1629
30. Norum JH, Andersen K, Sorlie T (2014) Lessons learned from the intrinsic subtypes of breast cancer in the quest for precision therapy. Br J Surg 101:925–938
31. Wang Y, Klijn JG, Zhang Y et al (2005) Gene-expression profiles to predict distant metastasis of lymph-node-negative primary breast cancer. Lancet 365:671–679
32. Paik S, Shak S, Tang G et al (2004) A multigene assay to predict recurrence of tamoxifen-treated, node-negative breast cancer. N Engl J Med 351:2817–2826
33. Paik S, Tang G, Skak S et al (2006) Gene expression and benefit of chemotherapy in women with node-negative, estrogen receptor-positive breast cancer. J Clin Oncol 24:3726–3734
34. Gianni L, Zambetti M, Clark K et al (2005) Gene expression profiles in paraffin-embedded core biopsy tissue predict response to chemotherapy in women with locally advanced breast cancer. J Clin Oncol 23:7265–7277
35. Buyse M, Loi S, van't Veer L et al (2006) Validation and clinical utility of a 70-gene prognostic signature for women with node-negative breast cancer. J Natl Cancer Inst 98:1183–1192
36. Ring BZ, Seitz RS, Beck R et al (2006) Novel prognostic immunohistochemical biomarker panel for estrogen receptor-positive breast cancer. J Clin Oncol 24:3039–3047
37. Perou CM, Sørlie T, Eisen MB et al (2000) Molecular portraits of human breast tumours. Nature 406:747–752
38. Sorlie T, Perou CM, Tibshirani R et al (2001) Gene expression patterns of breast carcinomas distinguish tumor subclasses with clinical implications. Proc Natl Acad Sci U S A 98:10869–10874

39. Sorlie T, Tibshirani R, Parker J et al (2003) Repeated observation of breast tumor subtypes in independent gene expression data sets. Proc Natl Acad Sci U S A 100:8418–8423
40. Cristofanilli M, Hayes DF, Budd GT et al (2005) Circulating tumor cells: a novel prognostic factor for newly diagnosed metastatic breast cancer. J Clin Oncol 23:1420–1430
41. Chang JC, Wooten EC, Tsimelzon A et al (2003) Gene expression profiling for the prediction of therapeutic response to docetaxel in patients with breast cancer. Lancet 362:362–369
42. Chang JC, Wooten EC, Tsimelzon A et al (2005) Patterns of resistance and incomplete response to docetaxel by gene expression profiling in breast cancer patients. J Clin Oncol 23:1169–1177
43. van de Vijver MJ, He YD, van't Veer LJ et al (2002) A gene-expression signature as a predictor of survival in breast cancer. N Engl J Med 347:1999–2009
44. van't Veer LJ, Dai H, van de Vijver MJ et al (2003) Expression profiling predicts outcome in breast cancer. Breast Cancer Res 5:57–58
45. Weichselbaum RR, Ishwaran H, Yoon T et al (2008) An interferon-related gene signature for DNA damage resistance is a predictive marker for chemotherapy and radiation for breast cancer. Proc Natl Acad Sci U S A A105:18490–18495
46. Sotiriou C, Powles TJ, Dowsett M et al (2002) Gene expression profiles derived from fine needle aspiration correlate with response to systemic chemotherapy in breast cancer. Breast Cancer Res 4:R3
47. Ayers M, Symmans WF, Stec J et al (2004) Gene expression profiles predict complete pathologic response to neoadjuvant paclitaxel and fluorouracil, doxorubicin, and cyclophosphamide chemotherapy in breast cancer. J Clin Oncol 22:2284–2293
48. Modlich O, Prisack HB, Munnes M et al (2004) Immediate gene expression changes after the first course of neoadjuvant chemotherapy in patients with primary breast cancer disease. Clin Cancer Res 10:6418–6431
49. Dewhirst MW, Chi J-T (2013) Understanding the tumour microenvironment and radioresistance by combining functional imaging with global gene expression. Sem Rad Oncol 23:296–305
50. Solin LJ, Gray R, Baehner FL et al (2013) A multigene expression assay topredict local recurrence risk for ductal carcinoma in situ of the breast. J Natl Cancer Inst 105:701–710
51. Eschrich SA, Fulp WJ, Pawitan Y (2012) Validation of a radiosensitivity molecular signature in breast cancer. Clin Cancer Res 18:5134–5143
52. Speers C, Zhao SG, Liu M et al (2015) Development and validation of a novel radiosensitivity signature in human breast cancer. Clin Cancer Res 21:3667–3677
53. Safwat S, Bentzen S, Turesson I et al (2002) Deterministic rather than stochastic factors explain most of the variation in the expression of skin telangiectasia after radiotherapy. Int J Rad Oncol Biol Phys 52:198–204
54. Russell NS, Grummels A, Hart AA et al (1998) Low predictive value of intrinsic fibroblast radiosensitivity in fibrosis development following radiotherapy for breast cancer. Int J Rad Oncol Biol Phys 73:661–670
55. Rattay T, Talbot CJ (2014) Finding the genetic determinants of adverse reactions to radiotherapy. Clin Oncol 26:301–308
56. Andreassen CN, Alsner J (2009) Genetic variants and normal tissue toxicity after radiotherapy: a systematic review. Radiother Oncol 92:299–309
57. Guo Z, Shu Y, Zhou H et al (2015) Radiogenomics helps to achieve personalized therapy by evaluating patient responses to radiation treatment. Carcinogenesis 36:307–317
58. Kerns SL, West CML, Andreassen CN et al (2014) Radiogenomics: the search for genetic predictors of radiotherapy response. Future Oncol 10:2391–2406
59. Barnett GC, Coles CE, Elliott RM et al (2012) Independent validation of genes and polymorphisms reported to be associated with radiation toxicity: a prospective analysis study. Lancet Oncol 105:289–295

60. Li C, Wilson PB, Levine E et al (1999) TGF-beta1 levels in pre-treatment plasma identify breast cancer patients at risk of developing post-radiotherapy fibrosis. Int J Cancer 84:155–159
61. West CML, Dunning AM, Rosenstein BS (2012) Genome-wide association studies and the prediction of normal tissue toxicity. Sem Rad Oncol 22(2):91–99
62. Barnett GC, West CM, Dunning AM et al (2009) Normal tissue reactions to radiotherapy: towards tailoring treatment dose by genotype. Nat Rev Cancer 9:34–42
63. Barnett GC, Wilkinson JS, Moody AM et al (2011) The Cambridge breast intensity-modulated radiotherapy trial: patient and treatment related factors that influence late toxicity. Clin Oncol 23:652–673
64. Pignol J-P, Olivotto I, Rakovitch E et al (2008) A multicentre randomised trial of breast intensity modulated radiation therapy to reduce acute radiation dermatitis. J Clin Oncol 26:2085–2092
65. Mukesh B, Mukesh G, Barnett JS et al (2013) Randomised controlled trial of intensity modulated radiotherapy for early breast cancer: 5-year results confirm superior overall cosmesis. J Clin Oncol 31:1–10
66. Early Breast Cancer Trialists' Collaborative Group (EBCTCG) (2000) Favourable and unfavourable effects on long-term survival of radiotherapy for early breast cancer: an overview of the randomised trials. Lancet 355:1757–1770
67. Darby SC, Ewertz M, McGale P et al (2013) Risk of ischaemic heart disease in women after radiotherapy of breast cancer. N Engl J Med 368:987–998
68. Elredge-Hindy H, Lockarny L, Crawford A et al (2015) Acting breathing coordinator; reduced radiation dos to the heart and preserves local control in patients with left breast cancer: report of a prospective trial. Pract Rad Oncol 5:4–10
69. Navin N, Kendall J, Troge J et al (2011) Tumour evolution inferred by single-cell sequencing. Nature 472:90–94
70. Morgan MA, Parsels LA, Zhao L et al (2010) Mechanism of radiosensitization by the Chk1/2 inhibitor AZD7762 involves abrogation of the G2 checkpoint and inhibition of homologous recombinational DNA repair. Cancer Res 70:4972–4981
71. DeRose YS, Wang G, Lin YC et al (2011) Tumor grafts derived from women with breast cancer authentically reflect tumor pathology, growth, metastasis and disease outcomes. Nat Med 17:1514–1520
72. Dean JL, McClendon AK, Hickey TE et al (2012) Therapeutic response to CDK4/6 inhibition in breast cancer defined by ex vivo analyses of human tumors. Cell Cycle 11:2756–2761
73. Siolas D, Hannon GJ (2013) Patient-derived tumor xenografts: transforming clinical samples into mouse models. Cancer Res 73:5315–5319
74. Yamada KM, Cukierman E (2007) Modeling tissue morphogenesis and cancer in 3D. Cell 130:601–610
75. Moding EJ, Kastan MB, Kirsch DG (2013) Strategies for optimizing the response of cancer and normal tissuesto radiation. Nat Rev Drug Discov 12:526–542
76. Katz E, Sims AH, Sproul D et al (2012) Targeting of Rac GTPases blocks the spread of intact human breast cancer. Oncotarget 3:608–619
77. Ward C, Harrison DJ, Kunkler IH et al (2013) An ex-vivo tumour model using core biopsy explants validate Carbonic Anhydrase IX (CAIX) as a therapeutic target in breast cancer. J Pathol 231:1
78. van der Kuip H, Murdter TE, Sonnenberg M et al (2006) Short term culture of breast cancer tissues to study the activity of the anticancer drug taxol in an intact tumor environment. BMC Cancer 6:86
79. Vaupel P, Breist S, Hockel M (2003) Hypoxia in breast cancer: pathogenesis, characterization and biological/therapeutic implications. Wien Med Wochenschr 152:334–342
80. Ward C, Langdon SP, Mullen P et al (2013) New strategies for targeting the hypoxic tumour microenvironment in breast cancer. Can Treat Rev 30:171–179

81. Hanahan D, Weinberg RA (2011) Hallmarks of cancer: the next generation. Cell 144:646–674
82. Gatenby RA, Smallbone K, Maini PK et al (2007) Cellular adaptation to hypoxia and acidosis during somatic evolution of breast cancer. Br J Cancer 5:646–653
83. Sattler UG, Meyer S, Quennet V et al (2010) Glycolytic metabolism and tumour response to fractionated irradiation. Radiother Oncol 94:102–109
84. Groussard C, Morel I, Chevanne M et al (2000) Free radical scavenging and antioxidant effects of lactate ion: an in vitro study. J Appl Physiol 89:169–175
85. Pettersen EO, Ebbesen P, Gieling RG et al (2014) Targeting tumour hypoxia to prevent cancer metastasis. From biology, biosensing and technology to drug development: the METOXIA consortium. J Enzym Inhib Med Chem 27:1–33
86. Dubois L, Peeters S, Lieuwes NG et al (2011) Specific inhibition of carbonic anhydrase IX activity enhances the in vivo therapeutic effect of tumor irradiation. Radiother Oncol 99:424–431
87. Dubois L, Peeters SG, van Kuijk SJ et al (2013) Targeting carbonic anhydrase IX by nitroimidazole based sulfamides enhances the therapeutic effect of tumor irradiation: a new concept of dual targeting drugs. Radiother Oncol 108:523–528
88. Theroux P, Chaitman BR, Danchin N et al (2002) Inhibition of the sodium-hydrogen exchancer with cariporide to prevent myocardial infarction in high-risk ischemic situations. Main results of the GUARDIAN trial. Circulation 102:3032–3038
89. Bola BM, Chadwick AL, Michopoulos F et al (2014) Inhibition of monocarboxylate transporter-1 by AZD3965 enhances radiosensitivity by reducing lactate transport. Mol Cancer Ther 13:2805–2816
90. Sonveaux P, Vegran F, Schroeder T et al (2008) Targeting lactate-fueled respiration selectively kills hypoxic tumor cells in mice. J Clin Invest 118:3930–3942
91. Slomiany MG, Grass GD, Robertson AD et al (2009) Hyaluronan, CD44, and emmprin regulate lactate efflux and membrane localization of monocarboxylate transporters in human breast carcinoma cells. Cancer Res 69:1293–1301
92. Grotius J, Dittfield C, Huether M et al (2009) Impact of exogenous lactate on survival and radioresponse of carcinoma cells in vitro. Int J Radiat Biol 85:989–1001
93. Huang XQ, Chen X, Xie XX et al (2014) Co-expression of CD147 and GLUT-1 indicates radiation resistance and poor prognosis in cervical squamous cell carcinoma. Int J Clin Exp Pathol 7:1651–1666
94. Hendrix A, Sormunen R, Westbroek W et al (2013) Vacuolar H+ATPase expression and activity is required for Rab27B-dependent invasive growth and metastasis of breast cancer. Int J Cancer 133:843–854
95. Graham RM, Thompson JW, Webster KA (2014) Inhibition of the vacuolar ATPase induces Bnip-dependent death of cancer cells and a reduction in tumor burden and metastasis. Oncotarget 5:1162–1173
96. Der G (2003) An overview of proton pump inhibitors. Gastroenterol Nurs 26:182–190
97. Paglin S, Hollister T, Delohery T et al (2001) A novel response of cancer cells to radiation involves autophagy and formation of acidic vesicles. Cancer Res 61:439–444
98. Chia SK, Wykoff CC, Watson PH et al (2001) Prognostic significance of a novel hypoxia-regulated marker, carbonic anhydrase IX, in invasive breast carcinoma. J Clin Oncol 19:3660–3668
99. Gut MO, Parkkila S, Vernerova Z et al (2002) Gastric hyperplasia in mice with targeted disruption of the carbonic anhydrase gene Car9. Gastroenterology 123:1889–1903
100. Leppilampi M, Karttunen J, Kivela J et al (2005) Gastric pit cell hyperplasia and glandular atrophy in carbonic anhydrase IX knockout mice: studies on two strains C57/BL6 and BALB/C. Transgenic Res 14:655–663
101. Doyen J, Parks SK, Marcie S et al (2012) Knock-down of hypoxia-inducible carbonic anhydrases IX and XII radiosensitises tumor cells by increasing intracellular acidosis. Front Oncol 2:199

Chapter 11
New Technologies in Radiation Therapy

Michio Yoshimura and Chikako Yamauchi

Abstract The evolution of radiation therapy in the treatment of breast cancer is remarkable in recent years. In the matter of dosing and schedule, shorter fraction schedules of whole-breast irradiation (WBI) have been admitted. Three randomized clinical trials comparing hypofractionated radiation therapy (RT) to standard fractionated RT have demonstrated equivalent local control and less adverse effect in the hypofractionated groups. Although there are still controversies for patient selection, hypofractionated RT is an effective and safe technique. Prone positioning technique for WBRT has developed for women with large and pendulous breasts. Prone technique decreases the inhomogeneity of a breast and dose of the lung and heart. Accelerated partial breast irradiation (APBI) is a hypofractionated radiation treatment with the use of limited and focused irradiation as alternatives to conventional WBI following breast-conserving surgery. There are various methods for APBI, and several clinical trials of each technique have been conducted. Some of the trials have demonstrated that APBI is tolerable and an effective treatment strategy. WBI with concurrent boost is also a new technique to shorten the overall treatment time. Ongoing clinical trials are expected to show the non-inferior control rate with tolerable toxicities, and WBI with concurrent boost could be an option of standard radiotherapy regimens.

Keywords Breast-conserving therapy • Breast radiotherapy • Hypofractionated radiation therapy • Accelerated partial breast irradiation

---

M. Yoshimura
Department of Radiation Oncology and Image-Applied Therapy, Kyoto University Graduate School of Medicine, Kyoto, Japan

C. Yamauchi (✉)
Department of Radiation Oncology, Shiga Medical Center for Adults, 5-4-30 Moriyama, Moriyama, Shiga 524-8524, Japan
e-mail: chikay1796@gmail.com

M. Toi et al. (eds.), *Personalized Treatment of Breast Cancer*,
DOI 10.1007/978-4-431-55552-0_11

11.1 Hypofractionated Radiation Therapy

11.1.1 Background

In whole breast irradiation (WBI) following breast-conserving surgery (BCS), a total dose of 45–50.4 Gy in 25–28 fractions (fr) over a period of 4.5–5.5 weeks has been conventionally used. Although that is considered as the standard radiation schedule, shorter hypofractionated (HF) schedules were examined in three randomized clinical trials (RCTs).

11.1.2 Clinical Trials

In an RTC conducted by the Ontario Clinical Oncology Group, a dose of 42.5 Gy in 16 fractions as an HF regimen and a standard dose of 50 Gy in 25 fractions were compared [1]. From 1993 to 1996, 1234 women with invasive breast cancer who were treated by lumpectomy and had pathologically negative margins and negative axillary lymph nodes were randomly assigned to receive WBI of 42.5 Gy in 16 fractions (HF arm) or 50 Gy in 25 fractions (standard arm). The risk of local recurrence in 10 years was 6.7 % in the standard arm as compared with 6.2 % in the HF arm (absolute difference, 0.5 %; 95 % CI, −2.5–3.5). In 10 years, the probability of survival was 84.4 % in the standard arm as compared with 84.6 % in the HF arm (absolute difference, −0.2 %; 95 % CI, −4.3–4.0), and no statistically significant difference was shown between the two arms. The cosmetic outcome has also shown that 71.3 % of women in the standard arm, as compared with 69.8 % of women in the HF arm, had an excellent or good cosmetic result (absolute difference, 1.5 %; 95 % CI, −6.9–9.8).

Moreover, two large RCTs, the Standardization of Breast Radiotherapy (START) A and START B, were conducted in the UK. The RCTs compared several HF RT schedules with standard schedules (50 Gy in 25 fractions over 5 weeks). Patients with both node-negative and node-positive breast cancer after BCS or mastectomy were included these RCTs. At first, the START A trial compared two different HF schedules and standard schedule [2]. In the trial, 2236 patients were randomly assigned to receive either 39 Gy or 41.6 Gy delivered in 13 fractions over 5 weeks or a standard regimen of 50 Gy in 25 fractions. After a median follow-up of 9.3 years, 10-year rates of local-regional recurrence did not differ significantly between the 41.6-Gy and 50-Gy regimen (6.3 %, 95 % CI 4.7–8.5 *vs* 7.4 %, 5.5–10.0; hazard ratio [HR] 0.91, 95 % CI 0.59–1· 38; $p=0.65$) or 39-Gy (8.8 %, 95 %CI 6.7–11.4) and 50-Gy regimen (HR 1.18, 95 % CI 0.79–1.76; $p=0.41$). However, normal tissue effect of moderate or marked breast induration, telangiectasia, and breast edema were significantly less common in the 39-Gy arm than in the 50-Gy arm. On the other hand, the normal tissue effects were equivalent in the 41.6-Gy and the 50-Gy group.

In the START B trial, 2215 women were enrolled and randomly assigned to the HF arm consisting of 40 Gy in 15 fractions over 3 weeks and the standard arm. With a median of 9.9 years, the local-regional relapse rates in 10 years were not significant in the difference between the HF group (4.3 %, 95 % CI 3.2–5.9) and standard group (5.5 %, 95 % CI 4.2–7.2; HR 0.77, 95 % CI 0.51–1· 16; $p = 0.21$). Moreover, breast shrinkage, telangiectasia, and breast edema were significantly less common in the HF group than the standard group. A meta-analysis of the UK START trials concluded that appropriately dosed hypofractionated radiotherapy is safe and effective for patients with early breast cancer [3]. On the other hand, there is still the controversy underlying the optimal selection of patients. The American Society for Therapeutic Radiology and Oncology (ASTRO) panel recommends HF WBI for patients older than 50 years old with pT1-2 N0, without chemotherapy, and with appropriate dose homogeneity. For the other patient, HF may be considered to use under taking care of reduction of irradiation to the heart [4]. In a Cochrane review evaluating these clinical trials, it was concluded that although the HF method for selected patients could reduce acute side effects without increasing local recurrence, a longer follow-up is required for a more complete assessment of the effect of altered fractionation [5]. Recently, more aggressive HF regimens with higher doses of radiation per fraction are evaluated. The FAST (faster radiotherapy for breast cancer patients) trial randomized women aged 50 years with node-negative breast cancer to standard group (50 Gy in 25 fractions) or HF (30 Gy in 5 fractions or 27.5 Gy in 5 fractions) over 5 weeks. At 3 years median follow-up, 28.5 Gy in 5 fractions is comparable to 50 Gy in 25 fractions, and significantly milder than 30 Gy in 5 fractions, in terms of adverse effects in the breast [6]. The Radiation Therapy Oncology Group (RTOG) conducted a non-inferiority phase III trial (RTOG 1005) comparing standard fractions (50 Gy in 25 fractions) or HF (42.7 Gy in 16 fractions) plus a sequential boost with an HF regimen that includes a concomitant boost to the tumor bed (40–48 Gy in 15 fractions). Furthermore, the long-term results of patients who do not meet the criteria of the ASTRO guideline and treated with HF regimen are expected to be reported.

11.2 Prone Technique

11.2.1 Background

Standard tangential WBI after breast-conserving surgery is predominantly performed in the supine position. Historically, supine position has been used in the important landmark clinical trials or clinical setting in breast-conserving therapy. However, it has been also noted that patients with large breast size experience increased acute and late adverse effects. An acute effect of increased skin toxicities, especially inframammary fold, was recognized. Late effects of increased fibrosis, retraction, and telangiectasia were often noted. Prone breast irradiation has been emerged for women with large, pendulous breasts for the purpose of reducing adverse effects in the early 1990s. It is expected to decrease dose inhomogeneity by prone positioning. The prone positioning has been used for MRI and stereotactic biopsy. In radiotherapy, its adoption was delayed, because it was needed that the special device for the patients to lie with the ill breast be suspended, and the lack of the setup accuracy was the problem.

11.2.2 Techniques

In 1994, investigators from the Memorial Sloan Kettering Cancer Center (MSKCC) reported prone breast radiotherapy [7]. In this study, the utility of the prone technique improved the dose distribution of the breast and reduced the volume of normal tissues irradiated during WBI. Especially irradiation of the heart, lungs, and contralateral breast are minimized in prone position irradiation. They developed a platform for prone breast irradiation to add to the treatment couch. The same group evaluated retrospectively, and the toxicity of WBI was delivered with prone positioning [8]. They analyzed 245 women with 248 early-stage invasive or in situ breast cancers treated between 1992 and 2004. WBI was carried out using a prone breast board with 46–50.4 Gy with standard fractionation by photon. Tumor bed boosts were administered in 85 % of cases, and adjuvant chemotherapy and hormonal therapy were delivered to 42 % and 62 % of patients, respectively. After a median follow-up of 4.9 years, the 5-year actuarial ipsilateral breast tumor recurrence rates were 4.8 % and 1.3 %, respectively. The 5-year actuarial rates of regional nodal recurrence and distant metastases were 1.6 % and 7.4 %. Actuarial disease-free, disease-specific, and overall survival rates in 5 years were 89.4 %, 97.3 %, and 93 %, respectively. Only 4.9 % of patients complained of acute chest wall discomfort. Regarding the acute adverse effects, grade 3 acute dermatitis was less than 2 % in patients, and chronic grade 2–3 skin and subcutaneous tissue toxicities were reported in 4.4 % and 13.7 % of patients, respectively.

Another group from New York University also researched prone breast irradiation with focus on designing a device adequate with prone positioning. They developed several types of the devices for prone position made of various materials and shapes and improved immobility, comfort, and convenience [9].

There were data suggesting feasibility of prone positioning, but almost all results of the studies used electronic portal imaging (EPI) to investigate inter-fractional variations. A randomized trial of supine versus prone breast radiotherapy (SuPr study) was conducted to compare setup errors and respiratory motion. It was designed to test a prone position against the standard supine position in terms of feasibility (including patient comfort, radiographer satisfaction, and treatment times), setup errors using cone-beam kV-CT (CBCT), and respiratory motion using 4D-CT. Twenty-five patients were randomized and a total of 365 fractions were analyzed. CBCT data were matched to planning CT data using the chest wall and clips, and systematic and random errors were calculated. Maximal displacement of the chest wall and clips with respiration was measured on 4D-CT. Patient comfort scores and treatment times were also evaluated. 3D population systematic errors were 1.3–1.9 mm in supine and 3.1–4.3 mm in prone ($p = 0.02$), and random errors were 2.6–3.2 mm in supine and 3.8–5.4 mm in prone ($p = 0.02$). Prone positioning reduced chest wall and clip motion in 0.5 ± 0.2 mm versus 2.7 ± 0.5 mm ($p < 0.001$) with respiration. Calculated CTV-PTV margins were greater for prone (12–16 mm) than for supine treatment (10 mm). Patient comfort scores and treatment times were comparable ($p = 0.06$).

Prone position breast radiation results in similar long-term disease control with a favorable toxicity profile compared with standard supine tangents and may contribute to improving the therapeutic ratio of WBI by improving dose homogeneity and minimizing cardiac and lung dose. One trade-off of the prone technique is lesser coverage of axillary lymph nodes [10].

A study was designed to compare the dosimetry of target and normal tissues. The CT images of 20 patients who had undergone simulation in supine and prone positions were used for planning, and the axillary lymph node regions (levels I–III), breast tissue, tumor bed, heart, and bilateral lungs were manually contoured. Although coverage of the LN regions was insufficient in either position, the mean dose to the nodal regions for levels I–III was approximately 50 % less on average in the prone as compared with the supine position.

11.3 Accelerated Partial Breast Irradiation (APBI)

11.3.1 Background and Rationale

Breast-conserving therapy has become a standard treatment option for stages I–II breast cancer patients. Several randomized trials showed the postoperative radiotherapy is essential after the breast-conserving surgery. The standard regimen of the radiotherapy is whole breast irradiation (WBI) at 45–50 Gy/1.8–2.0 Gy and, in some cases, is followed by a tumor bed boost in five to ten fractions (fr). But since it takes approximately 5–7 weeks to complete the whole course of radiotherapy, the patients, who live far from the radiotherapy facilities, are elderly with low performance status, are working with busy schedules, or have limited finance means, would not choose breast-conserving therapy due to the long treatment duration. Shortage of the radiotherapy duration will offer advantage for such patients.

The majority of recurrence in the ipsilateral breasts of the patients who did not receive radiotherapy after breast-conserving surgery is observed close to the tumor bed [11–15]. And the rate of new cancer development in the ipsilateral breast in the remote area from the tumor bed ("elsewhere failures") is similar to that in the contralateral breast [15]. These evidences suggested that whole-breast irradiation could be overtreatment and that partial breast irradiation could be enough. Partial breast irradiation can spare the normal tissue such as the lung and heart, resulting in the lower development of radiation pneumonia and ischemic heart failure.

Based on these rationales, several groups started short-course partial breast radiotherapy.

11.3.2 Patient Selection Criteria for APBI

In recent years many breast cancer patients have been treated with APBI after breast-conserving surgery, but few data were available to define which patients could be safely treated with APBI and which patients should receive WBI. From the viewpoint of these issues, the American Society for Radiation Oncology (ASTRO) published a consensus statement for proper patient selection regarding the use of APBI in 2009. The guideline classified the patients into three groups, "suitable," "cautionary," and "unsuitable" (Table 11.1).

11.3.3 APBI Techniques (Table 11.2)

11.3.3.1 Intraoperative Radiotherapy

Single-fraction intraoperative radiotherapy has been utilized for APBI with low-energy X-rays or electrons. The most common regimen for intraoperative radiotherapy is 20–21 Gy in one fraction. One of the advantages of this technique is that radiotherapy can be delivered to the accurate position of the tumor bed because radiotherapy is performed at the time of surgery. Another advantage is that radiotherapy can be completed at the same time of the lumpectomy and patients do not have to return to the hospital to receive radiotherapy after discharge. The disadvantage is the intraoperative radiotherapy must be delivered before the final pathological diagnosis.

11.3.3.2 Brachytherapy

Multicatheter Interstitial Brachytherapy

Multicatheter interstitial brachytherapy was initially developed for a tumor bed boost after whole-breast irradiation and then utilized for APBI. The catheters are placed around the lumpectomy cavity, and low-dose rate (Iodine-125) or high-dose rate (Iridium-192) radioactive sources are temporarily afterloaded into each

Table 11.1 ASTRO consensus: "suitable," "cautionary," and "unsuitable" patient groups for APBI [16]

Factors	"Suitable" group	"Cautionary" group	"Unsuitable" group
Patient factors			
Age, year	≧60	50–59	<50
BRCA1/2 mutation	Not present	NA	Present
Pathologic factors			
Tumor size	≦2 cm	2.1–3.0 cm	>3 cm
T stage	T1	T0 or T2	T3–T4
Margins	Negative by ≥2 mm	<2 mm	Positive
Grade	Any	–	–
LVSI	No	Limited/focal	Extensive
ER status	Positive	Negative	–
Multicentricity	Unicentric only	–	Present
Multifocality	Clinically unifocal with total size ≦2 cm	Clinically unifocal with total size 2.1–3.0 cm	Clinically multifocal or total size >3 cm
Histology	Invasive ductal or other favorable subtype	Invasive lobular	–
Pure DCIS	Not allowed	≦3 cm	>3 cm
EIC	Not allowed	≦3 cm	>3 cm
Associated LCIS	Allowed	–	–
N stage	pN0	–	pN1, pN2, pN3
Nodal surgery	SN biopsy or ALND	–	None performed
Neoadjuvant therapy	Not allowed	–	If used

LVSI lymph-vascular space invasion, *EIC* extensive intraductal component, *SN* sentinel node, *ALND* axillary lymph node dissection

multicatheters. Multicatheters enable radiation oncologists to deliver accurate irradiation to the tumor bed. The Radiation Therapy Oncology Group conducted the phase II trial of APBI using multicatheter brachytherapy after lumpectomy in early-stage breast cancers and reported excellent in-breast control rates (RTOG 95-17) [18].

Intracavitary Single-Lumen Brachytherapy

Proxima Therapeutics developed a single-lumen balloon catheter for intracavitary brachytherapy to reduce the technical difficulties of interstitial brachytherapy. The standard treatment dose is 34 Gy in ten fractions over 5 days using iridium-192 high-dose-rate brachytherapy [19, 20].

Table 11.2 Comparison of APBI techniques [17]

	3D CRT	Interstitial brachytherapy HDR, LDR, PDR	MammoSite	TARGIT, 50-kV X-rays	IORT, electrons
Coverage of target	Best	Variable	Good	Good	Good
Dose homogeneity	Best	Fair	Fair	Fair	Fair
Sparing of normal breast/other organs	Least	Good	Good	Best	Varies with location
Skin dose	Least	Least	Variable	Least (can shield)	Least
Technical feasibility for various size, shape, or location of cavity	Suitable for virtually all cases	Not suitable if inadequate tissue or near axilla	Not suitable for large/irregular cavities or at the periphery of the breast	Not suitable for large/irregular cavities or at the periphery of the breast	Not suitable for tumors near brachial plexus/axilla or skin
Expertise required	Average	High	Average	High	Very high
Potential for widespread use	Very good	Fair	Very good	Fair	Limited
Main drawback	Relatively higher dose to normal tissue and breathing motion	Adequacy of target coverage in some cases and wider applicability	Cavity shape and size. Although easy to use, stringent QA is required. Skin dose may be high	Very limited depth irradiated; cavity shape and size. Histology not available	Wider applicability. Histology not available. Based on quadrantectomy

Intracavitary Multi-lumen Brachytherapy

Since a single-lumen balloon catheter have limitation of target coverage, multi-lumen catheters such as SAVI, MammoSite ML, and Contura MLB have been developed to improve target coverage and utilized for APBI. These catheters are approved for use in the NSABP B-39/RTOG 0413.

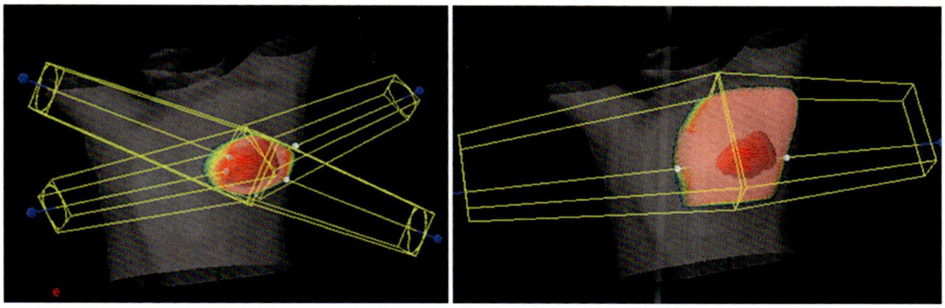

Fig. 11.1 3D CRT planning

3D Conformal External Beam Radiotherapy (EBRT)

Three-dimensional conformal external beam radiotherapy has been introduced to deliver APBI, because this technique is less invasive than interstitial brachytherapy. In general, three to five beams are used. The most common regimen is 38.5 Gy in ten fractions given twice daily over 5 days.

3D-CRT has many advantages over brachytherapy. First, this technique is noninvasive, because invasive surgery or anesthesia is not needed. Second, most radiotherapy centers have the radiotherapy facilities for 3D-CRT, and most radiation oncologists are familiar with the skills required for the planning of 3D-CRT. Finally, radiation oncologists can wait for the confirmation of pathological diagnosis regarding the surgical margin status before starting 3D-CRT (Fig. 11.1).

Several institutions reported the preliminary results of APBI with 3D-CRT. For example, the Radiation Therapy Oncology Group (RTOG) conducted RTOG 0319 trial, which utilized 3D-CRT with 38.5 Gy in ten fractions over 5 days and reported most patients enrolled in RTOG 0319 were satisfied with their treatment, and all would choose to have the 3D-CRT APBI again [21].

11.3.4 Clinical Trials

Several phase III clinical trials of APBI are now ongoing (Table 11.3).

11.3.4.1 TARGIT

The TARGIT-A trial compared single-dose targeted intraoperative radiotherapy (TARGIT) with fractionated external beam radiotherapy (EBRT) for breast cancer.

The 5-year risk for local recurrence in the conserved breast was 3 · 3 % for TARGIT versus 1 · 3 % for EBRT ($p = 0 \cdot 042$). Breast cancer mortality was much the same between groups 2 · 6 % for TARGIT versus 1 · 9 % for EBRT ($p = 0 \cdot 56$), but there were significantly fewer non-breast-cancer deaths with TARGIT,

Table 11.3 Phase III randomized trials of APBI

Trial	Techniques	Patients no.	WBI	APBI	Reference
TARGIT-A (IORT)	IORT	3451 (2000–2010)	40–56 Gy	20 Gy/1 fr	[22]
			±10–16 Gy		
ELIOT (IORT)	IORT	1305 (2000–2007)	50 Gy/25 fx	21 Gy/1 fr	[23]
			±10 Gy		
GEC-ESTRO (brachytherapy)	Brachytherapy	1233 (2004–2009)	50–50.4 Gy/25–28 fx	1. 2 Gy/8 f. HDR BID	[24]
			+10 Gy	2. 30.3 Gy/7 f. HDR BID	
				3. 50 Gy pulsed dose rate (0.6–0.8 Gy/h)	
NSABP B-39 /RTOG 0413	Brachytherapy/ MammoSite/3D-CRT	4300	50–50.4 Gy	1. Multicatheter 34 Gy/10 f. BID	[25]
			±10–16 Gy	2. MammoSite 34 Gy/10 f. BID	
				3. 3D-CRT 38.5 Gy/10 f. BID	
Ontario RAPID	3D-CRT	2128 (2006–2011)	42.5 Gy/16 fx	38.5 Gy/10 f. BID	[26]
			±10 Gy (larger breasts: 50 Gy/25 fx)		

attributable to fewer deaths from cardiovascular diseases and other cancers. Overall mortality was 3 · 9 % for TARGIT versus 5 · 3 % for EBRT ($p = 0 \cdot 099$) [27]. And grade 3 or 4 skin toxicities were significantly reduced with TARGIT ($p = 0 \cdot 029$).

11.3.4.2 ELIOT

The ELIOT trial compared intraoperative radiotherapy with electrons with whole-breast external radiotherapy after breast-conserving surgery with early-stage breast cancer.

With a median follow-up of 5.8 years, the 5-year recurrence rates for ELIOT versus external beam radiation therapy (EBRT) patients were 4.4 % and 0.4 %, respectively, ($p = 0.0001$). Five-year overall survival was 96 · 8 % in the intraoperative radiotherapy group and 96 · 9 % in the external radiotherapy group. Fewer acute or chronic skin side effects were observed in patients in the intraoperative radiotherapy group (8.0 %; 37/464) than in those in the external beam radiotherapy group (2.7 %; 11/412) ($p = 0 \cdot 0002$) [23].

11.3.4.3 NSABP B-39/RTOG

The NSABP B-39/RTOG 0413 trial allows the three radiotherapy options to be utilized (multicatheter interstitial brachytherapy, balloon intracavitary brachytherapy, and external beam 3D conformal therapy).

The definitive results from this trial will be reported many years later and useful to compare the outcome of these modalities and have the potential to expand the standard radiotherapy after breast-conserving surgery.

11.3.4.4 GEC-ESTRO

The GEC-ESTRO APBI trial is the phase III trial to compare interstitial brachytherapy with WBI. The regimens of APBI is HDR with 32.0 Gy/8 f. (twice/day), 30.3 Gy/7 f. (twice/day), or pulsed dose rate of 0.60–0.80 Gy/h to 50 Gy (1 pulse/h, 24 h/day). Between 2004 and 2009, 1233 patients have been randomized in 16 centers from seven European countries.

The results of the large multi-institutional, prospective, randomized trial that will define the long-term efficacy of APBI are eagerly anticipated.

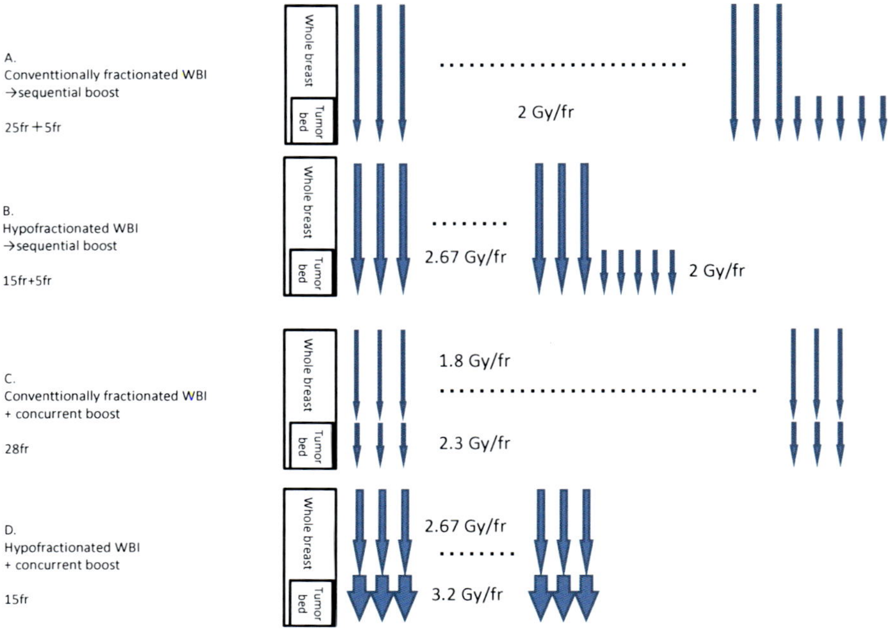

Fig. 11.2 Scheme of treatment regimen

11.4 Whole-Breast Irradiation (WBI) with Concurrent Boost (Fig. 11.2)

11.4.1 Background

11.4.1.1 Tumor Bed Boost

Two prospective randomized trials showed that a 10–16 Gy sequential boost after WBI reduced local recurrence rate even in breast cancer patients with negative resection margins after breast-conserving surgery [28, 29]. An international survey of physician members of the American Society for Therapeutic Radiology and Oncology (ASTRO) and the European Society for Therapeutic Radiology and Oncology (ESTRO) showed that 98 %/94 % of American/European respondents would offer a sequential boost with close margins, and 85 %/75 % of American/-European respondents would deliver a boost even in patients with negative margins [30].

11.4.1.2 Hypofractionated WBI

As was described in 11.1, several randomized trials showed hypofractionated WBI not inferior to conventionally fractionated WBI.

Hypofractionated WBI has become one of the standard radiotherapy regimens after breast-conserving surgery in several countries.

11.4.2 Conventionally Fractionated WBI with Concurrent Boost

The use of sequential boost of 1–2 weeks extends the radiotherapy treatment time, which is unfavorable for patients. To solve the disadvantage, the techniques of conventionally fractionated WBI with concurrent boost were introduced. McDonald et al. reported that conventionally fractionated WBI with concurrent boost reduced treatment duration by five fractions with a favorable acute toxicity profile and showed an excellent 3-year locoregional control rate [31]. Bantema-Joppe et al. reported that conventionally fractionated WBI with concurrent boost resulted in an excellent 3-year local control rate and did not impair toxicity and cosmetic outcome [32, 33].

The IMRT MC2 trial, which is a phase III randomized trial to compare intensity-modulated radiotherapy (IMRT) with simultaneous integrated boost (SIB) with conventional WBI plus a sequential boost after breast-conserving surgery, has opened in 2011. The regimen of WBI with a sequential boost is 50.4 Gy/1.8 Gy/28 f. for the whole breast, followed by a 16 Gy/2 Gy/8 f. boost, while the prescribed dose of the SIB-IMRT regimen is 50.4 Gy and 64.4 Gy/28 f. for the whole breast and tumor bed, respectively. The primary end point of the study is the evaluation of the cosmetic results of 6 weeks and 2 years and the 2- and 5-year local recurrence rates, and secondary objectives are long-term overall survival, disease-free survival, and quality of life [34].

11.4.3 Hypofractionated WBI with Concurrent Boost

Either a hypofractionated regimen or concurrent boost is very useful as a treatment strategy to shorten radiotherapy duration, respectively. To maximize the advantage, several institutions conducted the studies of hypofractionated WBI with concurrent boost for early breast cancer. Several groups have reported single institutional studies of hypofractionated WBI with concurrent boost resulted in favorable tumor control and tolerable side effects (Table 11.1).

Based on these studies, two groups started phase III randomized trials of hypofractionated WBI with concurrent boost (Table 11.2).

Table 11.4 Phases I and II trials of hypofractionated whole-breast irradiation (WBI) and concurrent boost in early-stage breast cancer

Study	Patients no.	Median f/u (year)	TN	WBI Total/daily (Gy)	WBI with concurrent boost Total/daily (Gy)	Local recurrence	Reference
NY University Formenti, 2003–2005	91	1.0 year	T1-2 N0-1	40.5/2.7	48/3.2	1 patient	[36]
Italy Morganti	99	2.6 years	T1-3 N0-2	40/2.5	44/2.75	0 %	[37]
National Institute for Cancer Research, Italy Corvo, 2007–2008	377	2.8 years	T1-2 N0-3	46/2.3	34.5/2.3 + 17.5/3.5	0 %	[38]
Ivrea Community Hp Cante, 2005–2009	463	2.3 years	Tis-2 N0-1	45/2.25	55/2.75	0 %	[39]
Princess Margaret Hp Teh, 2008–2009	15	1 year	Tis-3 N0-1	42.4/2.65	52.48/3.28	0 %	[40]
NY University	59	5 years	DCIS	42/2.8	49.5/3.3	4.1 % (5 years)	[41]
Ciervide, 2002–2009	86	–		40.5/2.7	48 Gy/3.2 Gy		
Pennsylvania University Freedman, 2003–2005	75	5.8 years	pTis-2 N0-1	45/2.25	56/2.8	2.7 % (5 years)	[42]
Beth Israel Medical Center Chadha, 2004–2010,	160	3.5 years	Tis-2 N0	40.5/2.7	45/3.0	99 % (5 years local relapse-free survival)	[43]
ARO study group ARO-2010–2011 Dellas, 2011–2012	151	–	Tis-3 N0-1	40/2.5	48/3.0	–	[44]

Table 11.5 Phase III randomized trials of WBI comparing sequential boost with concurrent boost in early-stage breast cancer

Trial	Sample size	Treatment fractionation Sequential boost	Treatment fractionation Concurrent boost
IMRT MC2	502	Control 50.4 Gy/1.8 Gy	WBI 50.4 Gy/1.8 Gy, concurrent boost 64.4 Gy/2.3 Gy
		→Sequential boost 16 Gy/2 Gy	
RTOG1005	2312	Control: 50 Gy/2 Gy	WBI 40 Gy/2.67 Gy, concurrent boost 48 Gy/3.2 Gy.
		→Sequential boost 12-14 Gy/2 Gy	
IMPORT high	2568	I: Control: 40 Gy/2.67 Gy	II: WBI 36 Gy/2.4 Gy, concurrent boost 48 Gy/3.2 Gy
		→Sequential boost 16 Gy/ 2 Gy	III: WBI 36 Gy/2.4 Gy, concurrent boost 53 Gy/3.53 Gy

The Radiation Oncology Group has opened a phase III trial of hypofractionated WBI plus concurrent boost versus standard WBI plus sequential boost after lumpectomy for early-stage breast cancer in 2011 (RTOG1005) [35]. The regimen of standard WBI for the control arm can be 50 Gy/2 Gy or 42.5 Gy/2.67 Gy plus sequential boost at 12–14 Gy/2 Gy. The WBI dose fractionation in the experimental arm is 40 Gy/2.67 Gy with the concurrent boost receiving 48 Gy/3.2 Gy. The primary objective is to determine whether hypofractionated WBI with concurrent boost will prove to be non-inferior in local control to standard WBI with a sequential boost. The secondary end points are examining local control, breast-related symptoms, cosmesis, cost, and toxicities (Tables 11.4 and 11.5).

The UK Intensity Modulated and Partial Organ Radiotherapy (IMPORT) high trial has opened in 2009. This trial will recruit 2568 participants and compare two hypofractionated concurrent boost regimens with sequential boost regimens. The fractionation of the control arm is 40 Gy WBI in 15 fractions with a sequential boost of 16 Gy/8 fr, while the treatment regimens of two experimental arms are 36 Gy for the whole breast, 40 Gy for the partial breast, and 48 Gy (test treatment 1) or 53 Gy (test treatment 2) for the tumor bed in 15 fractions. The primary end point is local tumor control and secondary end points include normal tissue toxicity [45].

We expect that the results from these two trials will show the non-inferior control rate with tolerable toxicities and that hypofractionated WBI with concurrent boost will be an option of standard radiotherapy regimens after breast-conserving surgery.

References

1. Whelan TJ, Pignol JP, Levine MN, Julian JA, MacKenzie R, Parpia S, Shelley W, Grimard L, Bowen J, Lukka H, Perera F, Fyles A, Schneider K, Gulavita S, Freeman C (2010) Long-term results of hypofractionated radiation therapy for breast cancer. N Engl J Med 362 (6):513–520. doi:362/6/513 [pii] 10.1056/NEJMoa0906260

2. Bentzen SM, Agrawal RK, Aird EG, Barrett JM, Barrett-Lee PJ, Bliss JM, Brown J, Dewar JA, Dobbs HJ, Haviland JS, Hoskin PJ, Hopwood P, Lawton PA, Magee BJ, Mills J, Morgan DA, Owen JR, Simmons S, Sumo G, Sydenham MA, Venables K, Yarnold JR (2008) The UK Standardisation of Breast Radiotherapy (START) trial B of radiotherapy hypofractionation for treatment of early breast cancer: a randomised trial. Lancet 371(9618):1098–1107
3. Haviland JS, Owen JR, Dewar JA, Agrawal RK, Barrett J, Barrett-Lee PJ, Dobbs HJ, Hopwood P, Lawton PA, Magee BJ, Mills J, Simmons S, Sydenham MA, Venables K, Bliss JM, Yarnold JR (2013) The UK Standardisation of Breast Radiotherapy (START) trials of radiotherapy hypofractionation for treatment of early breast cancer: 10-year follow-up results of two randomised controlled trials. Lancet Oncol 14(11):1086–1094. doi:10.1016/S1470-2045(13)70386-3
4. Smith BD, Bentzen SM, Correa CR, Hahn CA, Hardenbergh PH, Ibbott GS, McCormick B, McQueen JR, Pierce LJ, Powell SN, Recht A, Taghian AG, Vicini FA, White JR, Haffty BG (2011) Fractionation for whole breast irradiation: an American Society for Radiation Oncology (ASTRO) evidence-based guideline. Int J Radiat Oncol Biol Phys 81(1):59–68. doi:10.1016/j.ijrobp.2010.04.042
5. James ML, Lehman M, Hider PN, Jeffery M, Hickey BE, Francis DP (2010) Fraction size in radiation treatment for breast conservation in early breast cancer. Cochrane Database Syst Rev 11:CD003860. doi:10.1002/14651858.CD003860.pub3
6. Group FT, Agrawal RK, Alhasso A, Barrett-Lee PJ, Bliss JM, Bliss P, Bloomfield D, Bowen J, Brunt AM, Donovan E, Emson M, Goodman A, Harnett A, Haviland JS, Kaggwa R, Morden JP, Robinson A, Simmons S, Stewart A, Sydenham MA, Syndikus I, Tremlett J, Tsang Y, Wheatley D, Venables K, Yarnold JR (2011) First results of the randomised UK FAST Trial of radiotherapy hypofractionation for treatment of early breast cancer (CRUKE/04/015). Radiother Oncol 100(1):93–100. doi:10.1016/j.radonc.2011.06.026
7. Merchant TE, McCormick B (1994) Prone position breast irradiation. Int J Radiat Oncol Biol Phys 30(1):197–203
8. Stegman LD, Beal KP, Hunt MA, Fornier MN, McCormick B (2007) Long-term clinical outcomes of whole-breast irradiation delivered in the prone position. Int J Radiat Oncol Biol Phys 68(1):73–81. doi:10.1016/j.ijrobp.2006.11.054
9. Huppert N, Jozsef G, Dewyngaert K, Formenti SC (2011) The role of a prone setup in breast radiation therapy. Front Oncol 1:31. doi:10.3389/fonc.2011.00031
10. Alonso-Basanta M, Ko J, Babcock M, Dewyngaert JK, Formenti SC (2009) Coverage of axillary lymph nodes in supine vs. prone breast radiotherapy. Int J Radiat Oncol Biol Phys 73 (3):745–751. doi:10.1016/j.ijrobp.2008.04.040
11. Clarke M, Collins R, Darby S, Davies C, Elphinstone P, Evans E, Godwin J, Gray R, Hicks C, James S, MacKinnon E, McGale P, McHugh T, Peto R, Taylor C, Wang Y (2005) Effects of radiotherapy and of differences in the extent of surgery for early breast cancer on local recurrence and 15-year survival: an overview of the randomised trials. Lancet 366 (9503):2087–2106
12. Liljegren G, Holmberg L, Bergh J, Lindgren A, Tabar L, Nordgren H, Adami HO (1999) 10-year results after sector resection with or without postoperative radiotherapy for stage I breast cancer: a randomized trial. J Clin Oncol 17(8):2326–2333
13. Holli K, Saaristo R, Isola J, Joensuu H, Hakama M (2001) Lumpectomy with or without postoperative radiotherapy for breast cancer with favourable prognostic features: results of a randomized study. Br J Cancer 84(2):164–169. doi:10.1054/bjoc.2000.1571
14. Veronesi U, Marubini E, Mariani L, Galimberti V, Luini A, Veronesi P, Salvadori B, Zucali R (2001) Radiotherapy after breast-conserving surgery in small breast carcinoma: long-term results of a randomized trial. Ann Oncol 12(7):997–1003
15. Fisher B, Anderson S, Bryant J, Margolese RG, Deutsch M, Fisher ER, Jeong JH, Wolmark N (2002) Twenty-year follow-up of a randomized trial comparing total mastectomy, lumpectomy, and lumpectomy plus irradiation for the treatment of invasive breast cancer. N Engl J Med 347(16):1233–1241

16. Smith BD, Arthur DW, Buchholz TA, Haffty BG, Hahn CA, Hardenbergh PH, Julian TB, Marks LB, Todor DA, Vicini FA, Whelan TJ, White J, Wo JY, Harris JR (2009) Accelerated partial breast irradiation consensus statement from the American Society for Radiation Oncology (ASTRO). Int J Radiat Oncol Biol Phys 74(4):987–1001
17. Offersen BV, Overgaard M, Kroman N, Overgaard J (2009) Accelerated partial breast irradiation as part of breast conserving therapy of early breast carcinoma: a systematic review. Radiother Oncol J Eur Soc Ther Radiol Oncol 90(1):1–13. doi:10.1016/j.radonc.2008.08.005
18. Arthur DW, Winter K, Kuske RR, Bolton J, Rabinovitch R, White J, Hanson WF, Wilenzick RM, McCormick B (2008) A phase II trial of brachytherapy alone after lumpectomy for select breast cancer: tumor control and survival outcomes of RTOG 95-17. Int J Radiat Oncol Biol Phys 72(2):467–473. doi:10.1016/j.ijrobp.2007.12.056
19. Niehoff P, Polgar C, Ostertag H, Major T, Sulyok Z, Kimmig B, Kovacs G (2006) Clinical experience with the MammoSite radiation therapy system for brachytherapy of breast cancer: results from an international phase II trial. Radiother Oncol 79(3):316–320. doi:10.1016/j.radonc.2006.05.010
20. Shah C, Badiyan S, Ben Wilkinson J, Vicini F, Beitsch P, Keisch M, Arthur D, Lyden M (2013) Treatment efficacy with accelerated partial breast irradiation (APBI): final analysis of the American Society of Breast Surgeons MammoSite((R)) breast brachytherapy registry trial. Ann Surg Oncol 20(10):3279–3285. doi:10.1245/s10434-013-3158-4
21. Chafe S, Moughan J, McCormick B, Wong J, Pass H, Rabinovitch R, Arthur DW, Petersen I, White J, Vicini FA (2013) Late toxicity and patient self-assessment of breast appearance/satisfaction on RTOG 0319: a phase 2 trial of 3-dimensional conformal radiation therapy-accelerated partial breast irradiation following lumpectomy for stages I and II breast cancer. Int J Radiat Oncol Biol Phys 86(5):854–859. doi:10.1016/j.ijrobp.2013.04.005
22. Vaidya JS, Wenz F, Bulsara M, Tobias JS, Joseph DJ, Keshtgar M, Flyger HL, Massarut S, Alvarado M, Saunders C, Eiermann W, Metaxas M, Sperk E, Sütterlin M, Brown D, Esserman L, Roncadin M, Thompson A, Dewar JA, Holtveg HMR, Pigorsch S, Falzon M, Harris E, Matthews A, Brew-Graves C, Potyka I, Corica T, Williams NR, Baum M (2014) Risk-adapted targeted intraoperative radiotherapy versus whole-breast radiotherapy for breast cancer: 5-year results for local control and overall survival from the TARGIT-A randomised trial. Lancet 383(9917):603–613. doi:10.1016/s0140-6736(13)61950-9
23. Veronesi U, Orecchia R, Maisonneuve P, Viale G, Rotmensz N, Sangalli C, Luini A, Veronesi P, Galimberti V, Zurrida S, Leonardi MC, Lazzari R, Cattani F, Gentilini O, Intra M, Caldarella P, Ballardini B (2013) Intraoperative radiotherapy versus external radiotherapy for early breast cancer (ELIOT): a randomised controlled equivalence trial. Lancet Oncol 14(13):1269–1277. doi:10.1016/S1470-2045(13)70497-2
24. Polgar C, Van Limbergen E, Potter R, Kovacs G, Polo A, Lyczek J, Hildebrandt G, Niehoff P, Guinot JL, Guedea F, Johansson B, Ott OJ, Major T, Strnad V, group G-Ebcw (2010) Patient selection for accelerated partial-breast irradiation (APBI) after breast-conserving surgery: recommendations of the Groupe Europeen de Curietherapie-European Society for Therapeutic Radiology and Oncology (GEC-ESTRO) breast cancer working group based on clinical evidence (2009). Radiother Oncol J Eur Soc Ther Radiol Oncol 94(3):264–273. doi:10.1016/j.radonc.2010.01.014
25. (2006) NSABP B-39, RTOG 0413: a randomized phase III study of conventional whole breast irradiation versus partial breast irradiation for women with stage 0, I, or II breast cancer. Clin Adv Hematol Oncol 4(10):719–721
26. Olivotto IA, Whelan TJ, Parpia S, Kim DH, Berrang T, Truong PT, Kong I, Cochrane B, Nichol A, Roy I, Germain I, Akra M, Reed M, Fyles A, Trotter T, Perera F, Beckham W, Levine MN, Julian JA (2013) Interim cosmetic and toxicity results from RAPID: a randomized trial of accelerated partial breast irradiation using three-dimensional conformal external beam radiation therapy. J Clin Oncol 31(32):4038–4045. doi:10.1200/JCO.2013.50.5511
27. Vaidya JS, Wenz F, Bulsara M, Tobias JS, Joseph DJ, Keshtgar M, Flyger HL, Massarut S, Alvarado M, Saunders C, Eiermann W, Metaxas M, Sperk E, Sutterlin M, Brown D,

Esserman L, Roncadin M, Thompson A, Dewar JA, Holtveg HM, Pigorsch S, Falzon M, Harris E, Matthews A, Brew-Graves C, Potyka I, Corica T, Williams NR, Baum M, Group Tt (2014) Risk-adapted targeted intraoperative radiotherapy versus whole-breast radiotherapy for breast cancer: 5-year results for local control and overall survival from the TARGIT-A randomised trial. Lancet 383(9917):603–613. doi:10.1016/S0140-6736(13)61950-9

28. Romestaing P, Lehingue Y, Carrie C, Coquard R, Montbarbon X, Ardiet JM, Mamelle N, Gerard JP (1997) Role of a 10-Gy boost in the conservative treatment of early breast cancer: results of a randomized clinical trial in Lyon, France. J Clin Oncol 15(3):963–968
29. Bartelink H, Horiot JC, Poortmans PM, Struikmans H, Van den Bogaert W, Fourquet A, Jager JJ, Hoogenraad WJ, Oei SB, Warlam-Rodenhuis CC, Pierart M, Collette L (2007) Impact of a higher radiation dose on local control and survival in breast-conserving therapy of early breast cancer: 10-year results of the randomized boost versus no boost EORTC 22881-10882 trial. J Clin Oncol 25(22):3259–3265
30. Ceilley E, Jagsi R, Goldberg S, Grignon L, Kachnic L, Powell S, Taghian A (2005) Radiotherapy for invasive breast cancer in North America and Europe: results of a survey. Int J Radiat Oncol Biol Phys 61(2):365–373. doi:10.1016/j.ijrobp.2004.05.069
31. McDonald MW, Godette KD, Whitaker DJ, Davis LW, Johnstone PA (2010) Three-year outcomes of breast intensity-modulated radiation therapy with simultaneous integrated boost. Int J Radiat Oncol Biol Phys 77(2):523–530. doi:10.1016/j.ijrobp.2009.05.042
32. Bantema-Joppe EJ, van der Laan HP, de Bock GH, Wijsman R, Dolsma WV, Busz DM, Langendijk JA, Maduro JH (2011) Three-dimensional conformal hypofractionated simultaneous integrated boost in breast conserving therapy: results on local control and survival. Radiother Oncol 100(2):215–220. doi:10.1016/j.radonc.2011.05.027
33. Bantema-Joppe EJ, Schilstra C, de Bock GH, Dolsma WV, Busz DM, Langendijk JA, Maduro JH (2012) Simultaneous integrated boost irradiation after breast-conserving surgery: physician-rated toxicity and cosmetic outcome at 30 months' follow-up. Int J Radiat Oncol Biol Phys 83(4):e471–e477. doi:10.1016/j.ijrobp.2012.01.050
34. Askoxylakis V, Jensen AD, Hafner MF, Fetzner L, Sterzing F, Heil J, Sohn C, Husing J, Tiefenbacher U, Wenz F, Debus J, Hof H (2011) Simultaneous integrated boost for adjuvant treatment of breast cancer--intensity modulated vs. conventional radiotherapy: the IMRT-MC2 trial. BMC Cancer 11:249. doi:10.1186/1471-2407-11-249
35. Chen GP, Liu F, White J, Vicini FA, Freedman GM, Arthur DW, Li XA (2015) A planning comparison of 7 irradiation options allowed in RTOG 1005 for early-stage breast cancer. Med Dosim 40(1):21–25. doi:10.1016/j.meddos.2014.06.007
36. Formenti SC, Gidea-Addeo D, Goldberg JD, Roses DF, Guth A, Rosenstein BS, DeWyngaert KJ (2007) Phase I–II trial of prone accelerated intensity modulated radiation therapy to the breast to optimally spare normal tissue. J Clin Oncol 25(16):2236–2242. doi:10.1200/JCO.2006.09.1041
37. Morganti AG, Cilla S, Valentini V, Digesu C, Macchia G, Deodato F, Ferrandina G, Cece MG, Cirocco M, Garganese G, Di Lullo L, Traficante D, Scarabeo F, Panunzi S, De Gaetano A, Sallustio G, Cellini N, Sofo L, Piermattei A, Scambia G (2009) Phase I–II studies on accelerated IMRT in breast carcinoma: technical comparison and acute toxicity in 332 patients. Radiother Oncol J Eur Soc Ther Radiol Oncol 90(1):86–92. doi:10.1016/j.radonc.2008.10.017
38. Corvo R, Ricchetti F, Doino D, Torielli P, Agostinelli S, Cavagnetto F, Giannelli F, D'Alonzo A, Vagge S, Belgioia L, Guenzi M (2010) Adjuvant hypofractionated radiotherapy with weekly concomitant boost for women with early breast cancer: the clinical experience at Genoa university. Anticancer Res 30(11):4749–4753
39. Cante D, Rosa La Porta M, Casanova-Borca V, Sciacero P, Girelli G, Pasquino M, Franco P, Ozzello F (2011) Accelerated hypofractionated adjuvant whole breast radiotherapy with concomitant photon boost after conserving surgery for early stage breast cancer: a prospective evaluation on 463 patients. Breast J 17(6):586–593. doi:10.1111/j.1524-4741.2011.01159.x
40. Teh AY, Walsh L, Purdie TG, Mosseri A, Xu W, Levin W, Koch CA, Fyles A, Liu FF, Cho BC (2012) Concomitant intensity modulated boost during whole breast hypofractionated

radiotherapy – a feasibility and toxicity study. Radiother Oncol J Eur Soc Ther Radiol Oncol 102(1):89–95. doi:10.1016/j.radonc.2011.10.015

41. Ciervide R, Dhage S, Guth A, Shapiro RL, Axelrod DM, Roses DF, Formenti SC (2012) Five year outcome of 145 patients with ductal carcinoma in situ (DCIS) after accelerated breast radiotherapy. Int J Radiat Oncol Biol Phys 83(2):e159–e164. doi:10.1016/j.ijrobp.2011.11.025
42. Freedman GM, Anderson PR, Bleicher RJ, Litwin S, Li T, Swaby RF, Ma CM, Li J, Sigurdson ER, Watkins-Bruner D, Morrow M, Goldstein LJ (2012) Five-year local control in a phase II study of hypofractionated intensity modulated radiation therapy with an incorporated boost for early stage breast cancer. Int J Radiat Oncol Biol Phys 84(4):888–893. doi:10.1016/j.ijrobp.2012.01.091
43. Chadha M, Woode R, Sillanpaa J, Lucido D, Boolbol SK, Kirstein L, Osborne MP, Feldman S, Harrison LB (2013) Early-stage breast cancer treated with 3-week accelerated whole-breast radiation therapy and concomitant boost. Int J Radiat Oncol Biol Phys 86(1):40–44. doi:10.1016/j.ijrobp.2012.11.010
44. Dellas K, Vonthein R, Zimmer J, Dinges S, Boicev AD, Andreas P, Fischer D, Winkler C, Ziegler A, Dunst J, Group AROS (2014) Hypofractionation with simultaneous integrated boost for early breast cancer: results of the German multicenter phase II trial (ARO-2010-01). Strahlenther Onkol 190(7):646–653. doi:10.1007/s00066-014-0658-5
45. Donovan EM, Ciurlionis L, Fairfoul J, James H, Mayles H, Manktelow S, Raj S, Tsang Y, Tywman N, Yarnold J, Coles C (2011) Planning with intensity-modulated radiotherapy and tomotherapy to modulate dose across breast to reflect recurrence risk (IMPORT High trial). Int J Radiat Oncol Biol Phys 79(4):1064–1072. doi:10.1016/j.ijrobp.2009.12.052

Chapter 12
Radiotherapy Following Neoadjuvant Chemotherapy in Locally Advanced Breast Cancer

Nisha Ohri and Alice Ho

Abstract Neoadjuvant chemotherapy (NAC) is commonly used in patients with locally advanced breast cancer. Several challenges faced by radiation oncologists in treating these patients include the lack of an accurate pathologic stage to guide management and determining how response to NAC should affect further local therapy. In the postmastectomy setting, the available data demonstrates that both initial clinical stage and final pathologic stage independently predict for locoregional recurrence (LRR). Postmastectomy radiation therapy (PMRT) improves local control in patients with locally advanced clinical stage III disease, regardless of response to NAC, and in those with residual pathologic nodal disease. Patients with early-stage disease who respond well to NAC are at low risk for LRR. Within the intermediate risk groups, additional factors such as molecular subtype and presence of a complete pathologic response, both of which have been shown to predict for LRR, may help guide further management decisions. With regard to breast-conserving therapy after NAC, the available data demonstrates this is a safe and effective option in patients with minimal up-front nodal disease and small residual tumors after NAC. Additional contraindications for lumpectomy in any setting should also be considered. The role of regional nodal irradiation in patients who have received NAC is controversial, particularly among pathologically node-negative patients. There are two ongoing randomized trials open for accrual in the USA that aim to evaluate the benefits of adjuvant radiation therapy, including regional nodal irradiation, after NAC.

Keywords Breast cancer • Neoadjuvant chemotherapy • Postmastectomy radiation therapy • Pathologic complete response • Regional nodal irradiation

---

N. Ohri
Department of Radiation Oncology, Mount Sinai Hospital, 1184 Fifth Avenue, New York, NY 10029, USA

A. Ho (✉)
Department of Radiation Oncology, Memorial Sloan Kettering Cancer Center, 1250 First Avenue, SM-07, New York, NY 10011, USA
e-mail: HoA1234@mskcc.org

M. Toi et al. (eds.), *Personalized Treatment of Breast Cancer*,
DOI 10.1007/978-4-431-55552-0_12

12.1 Introduction

Neoadjuvant chemotherapy (NAC) is a common treatment modality for patients with locally advanced breast cancer. It can be used to facilitate surgery when up-front surgical resection is not feasible or to avoid mastectomy in cases where up-front breast conservation surgery may result in poor cosmetic outcome [1, 2]. Delivering preoperative systemic therapy may also treat micrometastatic disease and avoid delays due to postoperative healing issues after surgery.

The benefits of radiation therapy (RT) after breast conservation surgery with or without adjuvant chemotherapy have been well-established by the Early Breast Cancer Trialists' Collaborative Group (EBCTCG) meta-analysis [3]. Similarly, multiple randomized trials have demonstrated locoregional recurrence (LRR) and breast cancer survival benefits with postmastectomy radiation therapy (PMRT) in appropriately selected patients [4, 5]. The use of PMRT in general will likely increase, given that the most recent update of the EBCTCG meta-analysis showed significantly lower 10-year recurrence and 20-year breast cancer mortality rates with the addition of PMRT in patients with only one to three positive lymph nodes [6].

These trials included in the EBCTCG meta-analysis, however, did not enroll patients who received NAC. Neoadjuvant chemotherapy has been shown to change the extent of disease in 80–90 % of cases [2]. As a result, the pathologic indications for adjuvant radiation therapy after up-front surgical resection may be different in the setting of preoperative systemic therapy. Several common challenges faced by radiation oncologists when treating patients who have undergone NAC include the lack of an accurate pathologic stage to guide treatment decisions, assessing how the response to NAC should affect further local therapy, and formulating new treatment strategies for patients who demonstrate a poor response to NAC. To date, there is limited data from randomized trials to help answer these questions. This chapter will review the evolution of the role of radiation therapy in optimizing locoregional control in breast cancer patients who receive NAC.

12.2 LRR After NAC and Mastectomy Without PMRT

Available data from randomized studies comes from the National Surgical Adjuvant Breast and Bowel Project (NSABP) B-18 and B-27 trials. Mamounas et al. performed a retrospective combined analysis of these two trials to examine the rates and patterns of LRR after NAC as well as identify independent predictors of local failure. These trials were conducted in the late 1980s and 1990s before the benefits of PMRT were established [4, 5]. At that time, clinical trials did not allow postmastectomy chest wall or regional nodal RT, allowing the group to study LRR rates after NAC and mastectomy in patients who did not receive adjuvant radiation.

The NSABP B-18 trial randomly assigned 1523 patients with operable and palpable T1-3 and N0-1 breast cancer to receive either four cycles of neoadjuvant doxorubicin and cyclophosphamide (AC) or four cycles of adjuvant AC. Patients aged 50 or greater received hormonal therapy with tamoxifen for 5 years regardless of receptor status. The NSABP B-27 trial had similar enrollment criteria and randomly assigned 2411 patients to receive either four cycles of neoadjuvant AC or four cycles of neoadjuvant AC followed by four cycles of either neoadjuvant or adjuvant docetaxel. All patients received hormonal therapy with tamoxifen for 5 years regardless of age or receptor status. In both studies, patients who underwent breast conservation surgery received adjuvant radiation therapy. Patients who underwent mastectomy did not receive PMRT. The combined data set included 742 patients from the neoadjuvant AC arm of B-18 and 2346 patients from all three arms of B-27.

For the entire cohort, the 10-year cumulative incidence of LRR was 11.1 %. Among 1947 patients who underwent mastectomy, 12.6 % had a LRR (9.0 % local, 3.6 % regional). Several independent predictors of LRR were identified for all patients: age $\geq$50 years at randomization, clinical tumor size >5 cm before NAC, clinical nodal involvement before NAC, pathologic breast tumor response, and nodal status at surgery. For patients who underwent mastectomy, all factors except age remained significant on multivariate analysis. When LRR rates were examined according to the number of pathologically involved nodes at surgery, rates were higher with four or more positive lymph nodes than with one to three positive lymph nodes. However, LRR rates were above 10 % for all subsets of pathologically node-positive patients, indicating that residual nodal disease following NAC is an important negative prognostic factor for locoregional recurrence [7].

A series of retrospective reviews from the MD Anderson Cancer Center (MDACC) has also helped identify clinical and pathologic factors that predict for LRR after NAC and mastectomy without adjuvant radiation. The first study, published in 2002, analyzed outcomes from 150 breast cancer patients with early-stage to locally advanced disease treated on prospective institutional trials. With a median follow-up of 4.1 years, the 5- and 10-year actuarial rates of LRR were 27 %. Three factors independently predicted for LRR: (1) clinical stage IIIB or greater disease, (2) four or more positive lymph nodes, and (3) lack of tamoxifen. The pathologic complete response (pCR) rate was 10 % at the time of mastectomy. However, the LRR rate among those patients who achieved a pCR remained high at about 20 %, with pretreatment clinical stage ranging from IIA to IIIB. Patients who did not achieve a pCR had a similar rate of LRR (28 %). These results suggested that PMRT should be considered in patients who present with clinical stage III disease, even in the setting of a pCR. Clinical stage II disease is associated with a lower baseline risk of LRR, suggesting that the local control benefit of PMRT is also smaller [8].

To further study these lower-risk patients who undergo NAC and mastectomy, Garg et al. similarly analyzed a cohort of stage I and II patients from the same data set. The study included 132 patients, with 95 % of patients presenting with clinical stage II disease. All patients received either an anthracycline-based neoadjuvant regimen or single-agent paclitaxel followed by modified radical mastectomy. Nineteen percent of patients had no residual invasive disease at the primary site, 43 % had residual tumors ≤2 cm, and 26 % had residual tumors >2 cm. Among patients who presented with clinically involved lymph nodes, 36 % were pathologically node negative. The overall 5- and 10-year LRR rates were 10 %. Several factors associated with increased LRR were identified: (1) clinical stage T3N0 at presentation, (2) four or more positive lymph nodes at surgery, (3) age ≤40 at diagnosis, and (4) lack of tamoxifen. The 5-year LRR rate for patients with clinical T1-2 disease and one to three nodes positive at surgery was very low (5 %). This led investigators to conclude that among patients presenting with clinical stage II disease, PMRT is indicated for those who are young (defined as ≤40 years old), have T3 tumors, or have four or more positive lymph nodes at surgery. Conversely, patients with initial clinical T1-2 disease and one to three positive lymph nodes at surgery may have too low a risk of LRR to benefit from PMRT [9].

12.3 The Role of PMRT in Minimizing LRR After NAC and Mastectomy

Another series of retrospective studies from the MDACC investigated the role of PMRT in locally advanced breast cancer patients treated with NAC and mastectomy. In 2004, Huang et al. published a study including 676 patients treated from 1974 to 1998 with doxorubicin-based NAC and mastectomy ± PMRT. Ninety-five percent of patients also received adjuvant chemotherapy. Radiation therapy included 50 Gy to the chest wall and regional lymph nodes with an additional 10 Gy boost to the chest wall. About 30 % of patients received adjuvant hormonal therapy with tamoxifen.

At a median follow-up of 5.7 years, patients who received PMRT had a significantly lower 10-year rate of LRR compared to patients who did not (11 % vs. 22 %, $p = 0.0001$). Patients presenting with clinical stage I-IIA disease had similar rates of LRR with and without radiation, while those with stage IIB disease or greater had significantly lower rates of LRR with PMRT (11 % vs. 26 %, $p < 0.0001$). Stratifying by clinical T-stage and N-stage, patients with T3-4 tumors or N2-3 nodal disease benefited significantly from PMRT. Looking at posttreatment pathology, LRR rates were lower with PMRT for residual tumors >2 cm or with four or more positive lymph nodes ($p < 0.001$ for both parameters). In a subset of patients with clinical stage II disease and one to three positive lymph nodes after NAC, there was no difference in LRR rate with PMRT. Among patients who achieved a pCR, 10-year LRR rates were similar for patients with clinical stage I or II disease ($p = 0.22$) but were significantly improved with the addition of PMRT in patients with clinical stage III disease (33 % vs. 3 %, $p = 0.006$). PMRT significantly improved cause-specific survival (CSS) in patients with clinical stage IIIB disease or greater (44 % vs. 22 %, $p = 0.002$), clinical T4 tumors at presentation (45 %

vs. 24 %, $p = 0.007$), and four or more positive lymph nodes (45 % vs. 18 %, $p = 0.005$). Similar to prior studies, this review identified multiple pretreatment clinical factors and posttreatment pathologic factors that predicted for LRR after NAC and mastectomy. PMRT was highly effective in patients with significant residual disease burden after NAC and in patients who presented with locally advanced disease, even in the setting of a pCR [10].

A follow-up study analyzing clinical and pathologic predictors of LRR in the same cohort of 542 patients, all of whom received NAC, mastectomy, and PMRT, was subsequently published 1 year later. Over 70 % of the cohort had clinical stage IIIA or stage IIIB disease. Median follow-up was 70 months. The 5-year rate of LRR was 9 %, and the 10-year rate was 11 %. Over 60 % of failures occurred in the chest wall, and about 30 % occurred in the supraclavicular lymph nodes. On multivariate analysis, five factors were independently associated with LRR: (1) skin/nipple involvement, (2) supraclavicular lymph node involvement, (3) extracapsular extension, (4) estrogen-receptor-negative disease, and (5) lack of tamoxifen use. The 10-year LRR rate for patients with one or none of these factors was only 4 % compared to 8 % with two factors and 28 % with three or more factors ($p < 0.0001$). This data provided compelling evidence for the benefit of PMRT in patients receiving NAC with multiple high-risk features and also illuminated the need for alternative treatment strategies in such patients [11].

12.4 PMRT Following NAC for T3N0 Breast Cancer

The role of PMRT in patients with clinical T3N0 disease treated with NAC and mastectomy is controversial given the absence of nodal involvement upon disease presentation. An MDACC study specifically examined this question in a large retrospective series of 162 patients with cT3N0 breast cancer who received NAC followed by mastectomy. A substantial proportion of patients ($n = 119$; 73 %) received PMRT, which targeted the chest wall, high axilla, and supraclavicular fossa ± internal mammary node irradiation. The 5-year LRR rate for the irradiated group was 4 % compared to 24 % in the non-irradiated group ($p < 0.001$). However, more patients in the irradiated group had pathologically involved lymph nodes at surgery (52 % vs. 26 %, $p = 0.003$), which previous studies identified as a negative prognostic factor for LRR. Among all patients with pathologically involved lymph nodes, the 5-year LRR rate was lower with PMRT (5 % vs. 53 %, $p < 0.001$). Among pathologically node-negative patients, there was a trend toward improved 5-year LRR rate with PMRT (2 % vs. 14 %, $p = 0.06$). In the subset of patients who achieved a pCR ($n = 13$; 8 %), there were no locoregional recurrences. However, it is difficult to interpret these results given the limitations of a very small sample size. This study demonstrated a significant locoregional control benefit with PMRT after NAC and mastectomy in patients presenting with clinical T3N0 breast cancer who have pathologically involved lymph nodes. Even in patients who are pathologically node negative at surgery, the risk of LRR may be high enough to warrant consideration of PMRT [12].

12.5 Posttreatment Pathology and LRR

One of the biggest challenges in assessing patients who have received NAC is the lack of an accurate pathologic stage, as many patients are downstaged after treatment. From the NSABP B-18 trial, clinical breast tumor size was reduced in 80 % of patients ($n = 693$), and clinical nodal response was observed in 89 % of node-positive patients ($n = 185$) [2].

To explore how posttreatment pathology impacts LRR rate, Buchholz et al. from the MDACC performed a retrospective study of mastectomy patients treated with neoadjuvant vs. adjuvant chemotherapy without PMRT. The analysis included 1031 patients who received adjuvant chemotherapy and 150 patients treated with NAC. Most patients received a doxorubicin-containing regimen. Ninety-two percent of patients in the neoadjuvant group received additional chemotherapy after mastectomy. About 30 % of patients in both groups received tamoxifen.

Advanced clinical stage at presentation was significantly more common in the neoadjuvant group (55 % with clinical stage IIIA disease or greater vs. 9 %, $p < 0.001$). However, the pathologic size of primary tumor and nodal involvement was significantly less in the neoadjuvant group, suggesting favorable response to treatment. Fifty-six percent of patients had residual tumors measuring less than 2 cm, and 46 % were pathologically node negative (28 % presented as clinically node negative). The overall 5-year rate of LRR was higher in the neoadjuvant group (27 % vs. 15 %, $p = 0.001$). When stratified by primary tumor size (0–2 cm, 2.1–5.0 cm, >5.0 cm), the 5-year LRR rate remained significantly higher in the neoadjuvant group for each subset. Based on lymph node status, a significantly higher rate of LRR was seen in patients with four or more positive lymph nodes after NAC. For pathologically node-negative patients or those with one to three involved lymph nodes, the LRR rates were similar between both groups. While patients with T1N1 disease had similar rates of LRR (both <20 %), patients with T2N1 disease had higher rates of LRR with neoadjuvant chemotherapy (30 % vs. 15 %, $p = 0.016$). The group concluded that PMRT should be offered to all patients with pathologic N2 or T3 disease or clinical stage IIIA disease, regardless of preoperative or postoperative chemotherapy. There was insufficient information to assess LRR in patients with clinical stage II disease who received NAC, particularly in those with residual nodal involvement [13].

12.6 LRR After a Pathologic Complete Response

Previous retrospective series demonstrated that LRR rates in patients with locally advanced disease at presentation who achieved a pCR after NAC in the breast and axilla remained relatively high and were significantly reduced with the addition of PMRT [10]. As systemic therapy regimens continue to improve, the rate of pCR after neoadjuvant chemotherapy is expected to increase.

McGuire et al. from the MDACC performed a retrospective review specifically evaluating the outcomes of patients with locally advanced breast cancer who achieved a pCR after NAC. The study included 106 patients, with about 70 % presenting with clinical stage III disease. Over 90 % of patients received an anthracycline-based chemotherapy regimen before modified radical mastectomy. Seventy-two patients (68 %) received PMRT, which consisted of 50 Gy in 25 fractions to the chest wall and regional lymph nodes and an additional 10 Gy boost to the chest wall. The supraclavicular fossa and axillary apex were treated with a photon field, and the internal mammary nodes and medial chest wall were treated with an electron field.

Median follow-up was 5 years. While the irradiated group had a significantly higher proportion of patients who presented with advanced clinical stage (81 % vs. 35 % stage III, $p < 0.001$), the 10-year rates of LRR remained similar between the irradiated and non-irradiated groups (5 % vs. 10 %, respectively; $p = 0.40$). Stratifying by presenting clinical stage, there were no locoregional recurrences among patients with stage I or II disease, regardless of PMRT. Conversely, among patients with stage III disease, the use of PMRT was associated with a significantly lower 10-year LRR rate (7.3 % vs. 33.3 %, $p = 0.040$). No additional predictors of LRR were identified. Irradiated patients had significantly higher rates of 10-year distant metastasis-free survival (88 % vs. 41 %, $p = 0.0006$), CSS (87 % vs. 40 %, $p = 0.0014$), and OS (77 % vs. 33 %, $p = 0.0016$). This study confirmed that in locally advanced breast cancer patients who achieve a pCR after NAC, PMRT improves both local control and survival, again highlighting the significant impact of high disease burden at presentation [14].

12.7 Biology Subtype, pCR Rates, and Long-Term Outcomes

Over the past decade, multiple studies have determined that the likelihood of achieving a pathologic complete response (pCR) is associated with breast cancer subtype, with triple-negative (TN) and trastuzumab-treated Her2+ patients demonstrating a greater proclivity toward pCR compared to hormone-receptor-positive patients. Several studies have also demonstrated that a pathologic complete response to NAC can predict for improved long-term outcomes in breast cancer patients. A retrospective review by Kuerer et al. of 372 patients with locally advanced breast cancer treated on two prospective trials with anthracycline-based NAC examined pCR rates and survival outcomes. All patients underwent total mastectomy or segmental mastectomy with axillary dissection, additional adjuvant chemotherapy, and adjuvant radiation therapy. The pCR rate was 12 %. The 5-year OS and DFS rates were significantly higher in patients who achieved a pCR (89 % and 87 %, respectively) compared to the rest of the cohort (64 % and 58 %, respectively) [15].

More recently, von Minckwitz et al. from the German Breast Group performed a larger pooled analysis of 6377 patients from seven prospective neoadjuvant chemotherapy clinical trials. The group aimed to precisely define a pathologic complete response and determine its prognostic impact on long-term survival outcomes based on molecular subtype of breast cancer. All patients received neoadjuvant anthracycline-taxane-based chemotherapy. The median tumor size was 4.0 cm, and 12 % of patients presented with locally advanced disease. At a median follow-up of 46.3 months, there were 1466 relapses (23 %) and 775 deaths (12.2 %).

Various definitions of pCR were studied, including ypT0 ypN0 (15.0 %), ypTis ypN0 (4.8 %), and ypT0/is ypN+ (2.9 %). DFS was highest among patients with no residual invasive or in situ disease in the breast or lymph nodes or ypT0 ypN0, followed by ypTis ypN0, and finally ypT0/is ypN+ ($p < 0.001$). Patients were then stratified by the following molecular subtypes: luminal A, luminal B/Her2−, luminal B/Her2+, Her2+, and triple negative. Pathologic complete response rates ranged from 9 % (luminal A) to 50 % (Her2+ with trastuzumab). Both DFS and OS were significantly correlated with pCR only for the Her2+ (with and without trastuzumab) and triple-negative subtypes ($p < 0.001$). While DFS and OS rates were favorable for low-proliferating luminal A-like tumors, pCR was not predictive of survival outcomes in this molecular subtype. A mixed pattern was seen for luminal B-like tumors, with pCR appearing prognostic for Her2− tumors but not Her2+ tumors. This study demonstrated that to achieve the greatest prognostic value, pCR should be defined as no residual invasive or in situ disease in the breast or axilla. Additionally, pCR can serve as a surrogate marker for long-term outcomes in patients with Her2+, triple-negative, and luminal B/Her2− disease and may help guide treatment decisions for patients in whom the role of further local therapy remains unclear [16].

While pCR can be a reliable surrogate for DFS in certain patients, its relationship to LRR outcomes is less clearly defined. To address this question, another study from the MDACC by Caudle et al. aimed to identify patients at high risk for LRR after NAC and breast-conserving therapy based on response to NAC and molecular subtype. This study included 595 patients for analysis and used the following subtypes: ER+ or PR+ (HR+) and Her2−, HR+/Her2+, HR−/Her2+, and HR−/Her2−. All patients underwent lumpectomy with axillary node evaluation. Clinically node-negative patients underwent sentinel lymph node biopsy with completion axillary dissection if positive. Clinically node-positive patients underwent axillary dissection. Radiation therapy included 50 Gy in 25 fractions to the breast with an additional 10 Gy boost to the tumor bed. Regional nodal irradiation was delivered per physician discretion. Because this study was conducted before the routine use of neoadjuvant trastuzumab, patients who received trastuzumab were excluded.

Patients with HR− tumors had the greatest response to NAC. Pathologic complete response rates were lower in the HR+/Her2− (9 %) and HR+/Her2+ (18 %) subsets than in the HR−/Her2+ (36 %) and HR−/Her2− (38 %) subsets ($p < 0.001$). Additionally, HR− tumors had smaller pathologic tumor sizes and less residual nodal disease burden. However, 5-year LRR-free survival and OS rates were significantly higher for HR+/Her2− (97.0 % and 92.5 %, respectively) and HR+/Her2+ patients (95.9 % and 85.8 %, respectively) than for HR−/Her2+ (86.5 % and 84.4 %, respectively) and HR−/Her2− patients (89.5 % and 83.0 %, respectively). Among patients who did not achieve a pCR, those who were HR− had decreased 5-year LRR-free survival, while HR+ patients maintained high rates of LRR-free survival. While this study was limited by the lack of trastuzumab use in the neoadjuvant setting, it demonstrated high rates of local control in the HR+/Her2− and HR+/Her2+ subtypes, regardless of response to NAC. Although there are currently no alternative treatment strategies to improve locoregional control in patients with HR– subtypes who do not achieve a pCR after NAC, improving the efficacy of locoregional treatment in this subset of patients who are at high risk for LRR is an important research endeavor [17].

The most compelling evidence for the significance of a pathologic complete response and biologic subtype as independent predictors for LRR in patients receiving NAC comes from the pooled analysis of the CTNeoBC (Collaborative Trials in Neoadjuvant Breast Cancer) trials. In the final analysis, 5694 patients with data on biologic subtype and all covariates included in the multivariable analysis model were studied. Thirty-six percent of patients were HR+/grade 1, 11 % HR+/grade 3, 14 % HR−/Her2+, 18 % HR+/Her2+, and 21 % TN. The overall rate of LRR at 5 years was low (6.8 %). Biologic subtype (TN vs. HR+/grade 1: HR of 4.09 [3.01–5.55]) and pCR (ypN+ vs. pT0/isN0: HR 2.36 [1.62–4.34]) were the strongest predictors of LRR, with an overall LRR rate of 12.2 % in TN patients and 11.8 % in patients with residual positive lymph nodes following NAC. These results provided further evidence for the impact of biologic subtype and response to NAC on LRR risk [18].

12.8 Success of Breast Conservation Therapy After NAC

One significant advantage of NAC is the ability to potentially convert patients who would require up-front mastectomy to breast conservation candidates. The NSABP B-18 and EORTC 10902 trials compared locoregional control rates in patients who had preoperative chemotherapy with patients who had postoperative chemotherapy. Both studies demonstrated higher rates of breast conservation therapy in the preoperative chemotherapy arms [2, 19].

Long-term results of the NSABP B-18 trial showed similar rates of LRR in the preoperative chemotherapy and postoperative chemotherapy groups. For patients who underwent lumpectomy, the in-breast tumor recurrence (IBTR) rates were 13 % and 10 %, respectively ($p = 0.21$) [20]. Similarly, 10-year OS and LRR rates from the EORTC 10902 trial for patients who underwent breast conservation therapy were similar with preoperative chemotherapy and postoperative chemotherapy [21].

To study the patterns and predictors of local failure after NAC and breast-conserving therapy, Chen et al. from the MDACC performed a retrospective review of 340 patients with stage I–III breast cancer. A majority of patients (96 %) were clinical stage II–III at presentation. Lumpectomy included gross excision of the residual primary tumor with a margin of normal-appearing tissue. Re-excision was performed for positive margins, with 4 % of patients having focally positive final margins. About 80 % of patients underwent axillary level I–II dissection. Adjuvant radiation therapy included 50 Gy in 25 fractions to the whole breast with an additional 10 Gy electron boost to the tumor bed. Regional nodal irradiation was delivered at the discretion of the treating physician.

At a median follow-up of 60 months, 29 (8.5 %) patients developed LRR, and 16 were IBTRs. The 5-year LRR-free survival was 91 %, and the 5-year IBTR-free survival was 95 %. Four factors correlated with increased IBTR and LRR rates: (1) clinical N2 or N3 disease, (2) pathologic residual tumor >2 cm, (3) multifocal pattern of residual disease, and (4) lymphovascular space invasion (LVSI) [22]. The same group subsequently developed the MD Anderson Prognostic Index (MDAPI), which used the presence or absence of these four predictors of recurrence to establish an overall score ranging from 0 to 4. The actuarial 5-year IBTR-free survival rates were 97 % for a score of 0–1 ($n = 276$), 88 % for a score of 2 ($n = 43$), and 82 % for a score of 3–4 ($n = 12$), $p < 0.001$ [23]. These studies demonstrated that breast-conserving therapy after NAC in appropriately selected patients results in low rates of LRR and IBTR. This was confirmed by results from the recent large CTNeoBC pooled analysis (LRR rate of 6.0 % with a pCR after NAC and 6.3 % without a pCR) [18].

The available data demonstrates that breast-conserving therapy after NAC is a safe and effective option in patients with minimal nodal disease at presentation, residual T1 tumors or smaller after NAC without multicentric disease, and without LVSI. The contraindications for lumpectomy in any setting should also be considered, including up-front multicentric disease, diffuse microcalcifications, and persistently positive resection margins following lumpectomy. Finally, all patients should undergo whole-breast irradiation after breast-conserving surgery.

12.9 Regional Nodal Irradiation

The benefits of regional nodal irradiation (RNI) have been studied in both breast-conserved and postmastectomy patients, however in the setting of adjuvant chemotherapy delivery only. The National Cancer Institute of Canada Clinical Trials Group (NCIC-CTG) MA.20 trial was a randomized multicenter trial that included over 1800 patients with high-risk node-negative or node-positive breast cancer. All patients underwent breast-conserving surgery with axillary level I/II lymph node dissection. Patients were randomized to whole-breast irradiation (WBI) or WBI + RNI. The breast was treated to 50 Gy in 25 fractions with or without a 10 Gy boost to the tumor bed. The axillary apex, supraclavicular fossa, and internal mammary nodes were treated to 45 Gy in 25 fractions. Over 80 % of patients had one to three positive lymph nodes, and over 90 % received adjuvant chemotherapy.

Median follow-up was 62 months. The WBI + RNI group had a higher DFS (89.7 % vs. 84.0 %, $p = 0.003$), locoregional DFS (96.8 % vs. 94.5 %, $p = 0.02$), and distant DFS (92.4 % vs. 87.0 %, $p = 0.002$). There was a trend toward improved 5-year OS with WBI + RNI (92.3 % vs. 90.7 %, $p = 0.07$). While a longer follow-up may be required to establish an OS benefit with RNI, these results suggest that all patients undergoing breast-conserving surgery with node-positive disease should receive RNI in addition to WBI [24]. Coupled with the recent update of the EBCTCG meta-analysis demonstrating improved 10-year recurrence and 20-year breast cancer mortality rates with the addition of PMRT in patients with one to three positive lymph nodes, there appears to be a local control and survival benefit when these patients are treated more aggressively [6].

A recent meta-analysis by Budach et al. performed a pooled analysis of three large randomized trials (MA.20, EORTC 22922–10925, and the French trial) to further establish the benefits of regional nodal irradiation. Combining all three trials, there was a significant OS benefit with the addition of medial supraclavicular lymph node irradiation (HR 0.88, 95 % CI 0.80–0.97), with an absolute benefit of 1.6 % at 5 years from the MA.20 trial, 1.6 % at 10 years from the EORTC trial, and 3.3 % at 10 years from the French trial. Looking at the MA.20 and EORTC trials, medial supraclavicular and internal mammary lymph node irradiation was associated with a significant improvement in DFS (HR 0.85, 95 % CI 0.77–0.94) and distant metastasis-free survival (HR 0.82, 95 % CI 0.73–0.92). These combined results again indicate a statistically significant survival benefit with RNI [25].

There is little data to guide treatment decisions regarding regional nodal irradiation after NAC. A study from the Rene Huguenin Cancer Center in France looked specifically at patients who were pathologically node negative after NAC and breast-conserving surgery with axillary lymph node dissection. All patients ($n = 248$) received adjuvant whole-breast irradiation, with 64 % also receiving regional nodal irradiation. The 5-year LRR-free survival and OS rates were similar with regional nodal irradiation (89.4 % and 88.7 %, respectively) and without regional nodal irradiation (86.2 % and 92 %, respectively). However, the targeted lymph nodes varied significantly within the regional nodal irradiation group [26].

Similar results were seen in another retrospective study by the Korean Radiation Oncology Group (KROG 12-05). This study looked at the benefit of elective nodal irradiation in patients with clinical stage II–III breast cancer who received NAC followed by breast-conserving therapy and were pathologically node negative. The overall 5-year LRR-free survival and DFS rates were 95.5 % and 90.5 %, respectively. Elective nodal irradiation did not significantly affect survival outcomes [27].

While the necessity of regional RT or PMRT for ypN0 patients has been studied, data regarding the clinical benefits from treatment is conflicting. Internal mammary lymph node irradiation was not standardized in these studies. It is possible that exclusion of the IMNs from the radiation treatment volumes may have increased the risk of locoregional recurrence, consequently obscuring the benefit of PMRT [26–28].

12.10 Ongoing Trials Investigating the Role of RT After NAC

There are two ongoing randomized NAC trials that are open for accrual in the USA. The NSABP B-51/RTOG 1304 (NRG 9353) trial is enrolling patients with clinical stage II–III breast cancer (T1-3N1M0) with biopsy-proven axillary nodal disease (Fig. 12.1). Patients receive NAC with anti-Her2-targeted therapy if Her2+. Patients who are pathologically node negative at surgery (by axillary dissection or sentinel lymph node biopsy) are randomized to breast RT alone (lumpectomy) or no RT (mastectomy) vs. breast RT with regional nodal irradiation or PMRT with regional nodal irradiation. This study aims to evaluate the benefits of adjuvant radiation therapy, including regional nodal irradiation, in patients who are initially node positive and become node negative after NAC [29].

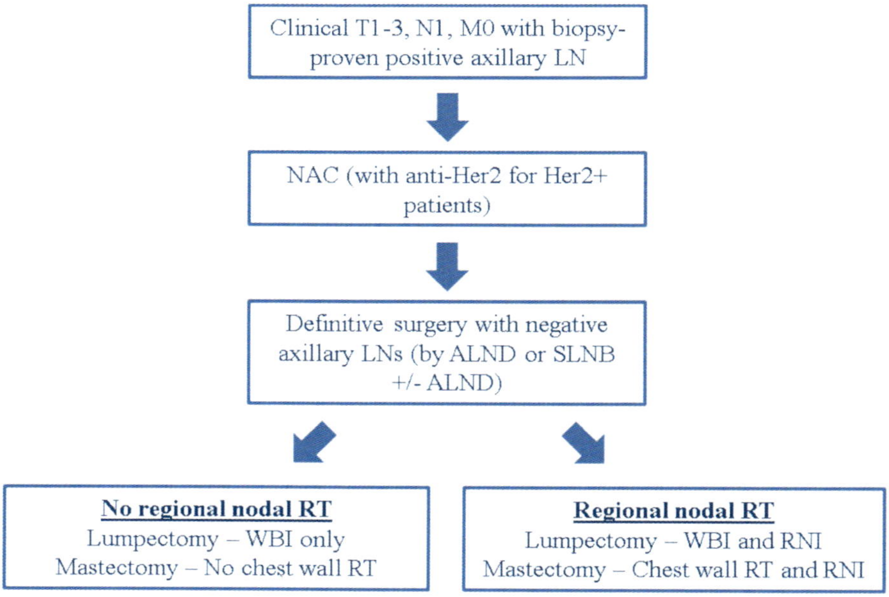

Fig. 12.1 NSABP B-51/RTOG 1304 (NRG 9353) schema. Abbreviations: *NAC* neoadjuvant chemotherapy, *ALND* axillary lymph node dissection, *SLNB* sentinel lymph node biopsy, *WBI* whole-breast irradiation, *RNI* regional nodal irradiation

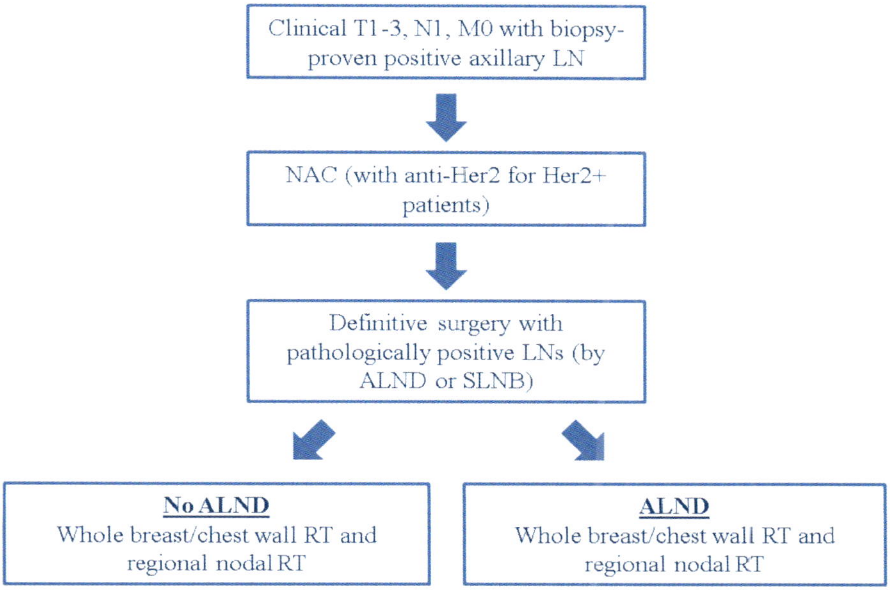

Fig. 12.2 Alliance A11101 schema. Abbreviations: *NAC* neoadjuvant chemotherapy, *ALND* axillary lymph node dissection, *SLNB* sentinel lymph node biopsy

The Alliance A11101 trial (Fig. 12.2) is another randomized trial that is enrolling patients with clinical stage II–III breast cancer (T1-3N1M0). Patients receive NAC with anti-Her2-targeted therapy if Her2+. Patients who are pathologically node positive by sentinel lymph node biopsy after NAC are randomized to breast/chest wall and regional nodal RT vs. axillary lymph node dissection and breast/chest wall and regional nodal RT. This study aims to compare axillary lymph node dissection to axillary radiation therapy in patients who remain node positive after NAC [30].

12.11 Conclusions

While we await the results of ongoing randomized trials, there is a lack of randomized data to guide treatment decisions for local therapy after NAC. Based on the available data, which is mostly retrospective, the initial clinical stage at presentation and the final pathologic stage after NAC both independently predict for LRR. A suggested treatment algorithm for PMRT after NAC is shown in Fig. 12.3. Following NAC, PMRT is indicated for patients who initially present with clinical stage III disease or greater regardless of response to NAC. It is also indicated for patients with residual pathologic nodal disease at the time of mastectomy. Clinical T3N0 disease has been associated with high LRR rates as well,

Pathologic Stage

Clinical Stage — LRR Rates	ypN+	ypN-/no breast pCR	pCR
T1-2 N0	11%	6%	7%
T3 N0	14-53%	13%	0-8%
T1-2 N1	15-27%	11%	0-9%
N2 or T3 N1 or T4 N0-1	16-40%		

Fig. 12.3 Estimated rates of locoregional recurrence in breast cancer patients after neoadjuvant chemotherapy (NAC) and mastectomy based on initial clinical stage and pathologic response to NAC. *Red* – PMRT recommended; *green* – no PMRT; *orange* – consider PMRT. Abbreviations: *LRR* locoregional recurrence, *pCR* pathological complete response

warranting further local therapy in the absence of a pCR. Even with a pCR, PMRT can be considered. Patients who present with early-stage clinically node-negative disease and remain pathologically node negative at the time of surgery do not seem to benefit from PMRT. The remaining groups of patients with clinical stage II disease may not require further therapy, as suggested by the reviewed data. However, this is largely based on results from small retrospective series. Additional factors such as age and molecular subtype can be considered for these patients.

References

1. Bonadonna G et al (1990) Primary chemotherapy to avoid mastectomy in tumors with diameters of three centimeters or more. J Natl Cancer Inst 82(19):1539–1545
2. Fisher B et al (1997) Effect of preoperative chemotherapy on local-regional disease in women with operable breast cancer: findings from National Surgical Adjuvant Breast and Bowel Project B-18. J Clin Oncol 15(7):2483–2493
3. Early Breast Cancer Trialists' Collaborative, G et al (2011) Effect of radiotherapy after breast-conserving surgery on 10-year recurrence and 15-year breast cancer death: meta-analysis of individual patient data for 10,801 women in 17 randomised trials. Lancet 378 (9804):1707–1716
4. Overgaard M et al (1997) Postoperative radiotherapy in high-risk premenopausal women with breast cancer who receive adjuvant chemotherapy. Danish Breast Cancer Cooperative Group 82b Trial. N Engl J Med 337(14):949–955
5. Overgaard M et al (1999) Postoperative radiotherapy in high-risk postmenopausal breast-cancer patients given adjuvant tamoxifen: Danish Breast Cancer Cooperative Group DBCG 82c randomised trial. Lancet 353(9165):1641–1648

6. Ebctcg et al (2014) Effect of radiotherapy after mastectomy and axillary surgery on 10-year recurrence and 20-year breast cancer mortality: meta-analysis of individual patient data for 8135 women in 22 randomised trials. Lancet 383(9935):2127–2135
7. Mamounas EP et al (2012) Predictors of locoregional recurrence after neoadjuvant chemotherapy: results from combined analysis of National Surgical Adjuvant Breast and Bowel Project B-18 and B-27. J Clin Oncol 30(32):3960–3966
8. Buchholz TA et al (2002) Predictors of local-regional recurrence after neoadjuvant chemotherapy and mastectomy without radiation. J Clin Oncol 20(1):17–23
9. Garg AK et al (2004) T3 disease at presentation or pathologic involvement of four or more lymph nodes predict for locoregional recurrence in stage II breast cancer treated with neoadjuvant chemotherapy and mastectomy without radiotherapy. Int J Radiat Oncol Biol Phys 59(1):138–145
10. Huang EH et al (2004) Postmastectomy radiation improves local-regional control and survival for selected patients with locally advanced breast cancer treated with neoadjuvant chemotherapy and mastectomy. J Clin Oncol 22(23):4691–4699
11. Huang EH et al (2005) Predictors of locoregional recurrence in patients with locally advanced breast cancer treated with neoadjuvant chemotherapy, mastectomy, and radiotherapy. Int J Radiat Oncol Biol Phys 62(2):351–357
12. Nagar H et al (2011) Local-regional recurrence with and without radiation therapy after neoadjuvant chemotherapy and mastectomy for clinically staged T3N0 breast cancer. Int J Radiat Oncol Biol Phys 81(3):782–787
13. Buchholz TA et al (2002) Pathologic tumor size and lymph node status predict for different rates of locoregional recurrence after mastectomy for breast cancer patients treated with neoadjuvant versus adjuvant chemotherapy. Int J Radiat Oncol Biol Phys 53(4):880–888
14. McGuire SE et al (2007) Postmastectomy radiation improves the outcome of patients with locally advanced breast cancer who achieve a pathologic complete response to neoadjuvant chemotherapy. Int J Radiat Oncol Biol Phys 68(4):1004–1009
15. Kuerer HM et al (1999) Clinical course of breast cancer patients with complete pathologic primary tumor and axillary lymph node response to doxorubicin-based neoadjuvant chemotherapy. J Clin Oncol 17(2):460–469
16. von Minckwitz G et al (2012) Definition and impact of pathologic complete response on prognosis after neoadjuvant chemotherapy in various intrinsic breast cancer subtypes. J Clin Oncol 30(15):1796–1804
17. Caudle AS et al (2012) Local-regional control according to surrogate markers of breast cancer subtypes and response to neoadjuvant chemotherapy in breast cancer patients undergoing breast conserving therapy. Breast Cancer Res 14(3):R83
18. Mamounas EP et al (2014) Locoregional recurrence (LRR) after neoadjuvant chemotherapy (NAC): pooled-analysis results from the Collaborative Trials in Neoadjuvant Breast Cancer (CTNeoBC). ASCO Meeting Abstracts. 32(26_suppl): p 61
19. van der Hage JA et al (2001) Preoperative chemotherapy in primary operable breast cancer: results from the European Organization for Research and Treatment of Cancer trial 10902. J Clin Oncol 19(22):4224–4237
20. Rastogi P et al (2008) Preoperative chemotherapy: updates of National Surgical Adjuvant Breast and Bowel Project Protocols B-18 and B-27. J Clin Oncol 26(5):778–785
21. van Nes JG et al (2009) Preoperative chemotherapy is safe in early breast cancer, even after 10 years of follow-up; clinical and translational results from the EORTC trial 10902. Breast Cancer Res Treat 115(1):101–113
22. Chen AM et al (2004) Breast conservation after neoadjuvant chemotherapy: the MD Anderson cancer center experience. J Clin Oncol 22(12):2303–2312
23. Chen AM et al (2005) Breast conservation after neoadjuvant chemotherapy. Cancer 103 (4):689–695
24. Whelan TJ, Olivotto I, Ackerman I, Chapman JW, Chua B, Nabid A, Vallis KA, White JR, Rousseau P, Fortin A, Pierce LJ, Manchul L, Craighead P, Nolan MC, Bowen J, McCready DR,

Pritchard KI, Levine MN, Parulekar W (2011) NCIC-CTG MA.20: an intergroup trial of regional nodal irradiation in early breast cancer. J Clin Oncol 29:p supp 15: p LBA1003
25. Budach W et al (2013) Adjuvant radiotherapy of regional lymph nodes in breast cancer – a meta-analysis of randomized trials. Radiat Oncol 8:267
26. Daveau C et al (2010) Is regional lymph node irradiation necessary in stage II to III breast cancer patients with negative pathologic node status after neoadjuvant chemotherapy? Int J Radiat Oncol Biol Phys 78(2):337–342
27. Noh JM et al (2014) Is elective nodal irradiation beneficial in patients with pathologically negative lymph nodes after neoadjuvant chemotherapy and breast-conserving surgery for clinical stage II-III breast cancer? A multicentre retrospective study (KROG 12-05). Br J Cancer 110(6):1420–1426
28. Shim SJ et al (2014) The role of postmastectomy radiation therapy after neoadjuvant chemotherapy in clinical stage II-III breast cancer patients with pN0: a multicenter, retrospective study (KROG 12-05). Int J Radiat Oncol Biol Phys 88(1):65–72
29. Mamounas EP, White JR, Bandos H, Julian TB, Kahn AJ, Shaitelman SF, Torres MA, McCloskey SA, Vicini FA, Ganz PA, Paik S, Gupta N, Costantino JP, Curran WJ (2014) NSABP B-51/RTOG 1304: randomized phase III clinical trial evaluating the role of postmastectomy chest wall and regional nodal XRT (CWRNRT) and post-lumpectomy RNRT in patients (pts) with documented positive axillary (Ax) nodes before neoadjuvant chemotherapy (NC) who convert to pathologically negative Ax nodes after NC. J Clin Oncol 32:5s
30. Clinicaltrials.gov (2014) Comparison of axillary lymph node dissection with axillary radiation for patients with node-positive breast cancer treated with chemotherapy. [cited 2014 16 Nov]. Available from: http://clinicaltrials.gov/show/NCT01901094

Part IV
Preoperative Hormone Therapy

Chapter 13
Novel Translational Research of Neo-adjuvant Endocrine Therapy

Alexey A. Larionov

Abstract Neo-adjuvant endocrine therapy has an established place in the treatment of post-menopausal oestrogen-receptor positive breast cancers. However, a number of clinical questions still need to be addressed to realise the full potential of the neo-adjuvant endocrine treatment. Thus, there is a shortage of data about direct comparison between endocrine and cytotoxic neo-adjuvant treatments in ER+ve patients. Other questions under investigation include optimal duration of therapy, utility of neo-adjuvant endocrine therapy in pre-menopause, selection between different endocrine agents and predicting and overcoming resistance. The latter attracts most of the translational attention. Significant effort has been directed toward (i) development of response-predictive bio-markers, (ii) understanding molecular diversity of resistance in clinical samples and (iii) development of new treatments targeting the resistance mechanisms (such as combination of m-TOR and aromatase inhibitors). The recent response prediction studies included re-analysis of established molecular markers (ER, PgR, HER2, Ki67) and development of new multi-gene signatures. Some of the transcriptional signatures initially developed for the adjuvant setting are being studied in neo-adjuvant endocrine context (e.g. Oncotype DX). Despite being able to improve response prediction, these signatures still provide limited information about the individual mechanisms of resistance. New analytical methods, new trial designs and new bioinformatics resources are being employed to overcome this limitation and to develop a panel of mechanism-focused tests for guiding future neo-adjuvant endocrine therapies in breast cancer.

Keywords Breast cancer • Endocrine treatment • Neoadjuvant treatment • Response assessment • Response prediction • Biomarkers

A.A. Larionov (✉)
Academic Laboratory of Medical Genetics, School of Clinical Medicine, University of Cambridge, Box 238, Lv 6 Addenbrooske's Treatment Centre, Cambridge BioMedical Campus, Cambridge CB2 0QQ, UK

Statistics and Computational Biology Laboratory, CRUK Cambridge Institute, University of Cambridge, Li Ka Shing Centre, Robinson Way, Cambridge CB2 0RE, UK
e-mail: al720@medschl.cam.ac.uk

M. Toi et al. (eds.), *Personalized Treatment of Breast Cancer*,
DOI 10.1007/978-4-431-55552-0_13

Abbreviations

AI	Aromatase inhibitors
ER	Estrogen receptor
PgR	Progesterone receptor

13.1 Introduction

Neo-adjuvant treatment is indicated for large non-disseminated tumours to shrink them before potentially curative surgery. The reduction of tumour volume may either reduce the volume of surgery or allow mastectomy for previously inoperable tumours [1]. The term "neo-adjuvant" was introduced to distinguish it from the "adjuvant" therapies, which had been used after surgery to delay or prevent relapse [2]. On the other hand, neo-adjuvant treatment should be distinguished from primary systemic treatment of disseminated disease, when there is no possibility for a potentially curative surgery. The main endocrine agents used in neo-adjuvant, adjuvant and disseminated modalities are the same. However, the duration of treatment, response assessment and clinical objectives differ between these settings. Importantly, the biology of large non-disseminated primary tumours (the primary target in neo-adjuvant setting) may differ from biology of both micro- and macro- metastatic disease (which are the primary targets in adjuvant and disseminated settings respectively).

Initial trials of primary endocrine treatment for operable breast cancer were reported in the 1980s, shortly after the introduction of tamoxifen into breast cancer clinics. They were focused on elderly patients (over 70 years old) with the intention of saving these patients from surgery [3]. Twenty-year follow-ups have recently been reported for these studies [4, 5]. The analysis showed that the addition of surgery to tamoxifen in elderly patients does not improve overall survival. However, it has also been shown that primary endocrine treatment could not substitute surgery in operable patients for local control. The hazard ratio (HR) for progression-free survival in operable elderly patients favoured surgery over tamoxifen (HR $= 0.55$, $p = 0.0006$, 95 % CI 0.39–0.77), as well as addition of surgery to primary tamoxifen (HR $= 0.65$, $p = 0.0001$, 95 % CI 0.53–0.81) [6, 7]. Thus the focus shifted towards combination of primary endocrine treatments with surgery when shrinkage of tumour was desirable to improve surgical outcomes [1]. At the same time, it should be noted that neo-adjuvant treatment may also be considered as the earliest opportunity to restrain the occult micro-lesions, in addition to the main effects on the primary tumour [2].

In parallel to the clinical benefits, it was recognised early that neo-adjuvant setting provides a unique model to study tumour biology and response to endocrine treatment [8]. The large size of primary tumours allows for sequential biopsies during neo-adjuvant treatment. Coupled with modern methods of molecular analysis, this provides an opportunity to study biology and changes in individual tumours during treatment [9, 10]. In turn, the neo-adjuvant research informs new clinical approaches by devélopment of biomarkers for response prediction [11, 12] and personalised classification of tumours [13] and by suggesting rational targets to prevent or overcome resistance to endocrine treatment [14]. This chapter will review recent findings in translational research relating them to clinical challenges in neo-adjuvant endocrine treatment of breast cancer.

13.2 Hormonal vs Cytotoxic Treatment in Neo-adjuvant Setting

Endocrine treatment is not the only possible neo-adjuvant option in breast cancer. The other common alternatives include cytotoxic chemotherapy and HER2-targeting agents. It has been shown that HER2-positivity requires inclusion of HER2-targeting agents [15, 16], and ER-negativity excludes the use of endocrine treatment. In contrast, there is no definitive evidence supporting a choice between cytotoxic and endocrine neo-adjuvant treatment in ER-positive patients.

The field was initially shaped by numerous neo-adjuvant trials, which compared different cytotoxic regimens between each other. These trials established pathological complete response (pCR) as a surrogate end-point [17] and reported typical cytotoxic pCR response rates in a range 10–30 % [18]. At the same time, typical pCR rates reported for neo-adjuvant endocrine treatments ranged from 0 to 10 % [19]. This put into question the efficiency of neo-adjuvant endocrine treatments, suggesting that it should be used only when side effects of cytotoxic treatments are not acceptable. However, such indirect comparison may be flawed because (i) it does not take into account ER-status of patients, (ii) it assumes that pCR has prognostic value in endocrine treatment and (iii) it ignores that the initial endocrine neo-adjuvant studies often used sub-optimal duration and drug selection. In fact, the high pCR rates of cytotoxic treatments are mainly limited to ER-negative tumours [20–23], pCR is not prognostic in ER+ve tumours [24] and is not recommended for response assessment in endocrine treatments [17]. Furthermore, the extention of neo-adjuvant endocrine treatment beyond the initially practiced 3–4 month may improve the pCR response rates up to 17 % [25]. A direct trial with adequate treatment duration and response assessment is still needed to compare the efficacy of cytotoxic and endocrine neo-adjuvant treatment for ER+ve patients.

To date, there are only three reports about randomised comparison of neo-adjuvant endocrine and cytotoxic treatments in ER+ve patients [26–28] (Table 13.1). These studies are relatively small. The biggest of them randomised 239 postmenopausal patients with large non-disseminated (T2-4, N0-2, M0) non-treated tumours between endocrine (3 months of anastrozole or exemestane) and cytotoxic (a standard antracycline-containing regimen followed by taxanes) arms [27]. There was no difference in clinical response rates (64 % of clinical responses were reported for both arms), pCR was detected in 3 % and 6 %,

Table 13.1 Studies directly comparing efficacy of neo-adjuvant Endocrine and Cytotoxic treatments in breast cancer

Trial, number and reproductive status of patients	Endocrine treatment	Cytotoxic treatment	Results
Semiglazov [27] $n = 239$ Post-menopausal Randomised	Anastrazole or Exemestane for 3 months	Doxorubicin and Paclitaxel	No statistically significant differences in clinical response rates (64 % in both arms) and in pCR rates (3 % in endocrine and 6 % in cytotoxic arm) Numeric trend to better conservation rates in endocrine arm (33 % vs 24 %, $p = 0.06$)
Alba [26] $n = 95$ Pre- ($n = 51$) and post-menopausal ($n = 44$) Randomised	Exemestane (plus goserelin in pre-menopause) for 6 months	Epirubicin plus Cyclophosphamide followed by Docetaxel	*All patients*: no statistically significant differences in clinical response rates, numeric trend favouring cytotoxic treatment (objective response rates 66 % and 48 %, $p = 0.08$) *Pre-menopausal patients*: superiority of cytotoxic treatment (75 % vs 44 %, $p = 0.027$), *Post-menopausal patients*: no difference in response rates (57 % vs 52 %, $p = 0.78$)
Palmiery [28] $n = 44$ Post-menopausal Randomised	Letrozole 4–6 months	Fluorouracil, Epirubicin and Cyclophosphamide with optional switch to Docetaxel	NEOCENT trial, stopped because of the low accrual; radiological response: 54.5 % in the cytotoxic arm vs 59.1 % in the letrozole arm; the low sample size precluded a statistical inference
Thomas [29] $n = 103$ Non-randomised Retrospective	Letrozole 3 months	Non-specified	Non-balanced by age, ER, reproductive status and other clinical parameters Higher pCR rates in cytotoxic group (18 % vs 1.9 %, $p = 0.007$) No differences in clinical response rates (89 vs 85 %, $p = 0.8$)

respectively. A tendency to a better conservation rates in the endocrine arm has been observed (33 % vs 24 %, $p = 0.06$). The second randomised neo-adjuvant trial enrolled 95 patients to compare cytotoxic treatment (epirubicin plus cyclophosphamide followed by docetaxel) with exemestane [26]. Importantly, the authors enrolled both pre- and post-menopausal patients (combining exemestane with goserelin in the premenopause). Overall, there was no statistically significant difference between the arms; however, the authors highlighted a numerical trend favouring cytotoxic treatment (objective response rates 66 % and 48 %, $p = 0.08$). A sub-group analysis showed that the superiority of cytotoxic treatment was limited to pre-menopausal patients (75 % vs 44 %, $p = 0.027$), while in post menopause the response rates were virtually identical (57 % vs 52 %, $p = 0.78$). The third trial randomised 44 patients and stopped because of the low accrual [28]. Objective radiological response was reported as 54.5 % in the cytotoxic arm and as 59.1 % in the letrozole arm; the low sample size precluded a statistical inference. One non-randomised retrospective comparison reported similar clinical response rates in post-menopausal endocrine and cytotocic neo-adjuvant treatment (53 vs 50 patients, respectively; clinical response rates 89 % vs 85 %, $p = 0.8$) and superiority of the cytotoxic treatment in achieving pathological response (18 % vs 1.9 %, $p = 0.007$) [29]. However, this comparison was retrospective and unbalanced by age, reproductive status, ER, tumour sizes and other clinical parameters. No other studies have been reported so far to directly compare efficacy of endocrine and cytotoxic treatments in a neo-adjuvant setting [30]. Given the evidence available to date it could be suggested that the efficacy of neo-adjuvant endocrine treatment in ER-positive tumours is not inferior to cytotoxic chemotherapy, especially in ER-rich low-grade post-menopausal tumours [31]. At the same time, endocrine treatment allows to save ER+ve patients of the toxicity associated with cytotoxic agents.

The side effects of cytotoxic therapies limit their use in breast cancer for a large proportion of breast cancer patients. Thus, cytotoxic treatment is used in less than 3 % of patients older than 70 years [32]. Importantly, these elderly patients constitute more than 30 % of all breast cancers [33]. The cytotoxic agents typically used for neo-adjuvant breast cancer treatment include antracyclines, mitotic poisons (taxanes), antimetabolites (antifolites and pyrimidine analogues) and cross-linking agents (such as cyclophosphamide and platinum-containing compounds). Their side effects are frequent and may reach life-threatening levels [34]. Cardiotoxicity is most severe in antracyclines, which are the major component in most neo-adjuvant cytotoxic regimens used in breast cancer. Myelosuppression is observed in virtually all cytotoxic agents. It is quite common (up to 20–30 % in some regimens) and severe (up to febrile neutropenia). Gastrointestinal toxicity includes stomatitis (up to 10–15 % in some regimens) and diarrhoea. The latter is most common in combinations of antimetabolites with cross-linking agents (up to 5 %) and may be life-threatening. Nausea, vomiting and alopecia are common in most of the cytotoxic agents too. Such a combination of side effects, including the life-threatening ones, applies strict limitations for the use of cytotoxic agents in patients after 60, which is the majority of ER+ve breast cancers. None of these severe adverse effects are observed in endocrine treatments.

Another group of common side effects of cytotoxic agents include damage to the ovaries, which is especially characteristic for DNA-cross-linking agents [34–38]. Damage to the ovaries is reported in up to 70–80 % of patients treated with regimens that include cross-linking agents and antimetabolites. These cytotoxic drugs are designed to cause DNA damage in tumour cells, which may affect ovaries and oocytes along with the tumour, introducing a risk of long-term effects to fertility and genetic defects in children, which may be of concern for younger patients. Again, none of the endocrine agents cause irreversible damage to fertility. Moreover, GnRH agonists were suggested for fertility preservation in pre-menopausal patients undergoing cytotoxic treatments [39, 40], although their effectiveness is yet to be confirmed [37, 38, 41].

Adverse effects commonly reported for endocrine agents in the neo-adjuvant setting include hot flashes, arthralgia, myalgia, stiffness, fatigue, night sweats, nausea and headaches [1, 14, 27, 42–46]. Many studies highlight good tolerability of endocrine treatment with up to 95 % of treatment-related adverse events being mild (grade 1 or 2). These side effects are similar to ones reported for the adjuvant endocrine setting. However, a short duration of the neo-adjuvant treatment prevents development of other adverse effects, which could be observed in the long-term endocrine treatments (increased risk of cardio-vascular events, fractures, venous thrombosis or endometrial carcinoma) [47].

The comparison of side effects between cytotoxic and endocrine treatments makes it clear that, independently of the future outcome of direct comparison of their efficacy, neo-adjuvant endocrine treatment will be indicated to many breast cancer patients. Contrary to the common belief, the available evidence does not preclude a simultaneous administration of cytotoxic and endocrine drugs; however, the preliminary reports suggest that such combination may have efficacy similar to either of the therapies alone [48–51].

13.3 Clinical Context of Translational Studies in Neo-adjuvant Endocrine Treatment

Clinical context is very important for design and interpretation of translational studies. The key clinical aspects that should be considered when reviewing neo-adjuvant endocrine studies in breast cancer include (i) response assessment, (ii) differences between endocrine agents, (iii) duration of treatment and (iv) reproductive status of patients.

13.3.1 Response Assessment

There are multiple approaches to response assessment of breast cancer in the neo-adjuvant setting. Different studies report responses based on measurement of clinical, pathological, proliferative or molecular changes [52]. This may significantly influence the numerical representation of response rates and complicate comparison between studies [30, 53].

13.3.1.1 Clinical Response

Clinical response assessment is based on measuring the size and spread of the tumour. This approach is implemented in RECIST and WHO criteria, which categorise patients to complete, partial responders, and those having a stable or progressive disease [54, 55]. While setting the important reference framework, this categorisation may lack the sensitivity needed in translational research. Specifically, the stable disease category includes any response ranging from 50 % tumour reduction to 25 % tumour growth. While being meaningful for clinical purposes, this broad grouping may ignore important biological differences substantial in translational studies. Reporting and analysing actual tumour sizes may provide better resolution required for translational purposes. Several methods are used to measure tumour size including callipers, mammography and ultrasound [30, 56]. Calliper measurement is the simplest, but most subjective and least accurate method. Mammography provides an objective record; however, it is two-dimensional. Also, compression of mamma during mammography may influence response assessment, if the tumour responds by softening, rather than shrinking. CT and MRI provide the most accurate three-dimensional measurements and provide an objective record. However, these methods are expensive and they are not used in routine clinical practice. Therefore ultrasound is emerging as a balanced practical method of choice: it is simple, allows three-dimensional measurements and provides an accurate record, especially if measurements before and after treatment are taken by the same operator. It has been shown that ultrasound better reflects pathological size detected during the surgery than calliper or mammography [57]. In addition, the ultrasound can easily be performed many times during the neo-adjuvant course, allowing for dynamic interim measurements of tumour volume.

13.3.1.2 Pathological Response

Neo-adjuvant treatment provides a unique opportunity to have a sequential pathological assessment of tumour during treatment. This is an important part of many neo-adjuvant translational studies [9, 29, 52]. Complete disappearance of tumour cells on pathological sections in tumour and lymph nodes (pCR) has been intensively studied in the cytotoxic neo-adjuvant context because of its prognostic value in ER-ve tumours [17, 18]. However, pCR assessment is less relevant to endocrine treatment because it is rarely detected in this treatment modality and it is not prognostic in ER+ve tumours [19, 24, 58]. Importantly, pathological changes during treatment are not limited by reduction of tumour cellularity. Thus, ~80 % of breast cancers display substantial morphological changes after 3 months of neo-adjuvant letrozole [29]. Along with significant reduction in tumour cellularity endocrine treatment tends to cause development of connective tissue at the centre of tumour. This has been described as a "central scar", which may occupy up to 30 % of tumour volume after the treatment. Formation of "central scar" is associated with total reduction in tumour volume. Cytotoxic therapy may also cause connective tissue rearrangement; however, in contrast to the endocrine treatment, it tends to be scattered, rather than centrally located [29]. Of the other commonly assessed pathological features it may be noted that neo-adjuvant treatment showed inconsistent effects on the expression of estrogen receptors, with stronger downregulation by tamoxifen than by AIs. In contrast, letrozole has been more effective than tamoxifen in reducing the expression of progesterone receptors [9]. The clinical relevance of changes in the expression of steroid receptors is not clear.

13.3.1.3 Proliferative Response

Reduction in proliferation has been established as the most clinically relevant pathological change detected during neo-adjuvant endocrine treatment. Multiple markers may reflect proliferation in breast cancer, including grade, mitotic count, S-phase fraction, PCNA, PHH3, thymidine or bromodeoxyuridine labelling index and some others [59–62]. Of them Ki 67 has been most widely accepted and becoming de-facto standard method for proliferation measurement in clinical specimens [63–65].

Ki67 was discovered about 30 years ago as a nuclear antigen expressed in proliferating lymphocytes [66]. Its expression is restricted to G1-S-G2-M phases of the cell cycle and Ki67 is not detectable in resting cells entering G0 [67–69]. The exact function of Ki67 in the cell is still poorly understood [70–72]. It is a large protein (>350 Kda) interacting with chromatin and forkhead-associated domains of other proteins [73, 74]. It can be phosphorylated [75]. It is associated with nucleoli, ribosome formation and protein biosynthesis [76, 77]. Because of its involvement in proliferation and protein biosynthesis, it has been even considered as a potential target for treatment [78]. Several antibodies have been developed to detect this Ki67 antigen; therefore in some studies it may be referred as MIB1 [79].

The earliest changes of Ki67 in a neo-adjuvant endocrine trial have been reported after 2–4 days of treatment [28]. However, most of the studies measure early changes of Ki67 after 2 weeks of treatment to allow sufficient time for proliferation to stop. This early Ki67 reduction is predictive of neo-adjuvant clinical response and is associated with prognosis in the adjuvant setting [80–82]. Residual post-neo-adjuvant Ki67 is also used for adjuvant prognosis

[11]. Interestingly, Ki67 changes in relatively small neo-adjuvant studies may be informative for planning of larger adjuvant trials. Thus, proliferative responses in the IMPACT trial showed higher efficiency of arimidex than tamoxifen or combination, which predicted the outcome of the ATAC trial [83–85]. Importantly, the neo-adjuvant design of the IMPACT study required only 330 patients, while the adjuvant ATAC trial needed 9366 participants.

Overall, the important role of proliferation in the biology of endocrine response and the well-documented association of Ki67 with prognosis and response to endocrine treatment suggested using Ki67 as a surrogate end-point in endocrine neo-adjuvant treatment resembling the use of pCR in cytotoxic studies [63, 65].

13.3.2 Comparison of Endocrine Agents

A series of trials established superiority of AIs over tamoxifen in all treatment settings in breast cancer [86, 87]. The key studies comparing AIs with tamoxifen in the neo-adjuvant setting included PO24, IMPACT and PROACT trials. PO24 trial compared neo-adjuvant tamoxifen with letrozole. The trial included patients non-suitable for breast conserving surgery before treatment. The end-points included clinical response and percent of breast conserving surgery after 4 months of treatment. In both end-points letrozole showed significantly better results, with 55 % vs 36 % of clinical responses ($p < 0.001$) and 45 % vs 35 % of breast conservation rate ($p = 0.022$) [42]. IMPACT and PROACT trials compared tamoxifen with anastrozole [88, 89]. In both trials, anastrozole showed no significant improvement in objective response. However, in PROACT trial anastrozole achieved better breast conservation rates (43.0 % vs 30.8 %, $p = 0.04$), and in IMPACT trial anastrazole showed significantly better proliferative response than tamoxifen (93 % vs 85 %, [83]). A meta-analysis of trials involving 1160 patients confirmed that preoperative AIs show superiority over tamoxifen in breast conserving surgery rate (relative risk 1.36, $p < 0.001$) and in objective responses detected either clinically or by ultrasound (relative risks 1.29, $p = 0.002$) [90].

Comparison between different aromatase inhibitors showed little difference in their neo-adjuvant clinical efficacy, with a possibility of a non-significant trend in favour of letrozole. There is experimental evidence suggesting that letrozole is more effective than other AIs in suppression of blood estrogens in breast cancer patients [91–94] with possible clinical implications in the advanced setting [95]. However, this translated to very subtle, if any, difference in the pre-operative treatment. Thus, ACOSOG Z1031 trial directly compared letrozole, anasrtozole and exemestane in the neo-adjuvant setting [43]. No differences were found between treatment arms with respect to proliferative responses measured by Ki67; although the numerical trend favoured the Ki67 response to letrozole. This numerical trend was also evident in the clinical response rates, reaching formal significance between letrozole and exemestane (95 % CI for difference in clinical response 0.5–23.3). The authors concluded that each AI markedly improved surgical outcomes and biomarker data suggested their biological equivalency.

The neo-adjuvant setting has been successfully used for establishing an adequate dose of fulvestrant in breast cancer. A phase II neo-adjuvant NEWEST study demonstrated that increasing fulvestrant's dose from 250 to 500 mg significantly reduces the residual proliferation [96]. Another pre-operative study even explored a further dose increase to 750 mg [46]. Experimental data on xenograft models suggested that combining fulvestrant with anastrozole may prevent the development of endocrine resistance [97]. This was consistent with some trials combining fulvestrant with anastrozole in the advanced setting (FIRST and SWOG-0226 trials) [98, 99]. However, a similar pre-operative study showed no difference in Ki67 reduction between the arms [100]. Overall, the available evidence suggests that fulvestrant may be at least as effective as anastrozole in the pre-operative setting. However, the use of fulvestrant in the pre-operative setting is still experimental.

13.3.3 Duration of Treatment

Historically, most neo-adjuvant endocrine studies tested 3–4 months of pre-operative treatment [30]. At the same time, accumulating evidence suggest that longer treatment might be better for most of the patients. Dixon with co-authors reported a study on 63 patients treated with neo-adjuvant letrozole in the Edinburgh Breast Unit. The average tumour volume reduction at 3 months was 52 %, with further reduction by 50 %, 37 % and 33 % at 6, 9 and 12 month of treatment, respectively [101]. Similarly, Allevi et al. compared 4, 8 and 12 months of pre-operative letrozole (40 patients in each group). Both clinical and pathological response rates significantly rose along with the duration of treatment: the clinical response rates were 12.5 %, 42.1 % and 57.5 % (p for trend <0.001) and the pCR rates were 2.5 %, 5 % and 17.5 % (p for trend 0.04) at 4, 8 and 12 months, respectively [25]. Another study on 32 patients also reported improved response rates when extending pre-operative letrozole from 4 to 8 months [102]. At the same time, the authors highlighted that most of the patients had become eligible for breast conservation after the initial 4 months of treatment, suggesting that further extension is indicated only on individual basis. This was consistent with the study on 56 patients treated with preoperative letrozole, which reported median time to objective response at 3.9 months (95 % CI 3.3–4.5), median time to maximal response at 4.2 months (95 % CI 4.0–4.5) and 37 % of patients achieving the maximal response after 6 months [103]. Importantly, patients on the extended treatment have to be carefully monitored because a small number of tumours may progress during the extension. For instance, 4 out of 116 patients treated with pre-operative exemestane progressed within the initial 4 months of treatment and 3 more patients progressed between 4 and 8 months; at the same time, 14 patients have achieved further tumour reduction during the treatment extension

[104]. Despite the relatively small sizes of the cited studies, the results are highly consistent. Thus, the emerging consensus with regard to neo-adjuvant endocrine treatment is that "If used, such treatment should be considered for a duration of 5–8 months or until maximum tumour response" [105].

13.3.4 Neo-adjuvant Endocrine Treatment in Pre-menopause

Reports about neo-adjuvant endocrine treatment in pre-menopause are scarce. Historically, neo-adjuvant endocrine treatment was avoided in pre-menopausal patients because the younger patients can tolerate the cytotoxic treatments, which showed good pCR rates. However, some young patients with ER+ve tumours may inquire about the possibility of endocrine alternatives because of the ovarian toxicity of cytotoxic drugs [37]. By analogy with the adjuvant and advanced settings, a combination of tamoxifen or anastrozole with goserelin has been explored by Masuda et al. in a neo-adjuvant pre-menopausal trial [45]. Expectedly, anastrozole showed superiority over tamoxifen (clinical response rates 70 % and 50 %, respectively; $p = 0.004$). Similar response rates have been shown by another trial for combination of letrozole with GnRH analogue [106].

As mentioned earlier, the only evidence to compare efficiency of cytotoxic and endocrine treatments in pre-menopause is available from a sub-analysis in a relatively small randomised trial [26]. This sub-analysis included 24 patients received epirubicin plus cyclophosphamide followed by docetaxel and 27 patients received exemestane plus goserilin for 6 months. The results showed the clear superiority of cytotoxic treatment: the objective response rates measured by MRI were 75 % (18/24) and 44 % (12/27) respectively, $p = 0.027$. While this result requires caution with regard to neo-adjuvant endocrine treatment in pre-menopause, it still awaits an independent confirmation. For instance, as discussed above, letrozole could show marginally better clinical response than exemestane in the neo-adjuvant setting [43]. Importantly, the study of Alba with co-authors [26] confirmed that, despite the potential overall inferiority to cytotoxics, a significant proportion of pre-menopausal patients with ER+ve tumours respond to endocrine treatment. This is consistent with the sited above studies, which showed the response rates in a range 50–70 % [45, 106]. Therefore, a biomarker-guided neo-adjuvant endocrine treatment may still be a viable choice in the future for some younger ER+ve patients willing to avoid risks to fertility.

13.4 Predicting Response and Outcome

The neo-adjuvant setting provides a unique opportunity to study markers and mechanisms of endocrine response and resistance in human breast tumours [8, 107]. Molecular analysis of sequential tumour biopsies taken during treatment has been successfully employed to study molecular changes caused by treatment [10, 52, 108], to predict neo-adjuvant response [12, 109] and to utilise data about neo-adjuvant response for optimising post-operative treatments [11, 110, 111].

13.4.1 Routinely Assessed Biomarkers

The biomarkers routinely assessed in breast cancer clinic include ER, PgR and HER2. Estrogen receptor is the main target and marker of endocrine treatment in breast cancer. No ER-ve tumours benefit from the treatment, while the majority of ER+ve do [112]. Several thresholds have been suggested for oestrogen-receptor positivity [113]. Of them, the 1 % threshold is most commonly used, assuming that patients may benefit from endocrine treatment if the tumour contains as little as 1 % of ER+ve cells [114, 115]. Along with the binary categorisation, routine pathological assessment can provide a semi-quantitative score. The most commonly used scoring system for semi-quantitative ER assessment in breast cancer is the Allred score, which splits tumours into eight categories according to the fraction of ER+ve cells and the intensity of staining. Scores 0 and 1 correspond to ER-ve tumours, and a score of 8 means that 100 % of tumour cells show strong ER expression [114]. A significant positive association between neo-adjuvant response and ER abundance have been observed for both tamoxifen and letrozole in P024 study [116]. IMPACT trial (anastrazole vs tamoxifene or combination) confirmed the association; however, it was confined to the combination arm only [89]. Importantly, this association is not absolute: despite the lower overall response rates in ER-poor tumours, many such tumours may still respond to neo-adjuvant endocrine treatment, especially to treatment with aromatase inhibitors. Data about the predictive utility of PgR are inconclusive: IMPACT study reported a positive association of PgR expression with proliferative response [83], while P024 reported no linear association of PgR expression with clinical response. Numerous experimental and clinical observations indicate that HER2-positivity may predispose for endocrine resistance in breast cancer [117]. However, in the same way as for the ER-poor and PgR-negative tumours, HER2-positivity does not preclude endocrine responses in many individual patients [116]. Taken together, these studies suggest that routinely assessed markers are not sufficient for accurate prediction of neo-adjuvant endocrine response within ER+ve patients. Therefore, a significant effort has been directed over the last decade to develop novel multigene biomarkers to predict response in the neo-adjuvant endocrine setting.

13.4.2 Multi-gene Signatures

Development of microarray technology enabled obtaining of genome-wide transcriptional profiles in clinical biopsies of breast cancer. A large number of studies have related these gene expression patterns to various phenotypic features.

13.4.2.1 Intrinsic Subtypes

In 2000, Perou and Sorlie with co-authors employed microarray technology to suggest the first clinically relevant multigene signature in breast cancer. The signature allowed separating breast tumours into five biologically distinctive groups: Luminal A and B, Basal-, Her2- and normal-like intrinsic subtypes of breast cancer [118, 119]. Overall, the intrinsic subtypes were broadly equivalent to the pathological classification used at the time (namely: ER+ve, ER-ve, HER2+ve and triple-negative tumours). At the same time, importantly for endocrine treatment, Perou and Sorlie subdivided ER+ve tumours into two sub-types: Luminal A and Luminal B.

Multiple later analyses highlighted the importance of proliferative component in separating luminal A and B tumours [120]. Addition of Ki67 to the standard clinical markers (ER, PgR and HER2) provided a practically convenient way to integrate intrinsic sub-types classification to the routine clinical practice [20, 121]. Alternatively, the PAM50 classification algorithm can be used to classify tumours using microarray data [122].

Initial studies of the intrinsic sub-types had been conducted in the adjuvant setting. However, because the PAM50 signature incorporates oestrogen-receptor and proliferation-associated genes, it could be expected to be informative for the neo-adjuvant endocrine setting too. This has been tested in a recent study by Dunbier with co-authors [123]. Somewhat counterintuitively, many of the studied ER+ve tumours showed biological features consistent with non-luminal intrinsic sub-types. Thus, of the 104 studied ER+ve tumours 36 % were classified as luminal A, 19 % as luminal B, 29 % as normal, 12 % as HER2 and 5 % as basal phenotype. Surprisingly, the highest proliferative response was observed in the normal-like subtype (83 % Ki67 suppression). Similar proliferative response was observed in luminal A and B tumours (75 % mean Ki67 suppression in both groups). As expected HER2 and basal phenotypes showed the lowest response rates (50 % and 15 % of Ki67 suppression, respectively). Because of unexpectedly high proportion of normal-like tumours and their high response to treatment an independent confirmation of these results is needed, possibly utilising different methods to detect the intrinsic sub-types (the study only used the PAM50 classifier). At the same time, the study highlights that a small proportion of ER+ve tumours may be biology similar to the basal intrinsic subtype despite the presence of oestrogen receptors. If confirmed, such tumours may be considered as candidates for exclusion from neo-adjuvant endocrine treatments.

13.4.2.2 Oncotype Dx

Oncotype Dx is a quantitative PCR test that measures the expression of 21 genes in paraffin-embedded samples of breast cancer. The gene list include five proliferation genes (Ki67, STK15, Survivin, CCNB1, MYBL2), four estrogen-related genes (ER, PgR, BCL2, SCUBE2), two HER2-related genes (HER2 and GRB7), two invasion-related genes (MMP11 and CTSL2), three additional genes (GSTM1, CD68, BAG1) and five reference genes (ACTB, GAPDH, RPLP0, GUS, TRFC) [124]. To date, this is the most thoroughly validated prognostic multi-gene test in breast cancer [125]. Its main clinical utility is to detect patients with a good prognosis, which do not need adjuvant cytotoxic chemotherapy after surgery [126, 127].

A recent study of Ueno et al. [109] has demonstrated that Oncotype Dx can be used to improve response prediction in the endocrine neo-adjuvant setting. The study showed that clinical responses and rates of conservation were much higher in low RS group than in the high RS group, as defined by Oncotype Dx (59.4 % vs 20.0 %, $p = 0.015$ for clinical responses and 90.6 % vs 46.7 %, $p = 0.028$ for the conservation rates). This is consistent with the results in adjuvant studies and with the biology behind the gene list. At the same time, because the gene list is closely related to the conventional clinical markers, it has been questioned how much of additional information is provided by Oncotype Dx to what is available from a routine quantitative assessment of ER and HER2 [128, 129].

13.4.2.3 Adjuvant Signatures of Endocrine Response

While the intrinsic sub-types and Oncotype Dx can provide additional information about endocrine responsiveness, they were not initially developed for this purpose. Multi-gene tests specifically focused on endocrine treatment include SET and EndoPredict signatures. So far both of these tests were validated for the adjuvant setting. However, it is reasonable to expect that in the near future they may be tested for neo-adjuvant setting too.

Development of the SET (Sensitivity to Endocrine Therapy) index was based on the hypothesis that expression of the oestrogen-related genes may better reflect functional activity of oestrogen signalling than the expression of ER itself [130]. The signature includes 165 genes. Importantly, the authors attempted to avoid proliferation-related genes to minimise the prognostic component of the signature. It has been shown that low SET index is associated with low ER expression [131], suggesting that it may also be associated with low neo-adjuvant endocrine response.

The EndoPredict test has been designed to assess prognosis in ER+ve HER2-negative tumours [132]. The test is based on quantitative PCR measurement of eight prognostic genes (BIRC5, UBE2C, DHCR7, RBBP8, IL6ST, AZGP1, MGP and STC2) normalised by three reference genes (CALM2, OAZ1 and RPL37A). It may be analysed together with tumour size and node status. It is the only multi-gene breast cancer test, except for Oncotype Dx, which has reached Level 1 of evidence for prognosis in ER+ve tumours [125]. Importantly, in contrast to Oncotype Dx, EndoPredict is focused on HER2-negative tumours and can be performed in a de-centralised manner. Like the SET test, EndoPredict has not yet been assessed in the neo-adjuvant setting.

13.4.2.4 Transcriptional Profiling of Neo-adjuvant Endocrine Treatment

A number of studies have performed whole-genome molecular profiling directly in the endocrine neo-adjuvant setting. The studies reported biological changes associated with endocrine treatment, elucidated mechanisms of response and resistance and suggested several signatures associated with response (although none of these signatures have yet been developed into a clinically validated test).

A series of studies conducted in Royal Marsden Hospital in London related transcriptional profiles to the proliferative response. McKay with co-authors reported that 2 weeks of treatment with letrozole caused changes in the expression of classical oestrogen-regulated genes, proliferation and stromal remodelling genes [133]. Recently, Dunbier et al. reported that early changes in a set of immune-related genes may be associated with changes in proliferation measured by Ki67 [134]. Potentially, these findings may be extrapolated to clinical response because the early changes in Ki67 are predictive to tumour shrinkage at 3 months [80].

The studies performed in Edinburgh Breast Research Unit directly related dynamic tumour molecular profiles to neo-adjuvant clinical response. Sequential frozen biopsies have been collected before, early on treatment and after treatment with letrozole (Fig. 13.1A). The tumours' volumes were measured by 3D ultrasound. The molecular profiles were analysed to identify what genes and pathways change during treatment [10] and which of them are predictive to clinical response [12]. A sub-analysis of non-responding tumours has been conducted to understand the diversity of resistance and to personalise strategies of tackling the resistance [135]. These studies confirmed that reduction in proliferation is the most prominent molecular change after 2 weeks of treatment (Fig. 13.1B). For the first time, it has been shown that early changes in genes encoding ribosomal proteins are strongly predictive of the clinical response (Fig. 13.1C) and that reduction in oxidative phosphorylation takes place after 3 month of treatment. Of the up-regulated pathways, it has been shown that post-treatment tumours exhibit features associated with epithelial-mesenchymal transition and stemness [136]. Other upregulated biological functions were associated with extracellular matrix rearrangement, local immune response and tumour-stroma interaction. Basing on these studies, the Edinburgh Breast Group has recently developed a four-genes test to predict neo-adjuvant response to letrozole [137]. Another recent study reported a multi-gene signature to select patients who benefit most from neo-adjuvant fulvestrant [138]. In contrast to some well-developed adjuvant multi-gene tests (such as

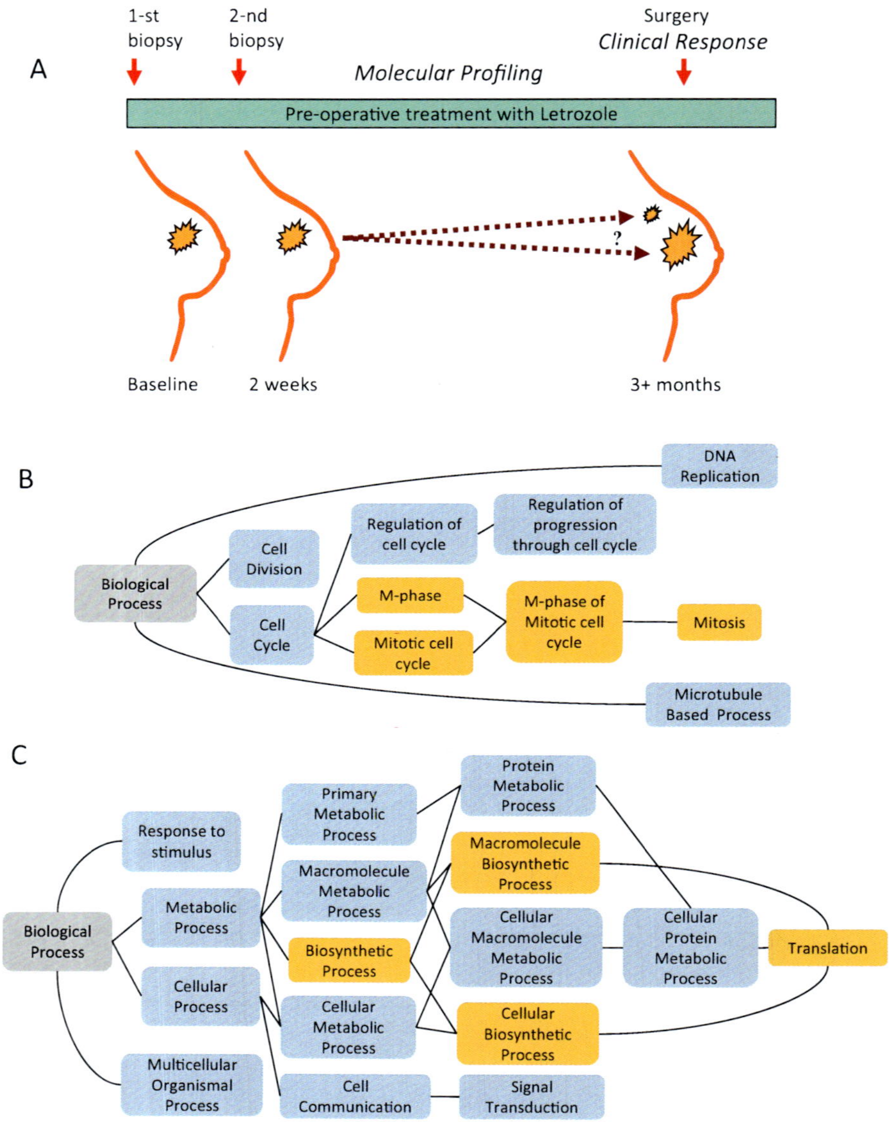

Fig. 13.1 Identifying molecular changes and predictive markers in a neo-adjuvant endocrine study. (**a**) Study design. Endocrine treatment was given for 3 months. Tumour size was monitored by ultrasound. Frozen biopsies were taken before therapy, after 2 weeks of treatment and at surgery (3+ months on treatment). Molecular profiles and their changes during treatment correlated with clinical response (Modified from [10, 12]). (**b**) Biological processes down-regulated after 2 weeks of treatment. (**c**) Biological processes, which changes after 2 weeks of treatment, are most predictive for response. Panels (**b**) and (**c**) show directed acyclic graphs for enriched Gene Ontology terms. Significantly enriched terms are highlighted in orange (Modified from [10, 12, 135])

OncotypeDx and EndoPredict), the currently suggested neo-adjuvant signatures are yet at early stages of development, reaching, at best, Level 2 of evidence [139].

13.4.3 *Using Neo-adjuvant Response to Guide Adjuvant Therapy*

Results of neo-adjuvant endocrine treatment may provide useful information to plan the post-operative adjuvant treatment. Similar to the cytotoxic drugs, good endocrine response in neo-adjuvant setting is associated with good prognosis after surgery [140, 141]. This allowed development of the Preoperative Endocrine Prognostic Index (PEPI) using data generated in P024 trial [11]. The design of PEPI was inspired by a point system utilised in cardiovascular clinic to predict outcomes for myocardial infarction. PEPI points are assigned for post-treatment tumour size, node status, ER and Ki67 levels. Each category can score from 0 to 3 points. Independent validation using data from the IMPACT study confirmed that low PEPI score can be used to select patients with an excellent prognosis, who may not need chemo-therapy after surgery. Therefore, the intended clinical utility of PEPI is similar to the Oncotype Dx or EndoPredict tests. What makes PEPI different is that this index incorporates information about the neo-adjuvant response, rather than rely solely on the pre-treatment features. A similar approach is being tested by a phase III multicentre Japanese trial (NEOS) which is evaluating whether a good neo-adjuvant response to letrozole can be used to select patients that do not need adjuvant cytotoxic chemotherapy after surgery [111].

13.5 Future Perspectives

Exciting new directions emerging in neo-adjuvant endocrine translational research include combining endocrine treatment with other targeted agents, employing novel multidrug adaptive trial designs, improving monitoring during treatment and adopting new research tools and bioinformatics resources.

13.5.1 *Targeted Treatments and New Trial Designs*

An example of successful combination of neo-adjuvant endocrine treatment with a new targeted agent has been reported by Baselga et al. [14]. They tested the effect of adding mTOR inhibitor everolimus to neo-adjuvant letrozole. Two hundred seventy postmenopausal ER+ve patients were randomised to letrozole + placebo or everolimus. The everolimus arm demonstrated significantly better anti-proliferative response (Ki67 reduction: 57 vs 30 %, $p < 0.01$) and a strong numerical trend toward better clinical response rate (68.1 % vs 59.1 %, $p = 0.062$). The improved efficacy was accompanied by a significantly higher rate of serious (grade 3 and 4) adverse effects (22.6 % vs 3.8 % in everolimus and placebo arms respectively). The trial incorporated an extensive biomarker analysis, including sequencing of PI3KCA and P53 genes, assessment of phospho-S6, cyclin D1, Ki67 and the routine biomarkers (ER and PgR). The patients with mutations in exon 9 of PIK3CA gene showed higher benefit from the addition of everolimus. Importantly, the study suggested that in the absence of everolimus this mutation may confer reduction of the anti-proliferative response to letrozole and a poor long-term outcome. This finding emphasises molecular diversity within breast cancers and illustrates the importance of companion-biomarkers for new drug combinations.

Because of the diversity of molecular features between individual patients, it may not be feasible to design trials focused solely on a specific rare molecular phenotype. To overcome this limitation, new multi-drug adaptive molecularly informed trial designs have been suggested [142]. The adaptive design allows "the eligibility criteria of a trial to be adaptively updated during the trial, restricting entry to patients likely to benefit from the new treatment" [143]. The molecularly informed multi-drug designs include "umbrella" and "basket" trials. The "umbrella" type includes multiple parallel branches when sequentially enrolled patients may be assigned to different treatments depending on results of the molecular tests. The "basket" type considers one drug for multiple molecular phenotypes, possibly within different tumour types. No such trials have yet been reported in the neo-adjuvant endocrine field; however, they may be expected in the near future.

13.6 Treatment Monitoring

The feasibility and importance of monitoring blood estrogens in AI trials have been demonstrated in a recent paper of Ingle with co-authors [144]. Aromatase inhibitors are indicated in post-menopause, when blood levels of estrogens are very low. Reliable monitoring of oestrogen suppression in post-menopause is technically challenging and may not be achievable with routinely used commercial radio-immuno-assay kits [145, 146]. Mass-spectrometry, an alternative sensitive technique for steroid measurements, was not affordable or feasible for the large studies at the time of AI development. Thus, all the major phase 3 AI trials did not report levels of oestrogens in the blood despite it being the main pharmacological end-point of AI action [84, 147, 148]. Until recently, the data about oestrogen suppression in blood by aromatase inhibitors was obtained only in a relatively small numbers of cases [91, 92, 94, 149, 150]. For the first time, Ingle with co-authors employed mass-spectrometry to measure blood oestrogens in a large multicentre adjuvant AI study on 649 patients [144]. In parallel they measured blood levels of anastrozole, the drug used in the trial. The measurements have been made before and after 1 month of treatment. Therefore they are directly relevant to the neo-adjuvant setting too. In 70 % of patients, oestrogens levels have been suppressed below the detection limit. However, the remaining 30 % demonstrated a very broad range of values, including the levels typical for pre-menopause women. Similarly, some patients showed much lower concentrations of anastrozole in the blood than others. If confirmed, these results may have important implications for our understanding of resistance to aromatase inhibitors. Such diversity in anastrozole and oestrogen concentrations on treatment could be explained by different factors. Biological explanations may include genetic variability in aromatase gene [162, 163] and individual variations in AI metabolism [164]. The other explanations may deal with treatment compliance and standards in assessment of post-menopausal status of patients. Either of these is important for future translational studies in the field.

13.6.1 New Genomics Methods and Bioinformatics Resources

Finally, future translational research in neo-adjuvant endocrine studies will be based on the new laboratory tools and bioinformatics resources. One of the most important recent developments is the fast progress of the massive parallel sequencing, which has revolutionised molecular profiling and has generated new datasets containing vast information about thousands of clinical cancer specimens.

Cancer Genome Atlas (TCGA project) is one of the largest novel molecular databases, which sets standards for translational bioinformatics resources [151, 152]. It has been established by NIH in an attempt to provide a comprehensive resource about genomic alterations in human tumours. It provides multi-layer molecular data on clinical cancer specimens matched with normal tissues from the same patient. The data is generated in several dedicated large-scale sequencing centres. The publically available files include genome-wide somatic mutations, copy-number variation data (generated by next generation sequencing and aCGH techniques) mRNA and miRNA expression data (RNA-seq and micro-array), methylation, proteomics data and clinical annotations of the specimens. Started in 2006 with a focus on lung, brain and ovarian cancers, in 2014 it provides data on more than 11,000 samples for 34 types of cancers, including more than a thousand samples for breast cancer. Bespoke analysis of TCGA data yet requires a significant bioinformatics expertise. However, new tools are being developed (e.g. www.cbioportal.org web portal) to enhance data access for a wider community.

Several groups have already reported analyses based on the breast sub-set of TCGA data. Thus, exploring the somatic mutation layer it has been possible to confirm that TP53 is the most commonly mutated gene in ER-ve cancers, while PIK3CA is the most common in ER+ve ones [20, 152]. This prompted an interest to potential clinical utility of PIK3CA somatic mutations in neo-adjuvant endocrine setting. Thus Baselga with co-authors included PIK3CA assessment in the biomarker program of the letrozole ± everolimus study described earlier [14]. Similarly, Lopez-Knowles et al. has recently studied potential role of PIK3CA mutations in neo-adjuvant response to anastrazole [153]. The results of these studies are inconsistent. While Baselga et al. suggested a poor proliferative response to letrozole in patients with mutated exon 9 of PIK3CA [14], Lopez-Knowles with co-authors reported association of PIK3CA mutations with favourable biomarkers and concluded that somatic mutations in PIK3CA do not preclude response to neo-adjuvant anastrozole [153].

PIK3CA has also been reported amongst the other genes reported by Ellis et al. in the recent study that employed massive parallel sequencing for the molecular profiling of pre-treatment biopsies from neo-adjuvant letrozole and anastrozole trials [13, 154]. The sequencing was performed on 77 samples: 46 were analysed by whole-genome sequencing and 31 underwent the whole-exome sequencing. The extensive bioinformatics analysis highlighted pathways and mechanisms associated with neo-adjuvant endocrine response and identified 18 genes predictive to response. Eight of the genes have already been implicated in breast cancer biology (PIK3CA, TP53, GATA3, CDH1, RB1, MLL3, MAP3K1 and CDKN1B). The other somatic mutations were not previously reported in breast cancer (TBX3, RUNX1, LDLRAP1, STNM2, MYH9, AGTR2, STMN2, SF3B1 and CBFB). However, four of them (RUNX1, CBFB, MYH9 and SF3B1) have been detected in haematopoietic malignancies. The authors highlight that MAP3K1 somatic mutations were associated with favourable biomarkers. In contrast, P53 was associated with high-grade and high proliferation in the studied samples. Mutations in GATA3 were associated with good proliferative response. Overall, the study demonstrated that new sequencing technologies are capable of finding new genes and pathways associated with response and resistance to neo-adjuvant endocrine treatments.

13.7 Conclusions

Neo-adjuvant endocrine therapy has an established place in the breast cancer clinic. A number of reviews traced the development of neo-adjuvant endocrine therapy over the last decade [19, 30, 33, 51, 56, 86, 87, 155–160]. Despite the wide use of neo-adjuvant cytotoxic and endocrine treatment, there is a shortage of evidence for direct comparison of these modalities in ER+ve patients. Extending duration of neo-adjuvant endocrine treatment to 6–8 months or until progression may increase the response rates. Application of neo-adjuvant endocrine treatment in pre-menopause is still experimental. Multiple markers based on gene expression patterns and somatic mutations are being developed to predict endocrine response in breast cancer, and new technologies are emerging to utilise translational opportunities provided by the preoperative treatment. However, the current clinical use of neo-adjuvant endocrine treatment is still based on conventional clinical parameters and biomarkers. The current consensus is that neo-adjuvant endocrine treatment is indicated for large ER+ve tumours with low grade and proliferation, which may be described as luminal A sub-type of breast cancer [31, 65, 121, 161].

References

1. Olson JA Jr et al (2009) Improved surgical outcomes for breast cancer patients receiving neoadjuvant aromatase inhibitor therapy: results from a multicenter phase II trial. J Am Coll Surg 208(5):906–914; discussion 915-6
2. Frei E 3rd (1982) Clinical cancer research: an embattled species. Cancer 50(10):1979–1992
3. Preece PE et al (1982) Tamoxifen as initial sole treatment of localised breast cancer in elderly women: a pilot study. Br Med J (Clin Res Ed) 284(6319):869–870
4. Chakrabarti J et al (2011) A randomised trial of mastectomy only versus tamoxifen for treating elderly patients with operable primary breast cancer-final results at 20-year follow-up. Crit Rev Oncol Hematol 78(3):260–264
5. Johnston SJ et al (2012) A randomised trial of primary tamoxifen versus mastectomy plus adjuvant tamoxifen in fit elderly women with invasive breast carcinoma of high oestrogen receptor content: long-term results at 20 years of follow-up. Ann Oncol 23(9):2296–2300
6. Hind D et al (2006) Surgery versus primary endocrine therapy for operable primary breast cancer in elderly women (70 years plus). Cochrane Database Syst Rev 1:CD004272
7. Bates T et al (1991) Breast cancer in elderly women: a Cancer Research Campaign trial comparing treatment with tamoxifen and optimal surgery with tamoxifen alone. The Elderly Breast Cancer Working Party. Br J Surg 78(5):591–594
8. Forrest AP et al (1986) A human tumour model. Lancet 2(8511):840–842
9. Miller WR et al (2003) Pathological features of breast cancer response following neoadjuvant treatment with either letrozole or tamoxifen. Eur J Cancer 39(4):462–468
10. Miller WR et al (2012) Sequential changes in gene expression profiles in breast cancers during treatment with the aromatase inhibitor, letrozole. Pharmacogenomics J 12(1):10–21
11. Ellis MJ et al (2008) Outcome prediction for estrogen receptor-positive breast cancer based on postneoadjuvant endocrine therapy tumor characteristics. J Natl Cancer Inst 100 (19):1380–1388
12. Miller WR et al (2009) Gene expression profiles differentiating between breast cancers clinically responsive or resistant to letrozole. J Clin Oncol 27(9):1382–1387
13. Ellis MJ et al (2012) Whole-genome analysis informs breast cancer response to aromatase inhibition. Nature 486(7403):353–360
14. Baselga J et al (2009) Phase II randomized study of neoadjuvant everolimus plus letrozole compared with placebo plus letrozole in patients with estrogen receptor-positive breast cancer. J Clin Oncol 27(16):2630–2637
15. Gianni L et al (2014) Neoadjuvant and adjuvant trastuzumab in patients with HER2-positive locally advanced breast cancer (NOAH): follow-up of a randomised controlled superiority trial with a parallel HER2-negative cohort. Lancet Oncol 15(6):640–647
16. Baselga J (2010) Treatment of HER2-overexpressing breast cancer. Ann Oncol 21(Suppl 7): vii36–vii40
17. FDA (2014) Guidance for industry: pathological complete response in neoadjuvant treatment of high-risk early-stage breast cancer: use as an endpoint to support accelerated approval. http://www.fda.gov/downloads/drugs/guidancecomplianceregulatoryinformation/guidances/ucm305501.pdf. Accessed 14 Jan 2016
18. Cortazar P et al (2014) Pathological complete response and long-term clinical benefit in breast cancer: the CTNeoBC pooled analysis. Lancet 384(9938):164–172
19. Abrial C et al (2006) Neoadjuvant endocrine therapy in breast cancer. Breast 15(1):9–19

20. Ades F et al (2014) Luminal B breast cancer: molecular characterization, clinical management, and future perspectives. J Clin Oncol 32(25):2794–2803
21. Carey LA et al (2007) The triple negative paradox: primary tumor chemosensitivity of breast cancer subtypes. Clin Cancer Res 13(8):2329–2334
22. Goldstein NS et al (2007) Molecular classification system identifies invasive breast carcinoma patients who are most likely and those who are least likely to achieve a complete pathologic response after neoadjuvant chemotherapy. Cancer 110(8):1687–1696
23. Colleoni M et al (2004) Chemotherapy is more effective in patients with breast cancer not expressing steroid hormone receptors: a study of preoperative treatment. Clin Cancer Res 10 (19):6622–6628
24. von Minckwitz G et al (2012) Definition and impact of pathologic complete response on prognosis after neoadjuvant chemotherapy in various intrinsic breast cancer subtypes. J Clin Oncol 30(15):1796–1804
25. Allevi G et al (2013) Increased pathological complete response rate after a long-term neoadjuvant letrozole treatment in postmenopausal oestrogen and/or progesterone receptor-positive breast cancer. Br J Cancer 108(8):1587–1592
26. Alba E et al (2012) Chemotherapy (CT) and hormonotherapy (HT) as neoadjuvant treatment in luminal breast cancer patients: results from the GEICAM/2006-03, a multicenter, randomized, phase-II study. Ann Oncol 23(12):3069–3074
27. Semiglazov VF et al (2007) Phase 2 randomized trial of primary endocrine therapy versus chemotherapy in postmenopausal patients with estrogen receptor-positive breast cancer. Cancer 110(2):244–254
28. Palmieri C et al (2014) NEOCENT: a randomised feasibility and translational study comparing neoadjuvant endocrine therapy with chemotherapy in ER-rich postmenopausal primary breast cancer. Breast Cancer Res Treat 148(3):581–590
29. Thomas JS et al (2007) Histopathology of breast carcinoma following neoadjuvant systemic therapy: a common association between letrozole therapy and central scarring. Histopathology 51(2):219–226
30. Charehbili A et al (2014) Neoadjuvant hormonal therapy for endocrine sensitive breast cancer: a systematic review. Cancer Treat Rev 40(1):86–92
31. Goldhirsch A et al (2013) Personalizing the treatment of women with early breast cancer: highlights of the St Gallen International Expert Consensus on the Primary Therapy of Early Breast Cancer 2013. Ann Oncol 24(9):2206–2223
32. Pierga JY et al (2004) Characteristics and outcome of 1755 operable breast cancers in women over 70 years of age. Breast 13(5):369–375
33. Dixon JM (2008) Prospects of neoadjuvant aromatase inhibitor therapy in breast cancer. Expert Rev Anticancer Ther 8(3):453–463
34. Shapiro CL, Recht A (2001) Side effects of adjuvant treatment of breast cancer. N Engl J Med 344(26):1997–2008
35. Sonmezer M, Oktay K (2004) Fertility preservation in female patients. Hum Reprod Update 10(3):251–266
36. Knobf MT (2006) The influence of endocrine effects of adjuvant therapy on quality of life outcomes in younger breast cancer survivors. Oncologist 11(2):96–110
37. Salama M et al (2013) Female fertility loss and preservation: threats and opportunities. Ann Oncol 24(3):598–608
38. Tomasi-Cont N et al (2014) Strategies for fertility preservation in young early breast cancer patients. Breast 23(5):503–510
39. Clowse ME et al (2009) Ovarian preservation by GnRH agonists during chemotherapy: a meta-analysis. J Women's Health (Larchmt) 18(3):311–319
40. Maltaris T, Beckmann MW, Dittrich R (2009) Review. Fertility preservation for young female cancer patients. In Vivo 23(1):123–130

41. Turner NH et al (2013) Utility of gonadotropin-releasing hormone agonists for fertility preservation in young breast cancer patients: the benefit remains uncertain. Ann Oncol 24 (9):2224–2235
42. Eiermann W et al (2001) Preoperative treatment of postmenopausal breast cancer patients with letrozole: a randomized double-blind multicenter study. Ann Oncol 12(11):1527–1532
43. Ellis MJ et al (2011) Randomized phase II neoadjuvant comparison between letrozole, anastrozole, and exemestane for postmenopausal women with estrogen receptor-rich stage 2 to 3 breast cancer: clinical and biomarker outcomes and predictive value of the baseline PAM50-based intrinsic subtype – ACOSOG Z1031. J Clin Oncol 29(17):2342–2349
44. Mustacchi G et al (2009) Neo-adjuvant exemestane in elderly patients with breast cancer: a phase II, multicentre, open-label. Ital Study Ann Oncol 20(4):655–659
45. Masuda N et al (2012) Neoadjuvant anastrozole versus tamoxifen in patients receiving goserelin for premenopausal breast cancer (STAGE): a double-blind, randomised phase 3 trial. Lancet Oncol 13(4):345–352
46. Young OE et al (2008) Effects of fulvestrant 750mg in premenopausal women with oestrogen-receptor-positive primary breast cancer. Eur J Cancer 44(3):391–399
47. Amir E et al (2011) Toxicity of adjuvant endocrine therapy in postmenopausal breast cancer patients: a systematic review and meta-analysis. J Natl Cancer Inst 103(17):1299–1309
48. Bottini A et al (2006) Randomized phase II trial of letrozole and letrozole plus low-dose metronomic oral cyclophosphamide as primary systemic treatment in elderly breast cancer patients. J Clin Oncol 24(22):3623–3628
49. Pico C et al (2004) Epirubicin-cyclophosphamide adjuvant chemotherapy plus tamoxifen administered concurrently versus sequentially: randomized phase III trial in postmenopausal node-positive breast cancer patients. A GEICAM 9401 study. Ann Oncol 15(1):79–87
50. Colleoni M et al (2005) Timing of CMF chemotherapy in combination with tamoxifen in postmenopausal women with breast cancer: role of endocrine responsiveness of the tumor. Ann Oncol 16(5):716–725
51. Colleoni M, Montagna E (2012) Neoadjuvant therapy for ER-positive breast cancers. Ann Oncol 23(Suppl 10):x243–x248
52. Miller WR (2010) Clinical, pathological, proliferative and molecular responses associated with neoadjuvant aromatase inhibitor treatment in breast cancer. J Steroid Biochem Mol Biol 118(4–5):273–276
53. Larionov AA, Miller WR (2009) Challenges in defining predictive markers for response to endocrine therapy in breast cancer. Future Oncol 5(9):1415–1428
54. Therasse P et al (2000) New guidelines to evaluate the response to treatment in solid tumors. European Organization for Research and Treatment of Cancer, National Cancer Institute of the United States, National Cancer Institute of Canada. J Natl Cancer Inst 92(3):205–216
55. Miller AB et al (1981) Reporting results of cancer treatment. Cancer 47(1):207–214
56. Chia YH, Ellis MJ, Ma CX (2010) Neoadjuvant endocrine therapy in primary breast cancer: indications and use as a research tool. Br J Cancer 103(6):759–764
57. Dixon JM et al (2000) The effects of neoadjuvant anastrozole (Arimidex) on tumor volume in postmenopausal women with breast cancer: a randomized, double-blind, single-center study. Clin Cancer Res 6(6):2229–2235
58. Tan MC et al (2009) Predictors of complete pathological response after neoadjuvant systemic therapy for breast cancer. Am J Surg 198(4):520–525
59. Keshgegian AA, Cnaan A (1995) Proliferation markers in breast carcinoma. Mitotic figure count, S-phase fraction, proliferating cell nuclear antigen, Ki-67 and MIB-1. Am J Clin Pathol 104(1):42–49
60. Lee LH, Yang H, Bigras G (2014) Current breast cancer proliferative markers correlate variably based on decoupled duration of cell cycle phases. Sci Rep 4:5122
61. Stuart-Harris R et al (2008) Proliferation markers and survival in early breast cancer: a systematic review and meta-analysis of 85 studies in 32,825 patients. Breast 17(4):323–334

62. Colozza M et al (2005) Proliferative markers as prognostic and predictive tools in early breast cancer: where are we now? Ann Oncol 16(11):1723–1739
63. Sheri A, Dowsett M (2012) Developments in Ki67 and other biomarkers for treatment decision making in breast cancer. Ann Oncol 23(Suppl 10):x219–x227
64. Luporsi E et al (2012) Ki-67: level of evidence and methodological considerations for its role in the clinical management of breast cancer: analytical and critical review. Breast Cancer Res Treat 132(3):895–915
65. Berruti A et al (2011) International expert consensus on primary systemic therapy in the management of early breast cancer: highlights of the Fourth Symposium on Primary Systemic Therapy in the Management of Operable Breast Cancer, Cremona, Italy (2010). J Natl Cancer Inst Monogr 2011(43):147–151
66. Gerdes J et al (1983) Production of a mouse monoclonal antibody reactive with a human nuclear antigen associated with cell proliferation. Int J Cancer 31(1):13–20
67. Gerdes J et al (1984) Cell cycle analysis of a cell proliferation-associated human nuclear antigen defined by the monoclonal antibody Ki-67. J Immunol 133(4):1710–1715
68. Gerdes J (1990) Ki-67 and other proliferation markers useful for immunohistological diagnostic and prognostic evaluations in human malignancies. Semin Cancer Biol 1(3):199–206
69. Lopez F et al (1991) Modalities of synthesis of Ki67 antigen during the stimulation of lymphocytes. Cytometry 12(1):42–49
70. Endl E, Gerdes J (2000) The Ki-67 protein: fascinating forms and an unknown function. Exp Cell Res 257(2):231–237
71. Scholzen T, Gerdes J (2000) The Ki-67 protein: from the known and the unknown. J Cell Physiol 182(3):311–322
72. Brown DC, Gatter KC (2002) Ki67 protein: the immaculate deception? Histopathology 40 (1):2–11
73. Cheutin T et al (2003) Three-dimensional organization of pKi-67: a comparative fluorescence and electron tomography study using FluoroNanogold. J Histochem Cytochem 51 (11):1411–1423
74. Li H et al (2004) Structure of human Ki67 FHA domain and its binding to a phosphoprotein fragment from hNIFK reveal unique recognition sites and new views to the structural basis of FHA domain functions. J Mol Biol 335(1):371–381
75. Byeon IJ et al (2005) Sequential phosphorylation and multisite interactions characterize specific target recognition by the FHA domain of Ki67. Nat Struct Mol Biol 12(11):987–993
76. Bullwinkel J et al (2006) Ki-67 protein is associated with ribosomal RNA transcription in quiescent and proliferating cells. J Cell Physiol 206(3):624–635
77. Rahmanzadeh R et al (2007) Chromophore-assisted light inactivation of pKi-67 leads to inhibition of ribosomal RNA synthesis. Cell Prolif 40(3):422–430
78. Rahmanzadeh R et al (2010) Ki-67 as a molecular target for therapy in an in vitro three-dimensional model for ovarian cancer. Cancer Res 70(22):9234–9242
79. van Diest PJ, van der Wall E, Baak JP (2004) Prognostic value of proliferation in invasive breast cancer: a review. J Clin Pathol 57(7):675–681
80. Bedard PL et al (2011) Low residual proliferation after short-term letrozole therapy is an early predictive marker of response in high proliferative ER-positive breast cancer. Endocr Relat Cancer 18(6):721–730
81. Dowsett M et al (2007) Prognostic value of Ki67 expression after short-term presurgical endocrine therapy for primary breast cancer. J Natl Cancer Inst 99(2):167–170
82. Urruticoechea A, Smith IE, Dowsett M (2005) Proliferation marker Ki-67 in early breast cancer. J Clin Oncol 23(28):7212–7220
83. Dowsett M et al (2005) Biomarker changes during neoadjuvant anastrozole, tamoxifen, or the combination: influence of hormonal status and HER-2 in breast cancer – a study from the IMPACT trialists. J Clin Oncol 23(11):2477–2492
84. Cuzick J et al (2010) Effect of anastrozole and tamoxifen as adjuvant treatment for early-stage breast cancer: 10-year analysis of the ATAC trial. Lancet Oncol 11(12):1135–1141

85. Howell A et al (2005) Results of the ATAC (Arimidex, Tamoxifen, Alone or in Combination) trial after completion of 5 years' adjuvant treatment for breast cancer. Lancet 365 (9453):60–62
86. Beresford MJ, Ravichandran D, Makris A (2007) Neoadjuvant endocrine therapy in breast cancer. Cancer Treat Rev 33(1):48–57
87. Mathew J et al (2009) Neoadjuvant endocrine treatment in primary breast cancer – review of literature. Breast 18(6):339–344
88. Cataliotti L et al (2006) Comparison of anastrozole versus tamoxifen as preoperative therapy in postmenopausal women with hormone receptor-positive breast cancer: the Pre-Operative "Arimidex" Compared to Tamoxifen (PROACT) trial. Cancer 106(10):2095–2103
89. Smith IE et al (2005) Neoadjuvant treatment of postmenopausal breast cancer with anastrozole, tamoxifen, or both in combination: the Immediate Preoperative Anastrozole, Tamoxifen, or Combined with Tamoxifen (IMPACT) multicenter double-blind randomized trial. J Clin Oncol 23(22):5108–5116
90. Seo JH, Kim YH, Kim JS (2009) Meta-analysis of pre-operative aromatase inhibitor versus tamoxifen in postmenopausal woman with hormone receptor-positive breast cancer. Cancer Chemother Pharmacol 63(2):261–266
91. Geisler J et al (2002) Influence of letrozole (Femara) and anastrozole (Arimidex) on total body aromatization and plasma estrogen levels in postmenopausal breast cancer patients evaluated in a randomized, cross-over-designed study. J Clin Oncol 20:751–757
92. Geisler J et al (2008) Letrozole is superior to anastrozole in suppressing breast cancer tissue and plasma estrogen levels. Clin Cancer Res 14(19):6330–6335
93. Elliott KM et al (2014) Effects of aromatase inhibitors and body mass index on steroid hormone levels in women with early and advanced breast cancer. Br J Surg 101(8):939–948
94. Dixon JM et al (2008) Letrozole suppresses plasma estradiol and estrone sulphate more completely than anastrozole in postmenopausal women with breast cancer. J Clin Oncol 26 (10):1671–1676
95. Rose C et al (2003) An open randomised trial of second-line endocrine therapy in advanced breast cancer. comparison of the aromatase inhibitors letrozole and anastrozole. Eur J Cancer 39(16):2318–2327
96. Kuter I et al (2012) Dose-dependent change in biomarkers during neoadjuvant endocrine therapy with fulvestrant: results from NEWEST, a randomized Phase II study. Breast Cancer Res Treat 133(1):237–246
97. Macedo LF et al (2008) Combination of anastrozole with fulvestrant in the intratumoral aromatase xenograft model. Cancer Res 68(9):3516–3522
98. Mehta RS et al (2012) Combination anastrozole and fulvestrant in metastatic breast cancer. N Engl J Med 367(5):435–444
99. Robertson JF et al (2009) Activity of fulvestrant 500 mg versus anastrozole 1 mg as first-line treatment for advanced breast cancer: results from the FIRST study. J Clin Oncol 27 (27):4530–4535
100. Robertson JF et al (2013) A randomized trial to assess the biological activity of short-term (pre-surgical) fulvestrant 500 mg plus anastrozole versus fulvestrant 500 mg alone or anastrozole alone on primary breast cancer. Breast Cancer Res 15(2):R18
101. Dixon JM et al (2009) Increase in response rate by prolonged treatment with neoadjuvant letrozole. Breast Cancer Res Treat 113(1):145–151
102. Krainick-Strobel UE et al (2008) Neoadjuvant letrozole in postmenopausal estrogen and/or progesterone receptor positive breast cancer: a phase IIb/III trial to investigate optimal duration of preoperative endocrine therapy. BMC Cancer 8:62
103. Llombart-Cussac A et al (2012) Phase II trial with letrozole to maximum response as primary systemic therapy in postmenopausal patients with ER/PgR[+] operable breast cancer. Clin Transl Oncol 14(2):125–131

104. Toi M et al (2011) Ki67 index changes, pathological response and clinical benefits in primary breast cancer patients treated with 24 weeks of aromatase inhibition. Cancer Sci 102 (4):858–865
105. Goldhirsch A et al (2009) Thresholds for therapies: highlights of the St Gallen International Expert Consensus on the primary therapy of early breast cancer 2009. Ann Oncol 20 (8):1319–1329
106. Torrisi R et al (2007) Antitumour and biological effects of letrozole and GnRH analogue as primary therapy in premenopausal women with ER and PgR positive locally advanced operable breast cancer. Br J Cancer 97(6):802–808
107. Dowsett M (2003) Preoperative models to evaluate endocrine strategies for breast cancer. Clin Cancer Res 9(1 Pt 2):502S–510S
108. Miller WR, Larionov AA (2012) Understanding the mechanisms of aromatase inhibitor resistance. Breast Cancer Res 14(1):201
109. Ueno T et al (2014) Evaluating the 21-gene assay Recurrence Score(R) as a predictor of clinical response to 24 weeks of neoadjuvant exemestane in estrogen receptor-positive breast cancer. Int J Clin Oncol 19(4):607–613
110. Dowsett M et al (2011) Endocrine therapy, new biologicals, and new study designs for presurgical studies in breast cancer. J Natl Cancer Inst Monogr 2011(43):120–123
111. Iwata H (2011) Neoadjuvant endocrine therapy for postmenopausal patients with hormone receptor-positive early breast cancer: a new concept. Breast Cancer 18(2):92–97
112. Early Breast Cancer Trialists' Collaborative, G (2005) Effects of chemotherapy and hormonal therapy for early breast cancer on recurrence and 15-year survival: an overview of the randomised trials. Lancet 365(9472):1687–1717
113. Brouckaert O et al (2013) A critical review why assessment of steroid hormone receptors in breast cancer should be quantitative. Ann Oncol 24(1):47–53
114. Harvey JM et al (1999) Estrogen receptor status by immunohistochemistry is superior to the ligand-binding assay for predicting response to adjuvant endocrine therapy in breast cancer. J Clin Oncol 17(5):1474–1481
115. Hammond ME et al (2010) American Society of Clinical Oncology/College Of American Pathologists guideline recommendations for immunohistochemical testing of estrogen and progesterone receptors in breast cancer. J Clin Oncol 28(16):2784–2795
116. Ellis MJ et al (2001) Letrozole is more effective neoadjuvant endocrine therapy than tamoxifen for ErbB-1- and/or ErbB-2-positive, estrogen receptor-positive primary breast cancer: evidence from a phase III randomized trial. J Clin Oncol 19(18):3808–3816
117. Nahta R, O'Regan RM (2012) Therapeutic implications of estrogen receptor signaling in HER2-positive breast cancers. Breast Cancer Res Treat 135(1):39–48
118. Perou CM et al (2000) Molecular portraits of human breast tumours. Nature 406 (6797):747–752
119. Sorlie T et al (2001) Gene expression patterns of breast carcinomas distinguish tumor subclasses with clinical implications. Proc Natl Acad Sci U S A 98(19):10869–10874
120. Wirapati P et al (2008) Meta-analysis of gene expression profiles in breast cancer: toward a unified understanding of breast cancer subtyping and prognosis signatures. Breast Cancer Res 10(4):R65
121. Goldhirsch A et al (2011) Strategies for subtypes – dealing with the diversity of breast cancer: highlights of the St. Gallen International Expert Consensus on the Primary Therapy of Early Breast Cancer. Ann Oncol 22(8):1736–1747
122. Parker JS et al (2009) Supervised risk predictor of breast cancer based on intrinsic subtypes. J Clin Oncol 27(8):1160–1167
123. Dunbier AK et al (2011) Association between breast cancer subtypes and response to neoadjuvant anastrozole. Steroids 76(8):736–740
124. Paik S et al (2004) A multigene assay to predict recurrence of tamoxifen-treated, node-negative breast cancer. N Engl J Med 351(27):2817–2826

125. Harbeck N et al (2014) Molecular and protein markers for clinical decision making in breast cancer: today and tomorrow. Cancer Treat Rev 40(3):434–444
126. Paik S et al (2006) Gene expression and benefit of chemotherapy in women with node-negative, estrogen receptor-positive breast cancer. J Clin Oncol 24(23):3726–3734
127. Carlson JJ, Roth JA (2013) The impact of the Oncotype Dx breast cancer assay in clinical practice: a systematic review and meta-analysis. Breast Cancer Res Treat 141(1):13–22
128. Milburn M et al (2013) Is oncotype DX recurrence score (RS) of prognostic value once HER2-positive and. low-ER expression patients are removed? Breast J 19(4):357–364
129. Allison KH et al (2012) Routine pathologic parameters can predict Oncotype DX recurrence scores in subsets of ER positive patients: who does not always need testing? Breast Cancer Res Treat 131(2):413–424
130. Symmans WF et al (2010) Genomic index of sensitivity to endocrine therapy for breast cancer. J Clin Oncol 28(27):4111–4119
131. Harbeck N, Rody A (2012) Lost in translation? Estrogen receptor status and endocrine responsiveness in breast cancer. J Clin Oncol 30(7):686–689
132. Filipits M et al (2011) A new molecular predictor of distant recurrence in ER-positive, HER2-negative breast cancer adds independent information to conventional clinical risk factors. Clin Cancer Res 17(18):6012–6020
133. Mackay A et al (2007) Molecular response to aromatase inhibitor treatment in primary breast cancer. Breast Cancer Res 9(3):R37
134. Dunbier AK et al (2013) Molecular profiling of aromatase inhibitor-treated postmenopausal breast tumors identifies immune-related correlates of resistance. Clin Cancer Res 19 (10):2775–2786
135. Miller WR, Larionov A (2010) Changes in expression of oestrogen regulated and proliferation genes with neoadjuvant treatment highlight heterogeneity of clinical resistance to the aromatase inhibitor, letrozole. Breast Cancer Res 12(4):R52
136. Creighton CJ et al (2009) Residual breast cancers after conventional therapy display mesenchymal as well as tumor-initiating features. Proc Natl Acad Sci U S A 106(33):13820–13825
137. Turnbull AK et al (2015) Accurate prediction and validation of response to endocrine therapy in breast cancer. J Clin Oncol 33(20):2270–2278
138. Knudsen S et al (2014) Development and validation of a gene expression score that predicts response to fulvestrant in breast cancer patients. PLoS One 9(2):e87415
139. Simon RM, Paik S, Hayes DF (2009) Use of archived specimens in evaluation of prognostic and predictive biomarkers. J Natl Cancer Inst 101(21):1446–1452
140. Akashi-Tanaka S et al (2007) Favorable outcome in patients with breast cancer in the presence of pathological response after neoadjuvant endocrine therapy. Breast 16(5):482–488
141. Cleator SJ et al (2005) Good clinical response of breast cancers to neoadjuvant chemoendocrine therapy is associated with improved overall survival. Ann Oncol 16 (2):267–272
142. Menis J, Hasan B, Besse B (2014) New clinical research strategies in thoracic oncology: clinical trial design, adaptive, basket and umbrella trials, new end-points and new evaluations of response. Eur Respir Rev 23(133):367–378
143. Simon N, Simon R (2013) Adaptive enrichment designs for clinical trials. Biostatistics 14 (4):613–625
144. Ingle JN et al (2015) Estrogens and their precursors in postmenopausal women with early breast cancer receiving anastrozole. Steroids 99:32–38
145. Lønning PE, Ekse D (1995) A sensitive assay for measurement of plasma estrone sulphate in patients on treatment with aromatase inhibitors. J Steroid Biochem Mol Biol 55(3/4):409–412
146. Geisler J et al (2008) An optimised, highly sensitive radioimmunoassay for the simultaneous measurement of estrone, estradiol and estrone sulfate in the ultra-low range in human plasma samples. J Steroid Biochem Mol Biol 109:90–95
147. Regan MM et al (2011) Interpreting Breast International Group (BIG) 1–98: a randomized, double-blind, phase III trial comparing letrozole and tamoxifen as adjuvant endocrine therapy

for postmenopausal women with hormone receptor-positive, early breast cancer. Breast Cancer Res 13(3):209
148. van de Velde CJ et al (2011) Adjuvant tamoxifen and exemestane in early breast cancer (TEAM): a randomised phase 3 trial. Lancet 377(9762):321–331
149. Iveson TJ et al (1993) Phase I study of the oral nonsteroidal aromatase inhibitor CGS 20267 in postmenopausal patients with advanced breast cancer. Cancer Res 53:266–270
150. Geisler J et al (1996) Influence of anastrozole (Arimidex), a selective, non-steroidal aromatase inhibitor, on in vivo aromatisation and plasma oestrogen levels in postmenopausal women with breast cancer. Br J Cancer 74(8):1286–1291
151. Cancer Genome Atlas, N (2012) Comprehensive molecular portraits of human breast tumours. Nature 490(7418):61–70
152. Ma CX, Ellis MJ (2013) The Cancer Genome Atlas: clinical applications for breast cancer. Oncology (Williston Park) 27(12):1263–1269, 1274–9
153. Lopez-Knowles E et al (2014) Relationship of PIK3CA mutation and pathway activity with anti-proliferative response to aromatase inhibition. Breast Cancer Res 16(3):R68
154. Ellis MJ (2013) Mutational analysis of breast cancer: guiding personalized treatments. Breast 22(Suppl 2):S19–S21
155. Saleh RR et al (2014) Neoadjuvant endocrine treatment for breast cancer: from bedside to bench and back again? Curr Oncol 21(1):e122–e128
156. Dixon JM, Anderson TJ, Miller WR (2002) Neoadjuvant endocrine therapy of breast cancer: a surgical perspective. Eur J Cancer 38(17):2214–2221
157. Freedman OC, Verma S, Clemons MJ (2005) Using aromatase inhibitors in the neoadjuvant setting: evolution or revolution? Cancer Treat Rev 31(1):1–17
158. Barnadas A et al (2008) Neoadjuvant endocrine therapy for breast cancer: past, present and future. Anticancer Drugs 19(4):339–347
159. Macaskill EJ, Renshaw L, Dixon JM (2006) Neoadjuvant use of hormonal therapy in elderly patients with early or locally advanced hormone receptor-positive breast cancer. Oncologist 11(10):1081–1088
160. Huober J et al (2004) Neoadjuvant endocrine therapy in primary breast cancer. Clin Breast Cancer 5(5):341–347
161. Gralow JR, Zujewski JA, Winer E (2008) Preoperative therapy in invasive breast cancer: reviewing the state of the science and exploring new research directions. J Clin Oncol 26 (5):696–697
162. Sowers MR et al (2006) Aromatase gene (CYP 19) polymorphisms and endogenous androgen concentrations in a multiracial/multiethnic, multisite study of women at midlife. Am J Med 119(9 Suppl 1):S23–30
163. Wang L et al (2010) Functional genetic polymorphisms in the aromatase gene CYP19 vary the response of breast cancer patients to neoadjuvant therapy with aromatase inhibitors. Cancer Res 70(1):319–328
164. Sun D et al (2010) Characterization of 17-dihydroexemestane glucuronidation: potential role of the UGT2B17 deletion in exemestane pharmacogenetics. Pharmacogenet Genomics 20 (10):575–585

Chapter 14
Alterations of Biomarkers by Neoadjuvant Endocrine Therapy

Yukiko Shibahara and Hironobu Sasano

Abstract Endocrine therapies exert potent tumor-suppressing effects in breast cancer (BC). Estrogen receptor (ER) positivity is generally considered the most powerful biomarker to predict therapy response in a neoadjuvant setting. However, due to the heterogeneity of BCs, many ER-positive cases do not necessarily respond to treatment. Therefore, identification of new biomarkers is warranted to predict treatment response and to detect acquired resistance to therapy. In this chapter, we discuss clinical factors of BC to predict treatment response and identify available pathological and immunohistochemical factors. Histologically, shrinkage of tumors as well as diminished mitosis is evidence of response to endocrine therapy (ET). Immunohistochemically, ER abundance and the Ki-67 labeling index are used to predict response to ET. In addition, we assess the utility of miRNAs, especially circulating miRNAs, as previous studies have indicated that these molecules may be the next generation of biomarkers to assess treatment response. Acquired resistance to ET is a major clinical obstacle, especially since there is no established biomarker to predict treatment response or resistance to aromatase inhibitors in the neoadjuvant setting of ET before surgery.

Endocrine therapy (ET) for postmenopausal breast cancer (BC) is well established. At present, aromatase inhibitors (AIs) are first choice agents for adjuvant ET and are also gaining credibility for use in neoadjuvant ET. While it is generally assumed that all estrogen receptor (ER)-positive BCs are eligible for and respond to ET, the reality is different. Some ER-positive BCs do not respond to ET, and quite a few develop resistance after an initial response. Therefore, treatment resistance has become a major impediment in clinical practice. Thus, further research of biomarkers to predict response to ET is warranted.

BC is one of the most intensely studied cancers, and various biomarkers to predict prognosis or therapeutic response have been reported. However, in terms of ET, in particular AIs, there are relatively few established biomarkers with high sensitivity and specificity that reflect response or resistance to treatment. ER positivity and postmenopausal status seem to be the most reliable biomarkers

---

Y. Shibahara • H. Sasano (✉)
Department of Pathology, Tohoku University, Graduate School of Medicine,
2-1 Seiryo-machi, Aoba-ku, Sendai, Miyagi 980-8575, Japan
e-mail: hsasano@patholo2.med.tohoku.ac.jp

M. Toi et al. (eds.), *Personalized Treatment of Breast Cancer*,
DOI 10.1007/978-4-431-55552-0_14

currently established to predict response to ET. However, the heterogeneity of luminal-type BC creates many exceptions, and therefore, monitoring these two biomarkers is insufficient to guarantee therapy efficacy. In this chapter, we discuss alterations of biomarkers by ET, mainly AIs, and scrutinize potential biomarkers to precisely predict response or resistance to ET.

Keywords Radiotherapy • Neoadjuvant • Pathological complete response • Regional node

14.1 Clinical Factors

Clinical factors, such as sex, age, hormone receptor status, menopausal status, family history, obesity, and dietary habits, are well-established biomarkers in BC. In this chapter, we discuss correlations between clinical factors and ET. First, BC mainly occurs in females, and most studies examine female BC as the major premise. Therefore, most issues examined in this chapter are based on female BC studies. But before going any further, we would like to note that male BC, although comparatively rare, is also of interest to BC researchers. Past studies indicated that response to and outcomes after ET in male BC may be considered comparable with female BC studies described in the literature [1].

As mentioned earlier, menopausal status is a major biomarker to predict response to AI therapy. Neoadjuvant AI therapy is often implemented in postmenopausal hormone receptor-positive BC, and its potent tumor-suppressing effects are well documented. However, some studies have indicated the usefulness of AIs in premenopausal BC in a neoadjuvant setting, and the current practice is shifting toward expanding the use of AIs. In premenopausal BC, one study indicated that neoadjuvant AI therapy plus ovarian suppression (e.g., luteinizing hormone-releasing hormone analogues) showed clinical as well as pathological responses, some better than that of tamoxifen therapy [2]. This is one example that the established biomarker of neoadjuvant ET, menopausal status, is changing, but further large cohort studies comparing neoadjuvant chemotherapy to ET are needed to assess the utility of menopausal status in clinical practice.

Body mass index (BMI) is another important biomarker among clinical factors. A recent study examined correlations between BMI and aromatase or plasma estrogen levels. Previous studies indicated that pre-AI treatment levels of aromatase were correlated to plasma estradiol (E2), estrone, and estrone sulfate levels but not BMI. Intra-treatment plasma estrone sulfate was correlated to BMI, but not aromatization levels, aromatase inhibition rates, or tumor estrogen levels, indicating that BMI is more of a biomarker of plasma estrogen levels rather than in tumor estrogen production by aromatase. Therefore, AIs are not influenced by BMI and the same effects of AIs can be expected for overweight patients as for normal-weight patients [3].

The impact of family history cannot be discussed without mentioning BRCA1/BRCA2 mutations. BRCA1/BRCA2 mutation is a potent biomarker of BC prognosis and response to therapy. Because the majority of BRCA1/BRCA2 mutations are related to ER-negative BC, most of these tumors may not seem to be candidates for ET. However, evidence indicates correlations between ER status and BRCA1/BRCA2, such as estrogen-dependent organ involvement in BRCA1/BRCA2 syndrome. Although the use of AIs could inhibit BC development among these patients, oral contraceptives increased the risk of BC development [4, 5]. Neoadjuvant ET is not an impractical choice for BRCA1/BRCA2-associated BCs, although future clinical trials are required to clarify the efficacy of this regimen.

Serum tumor markers such as carcinoembryonic antigen and cancer antigen 15-3 are commonly used in clinical practice for postoperative monitoring of BC [6] but are not sufficiently specific or sensitive for use in screening. The applicability of these tumor markers as biomarkers of ET efficacy has not been examined to date. Other factors, such as age and dietary habits, have not been established as biomarkers for ET.

14.2 Tumor Size and Tumor Imaging

Tumor size by clinical palpation is the easiest and most accessible noninvasive biomarker to assess therapeutic efficacy. Clinical response is measured by palpation in approximately half of the patients who receive neoadjuvant AI treatment. Of these, about 10 % achieve complete response, while 40 % show a partial response. Response rates are reportedly significantly lower for patients receiving tamoxifen, where one-third of the patients showed a clinical response [6]. Therefore, AIs are more effective in reducing tumor size and thus avoiding total mastectomy for patients with large initial tumors. Another study reported a clinical response rate of nearly 60 %, with a decrease in the mean tumor size of >50 % (39.1–16.7 mm). Ultrasound and mammography are also noninvasive methods to assess efficacy, and the clinical response rate was 33 % for AI and 25 % for tamoxifen [6].

14.3 Pathological Features

Pathologically, the main feature of neoadjuvant treatment is a decrease in mitotic figures [7]. Tubule formation by tumor cells and nuclear atypia often remain unchanged. Consequently, pathological grade (total score of tubule formation, 0–3; nuclear pleomorphism, 0–3; mitotic counts, 0–3) is often unchanged or decreased as shown in Fig. 14.1 [8]. Nuclear atypia must be carefully evaluated by experienced pathologists because treatment-induced degeneration can be mistaken for higher-grade atypia. The characteristics of treatment effect include

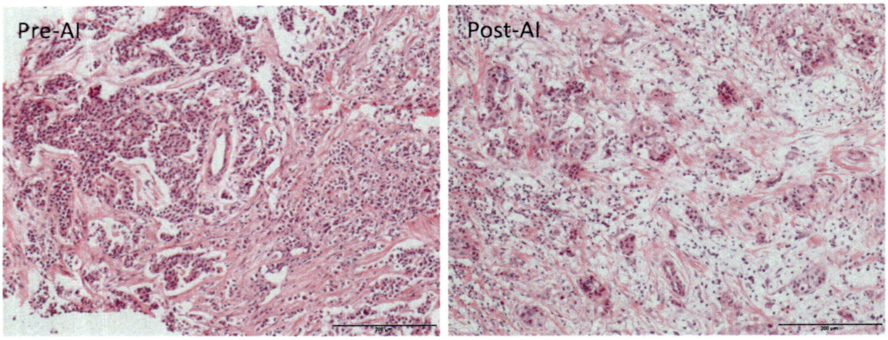

Fig. 14.1 Hematoxylin-eosin staining of the same tumor before (*left*, needle biopsy) and after (*right*, mastectomy) treatment with exemestane (original magnification × 100). Tubule formation and nuclear pleomorphism remained unchanged, while mitotic figures decreased. Note the inflammatory changes detected in posttreatment tumor, with fibrosis and scarring. Also, foamy macrophages were abundant

eosinophilic cytoplasm, bulky or disintegrated nuclei without prominent nucleoli, and apoptosis, while nuclei with diameters of often twice the size of red blood cells, coarse to vesicular chromatin, prominent nucleoli, and mitosis suggest high nuclear grade. Necrosis and fibrosis with scattered cancer cells are more frequently observed in specimens following chemotherapy. Central scarring is a common characteristic of AI-treated specimens [9].

14.4 ER and Enzymes Involved in Intratumoral Estrogen Production

Immunohistochemical detection of ERα expression is the most important indicator and determinant of ET efficacy. Lack of ERα expression initially disqualifies a case from ET, and this phenotype is the most powerful biomarker to predict ET failure. Therefore, BCs must be ERα positive before administration of ET [10]. However, ER positivity does not guarantee a response to ET. Initial, as well as acquired, resistance occurs, and while one ET may be efficacious, others may not [11]. The St. Gallen International Expert Consensus in 2009 indicated that although any level of ER positivity qualifies for ET, cancers that show a strong response to ET have 50 % or more ER-positive cells immunohistochemically [12].

Our data and those from other studies show that ER is generally unchanged by AI treatment [7]. Overall, AI does not affect ER positivity during the treatment course, as shown in Fig. 14.2. Interestingly, cases treated with adjuvant AI therapy that have later acquired resistance also continue to express ERs, indicating that ET may be effective by other mechanisms after acquiring AI resistance [12]. This is contrary to tamoxifen-treated specimens, in which ER positivity is decreased. Also,

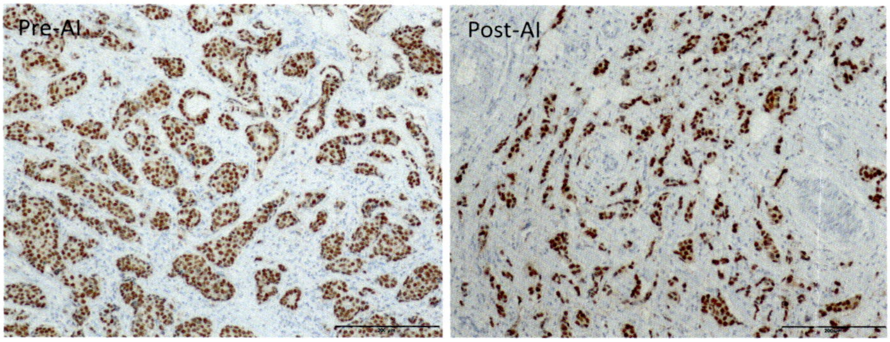

Fig. 14.2 Estrogen receptor immunostaining of the same tumor before (*left*) and after (*right*) treatment with exemestane, exhibiting marked immunopositivity (Allred score PS5+IS3=TS8) despite treatment (original magnification × 100)

levels of enzymes involved in intratumoral estrogen production (steroid or estrogen sulfatase, STS; and 17b-hydroxysteroid dehydrogenase type 1, 17b-HSD1) are also reduced by AI, as indicated by immunohistochemical analysis [13]. This phenomenon implies a compensatory reaction to estrogen depletion by AIs in BC by attempting to increase intratumoral estrogen via pathways other than aromatase. Also, STS levels are decreased in clinical and pathological responders as well as in cases with a low Ki-67 labeling index post-AI. 17b-HSD1 was increased despite response to changes in AIs or Ki-67 [13].

Yamashita et al. [15] examined aromatase expression levels before and after AI treatment and found that aromatase expression in cancer stromal cells was significantly decreased post-AI, but the changes were not significant in cancer cells. Therefore, ER is suitable as a biomarker to predict initial response to ET, while a difference in ER levels seems to be the key factor in predicting initial response.

14.5 Progesterone Receptor

AI greatly affects progesterone receptor (PR) status, as demonstrated by a substantial decrease in the ratio of PR-positive cells, resulting in a switch from PR positivity to negativity in most cases. This is due to the inhibition of aromatase activity and estrogen production, which affects PR expression downstream from the ER signaling pathway [14]. This phenomenon was observed regardless of response to AI or types/doses of AI; thus, PR status is not a biomarker of AI response [7, 14]. For cases in which the tumor has a negative PR status pretreatment, PR status remained unchanged post-treatment. Also, this phenomenon was observed regardless of the human epidermal growth factor receptor 2 (HER2) status of the tumors [15]. Figure 14.3 shows a representative scheme of PR status of BC cells turning negative.

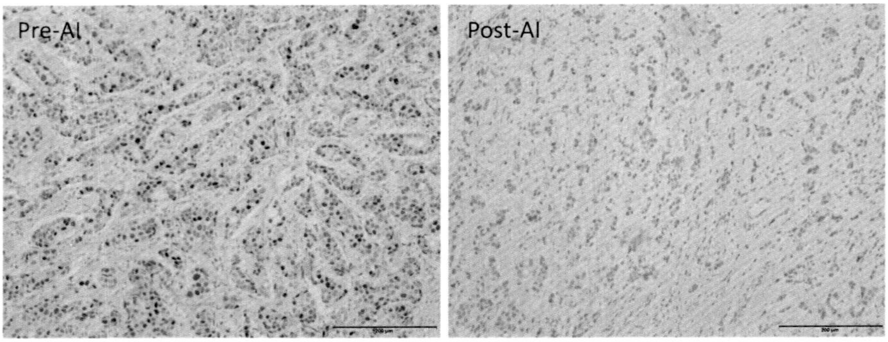

Fig. 14.3 Progesterone receptor immunostaining of the same tumor before (*left*) and after (*right*) treatment with exemestane, demonstrating major reduction in staining after treatment (original magnification × 100)

14.6 HER2

HER2 expression levels are not significantly changed by AI treatment [14]. HER2-negative tumors tend to show a greater decrease in the Ki-67 index compared with HER2-positive tumors following AI therapy (12 weeks of anastrozole) [16], but this may be due to the higher pre-therapy Ki-67 labeling index value in HER2-positive tumors.

HER2 status is not a factor affecting short-term treatment response; however, in the long term, continued growth via activation of the HER2 pathway is a negative biomarker for response to neoadjuvant AI therapy in ER- and HER2-positive tumors that escape the tumor-suppressing properties of AI therapy [17].

14.7 Ki-67

Quantification of Ki-67 antigen expression is a well-established method to routinely assess cell proliferation in the clinical setting [18]. Anti-Ki-67 antibody is expressed in the nucleus and is an established biomarker to distinguish luminal type A from type B BC [19]. AI treatment greatly reduces the Ki-67 positivity index, inferring that luminal B-type tumors, which initially have poorer prognosis than luminal A types, may convert to luminal A types by means of AI treatment. This phenomenon was observed across different AIs, including exemestane [20], anastrozole [21], and letrozole [15], in a neoadjuvant setting.

Contrary to PR expression, for which a decrease merely reflects the expression of basic AI mechanisms, the Ki-67 index can act as a biomarker of response to AIs in a neoadjuvant setting. The Ki-67 labeling index was more reduced in the post-AI surgical specimens of responders than in those of nonresponders [14]. Even for patients who received short-term treatment (2 weeks of AI treatment),

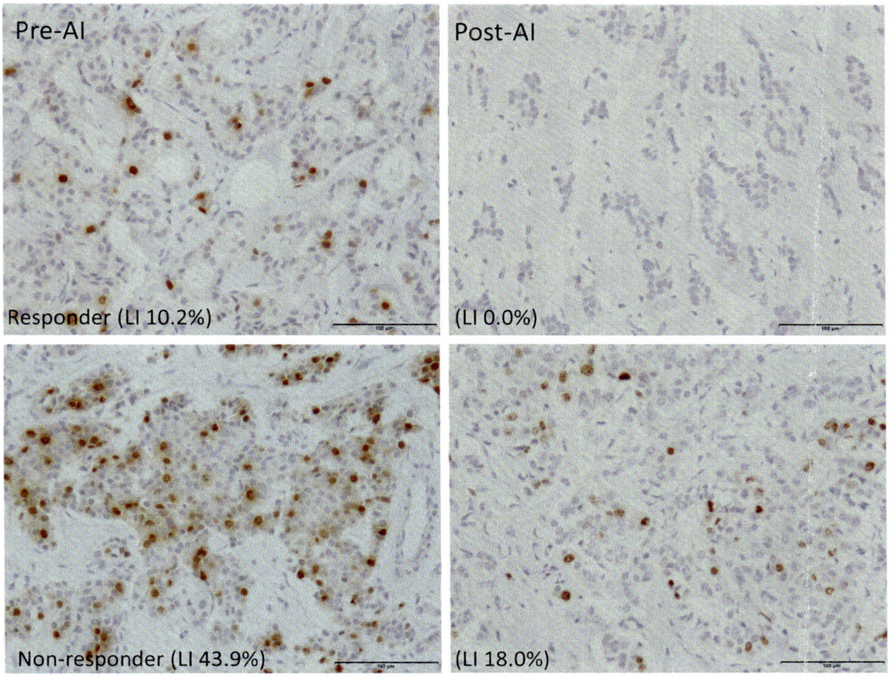

Fig. 14.4 Ki-67 immunostaining of the same tumor before (*left*) and after (*right*) treatment with exemestane. *Upper panels* demonstrate the immunostaining of a responder showing major reduction in labeling index (LI) following treatment. *Lower panels* demonstrate the immunostaining of a nonresponder, showing a mild reduction compared to those of the responder (original magnification × 200 upper panels)

posttreatment AI was predictive of prognosis, and patients with a lower Ki-67 labeling index had better recurrence-free survival rates [22]. This evidence favors neoadjuvant AI therapy than adjuvant. It is easier to obtain post-AI specimens in a neoadjuvant setting than in an adjuvant setting; therefore, immunohistochemical evaluation of the Ki-67 index can be easily performed to predict patient prognosis. Also, AI may be used in a neoadjuvant setting not only because of its powerful effects and lower toxicity but as a measure to assess endocrine efficacy pre-op. AI lowers the Ki-67 labeling index by a greater degree than tamoxifen, which also supports a better clinical outcome of AI treatment [21]. Therefore, Ki-67 can be considered as one of the most important biomarkers of neoadjuvant AI treatment. Therefore, pre-op needle biopsies should be routinely stained for Ki-67. Figure 14.4 shows a marked decrease in Ki-67-positive cells after AI treatment.

A previous immunohistochemical study reported a decrease in other representative markers of tumor cell proliferation (cyclin D1, bcl-2, and p53) by AI treatment [14]. However, the changes were statistically insignificant, and therefore, these markers are not suitable to gauge AI response.

14.8 Tissue Concentrations of Sex Steroids

Even after menopause, E2 levels in BC tissues are maintained close to premenopausal levels [23]. At present, it is generally accepted that the aromatase pathway in the tumor microenvironment itself as well as the surrounding cancer-associated fibroblasts and adipose tissue is the major source of local estrogen production. First of all, plasma E2 levels are lowered to undetectable limits by AI treatment [24]. Liquid chromatography/electrospray tandem mass spectrometry is a useful tool to measure tissue concentrations of sex steroids, which are relatively difficult to precisely evaluate, due to the abundant fat and fibrous tissue in the breast. Intratumoral E2 concentration is suppressed by 90–100 % by AI (15 weeks of anastrozole [25] and 16 weeks of letrozole [26]).

A 2010 study by our group on intratumoral concentrations of androgens in AI-treated BC specimens found that intratumoral dihydrotestosterone (DHT) concentrations were increased by more than twofold, and the corresponding E_2:DHT ratio in each patient was decreased by >90 % following neoadjuvant exemestane treatment for 2 weeks [27].

14.9 RNA

Miller et al. [28] examined molecular changes following AI therapy using a microarray of tumor RNA and reported that 3 months of letrozole therapy did not induce specific molecular changes, where only a single gene was changed by > twofold in all 59 tumors following treatment. These findings indicated that every tumor responded in a different way as per its genetic signature following treatment. Cluster analysis indicated that tumors can be divided into four to seven groups, which indicated the difficulty in predicting AI response and resistance.

More recently, the same group reported changes in expression levels of markers of estrogen regulation (i.e., KIAA0101, TFF3, SERPINA3, IRS-1, and TFF1) and proliferation (i.e., CDC2, CKS-2, cyclin B1, thymidine synthetase, and PCNA) by AI and found that tumors could be separated into the three following subgroups: (i) both proliferation and estrogen signaling signatures are reduced by treatment; (ii) both proliferation and estrogen signaling are unaffected or increased by treatment; and (iii) expression of estrogen-regulated genes is decreased, whereas proliferation genes remained unchanged or increased [29]. Also, Mackay et al. [30] reported that expression levels of the aromatase gene itself were decreased by AI treatment. However, these findings were not in accordance with AI response or resistance patterns; thus, further investigations are warranted to clarify the molecular changes in response to AI treatment.

14.10 MicroRNAs

MicroRNAs (miRNAs) are very small (about 20 nucleotides in length), noncoding RNAs that base-pair with target mRNAs to regulate gene expression [31] and are frequently located in cancer-associated gene regions. Aberrant expression patterns of these molecules in various cancers have been established. Due to the characteristic of being well preserved in the form of circulating molecules, miRNAs are of particular interest as potential diagnostic markers [32]. We may assume the role of miRNAs in AI response, but evaluation of miRNAs to monitor neoadjuvant AI is still in a primary state. Maillot et al. [33] reported increased levels of several microRNAs 4 months after ET with a combination of exemestane and tamoxifen. The miRNAs monitored in this study included miR-21, miR-181b, miR-26a, miR-26b, miR-27b, and miR-23b, as well as estrogen-regulated miRNAs. Among these, expression levels of miR-21, miR-23b, and miR-181b were increased in an in vitro experiment using tamoxifen-resistant MCF-7 BC cell lines. The results of this study showed that ET affects miRNA expression and that miRNAs are suitable markers to predict AI response.

Masri et al. [34] identified hormone-responsive miRNAs using microarray analysis of hormone refractory BC cell lines. Among the identified miRNAs, miR-128a was shown to target TGF-β, which exhibits impaired sensitivity in letrozole-resistant cell lines. These results showed that hormone-sensitive miRNAs could be potential biomarkers to identify signs of AI resistance and also indicated the utility of miRNAs in the identification of complex mechanisms of AI resistance.

In 2012, our group performed an in vitro study of letrozole-treated MCF-7 cell lines to evaluate pre- and posttreatment miRNA alterations using a miRNA-PCR array. The results of this study indicated that several tumor suppressor miRNAs were upregulated by letrozole treatment. In particular, let-7f, a tumor-suppressing miRNA identified in various cancers [35], was also upregulated in letrozole-treated BC specimens. We further performed a luciferase assay to determine whether the aromatase gene was a direct target of let-7f and discovered that let-7f expression was negatively correlated to aromatase expression by immunohistochemical analysis [36]. Therefore, the immunohistochemical identification of target RNAs of AI-responsive miRNAs is useful to target RNAs and could be an alternative method to detect tissue or serum miRNAs.

A previous study identified variations in miRNA expression profiles in tamoxifen-sensitive as well as tamoxifen-resistant BC cell lines. This analysis revealed 97 miRNAs that were associated with tamoxifen resistance [37]. Further, another study indicated that miR-221 and miR-222 were upregulated in HER2(+) BC cells compared with HER2(−), and ectopic expression of miR-221/miR-222 using small interfering RNA resulted in acquired resistance to former tamoxifen-sensitive BC cells [38]. p27kip1 was identified as a target gene of miR-221/miR-222, and its overexpression induced enhanced cytotoxicity in tamoxifen-resistant breast tumors [38, 39]. miR-221/miR-222 deserves further attention, as Rao et al. [40] reported the same aberrant expression in AI (fulvestrant)-resistant cell lines. Therefore, miR-221/miR-222 seems to play an important role in the regulation of estrogen metabolism and ERα expression in ET.

In addition, miR-15a/miR-16 reportedly plays a role in endocrine resistance. The suppression of miR-15a/miR-16 and incrementally increased levels of the antiapoptotic protein BCL-2 were observed following tamoxifen treatment. Moreover, overexpression of these miRNAs suppressed BCL-2 expression and resensitized tamoxifen-resistant cell lines [41]. However, the role of miR-15a/miR-16 has not been examined in AI treatment of either BC specimens or cell lines.

Cittelly et al. [42] demonstrated that miR-342 was downregulated in tamoxifen-resistant BC cell lines and specimens and concluded that miR-342 was predictive of the initial response as well as acquired resistance to tamoxifen. Also, in vitro experiments indicated restoration of miR-342 in resensitized tamoxifen-resistant cells. Furthermore, miR-342 restoration inhibited cell proliferation and promoted cancer cell apoptosis. Other miRNAs reportedly implicated in ET resistance include miR-101, miR-210, and miR-301, which are involved with the tumor suppressor phosphatase and tensin homolog (PTEN) [43].

In summary, miRNAs seem to be more useful biomarkers than RNAs, due to the above reasons, and circulating miRNAs may have clinical implications. However, further studies are needed to clarify the involvement of miRNAs in AI treatment. Thus, deciphering the usefulness of miRNAs in predicting AI response will require more time.

14.11 Epigenetics

The use of epigenetics has recently gained popularity in BC research. DNA methylation and histone hypoacetylation are primary features that can be assessed by epigenetics. These posttranslational modifications continue to receive attention as new biomarkers for diagnosis, treatment, and prognosis of BC. DNA methylation is of particular interest in BC because of the frequent global DNA hypomethylation (up to 50 %) in BCs, compared with cancers of other sites. Hypomethylation in BC is associated with poor prognosis [44]. Also, BC-related genes, such as ER, HOXA5, Twist, E-cadherin, and RARβ, are hypermethylated and thus silenced compared to normal breast tissue [45]. A study of the methylation status of CDH1, DCR1, DAPK1, RASSF1A, DCR2APC, MGMT, GSTP1, and PTEN showed methylation of at least one of these genes in approximately 70 % of BC specimens [46].

A study of the prevalence of ER methylation reported that ER is unmethylated at the CpG island in normal breast tissues. A higher frequency of methylation was observed in ER-positive tumors compared to ER-negative tumors. Therefore, ER-positive tumors are indicated as a better target for epigenetic research and as a treatment target compared with ER-negative tumors. Also, methylation reversal at the ER promoter may resensitize ET-resistant BC tumors, although further studies are required to investigate this possibility. Furthermore, miRNA hypermethylation is a relatively new area of interest, which may lead to the loss of tumor-suppressing properties of miRNA by silencing [47]. However, further research is needed to address this issue.

14.12 Tumor-Infiltrating Lymphocytes

Tumor-infiltrating lymphocytes (TILs) are immune cell infiltrates in cancers that influence prognosis and are thought to have two different effects, a protective role and a tumor-promoting role. However, tumor-infiltrating $CD8^+$ TILs are reported to indicate improved prognosis in cancer [48]. Recently, we evaluated the role of TILs in BC cases receiving neoadjuvant AI therapy using double immunohistochemical staining of CD8+ and T regulatory cells (Tregs) or Foxp3−. Here, we found a significant increase in the CD8+/Treg ratio in cases that clinically respond to neoadjuvant AI, but not in cases with a poor response. This implies that AI may induce alterations in the host immune response to BC, which subsequently affects the response to AIs.

14.13 Changes in Angiogenesis

Angiogenesis is also altered by AI treatment. We recently reported that neovascularization, as analyzed by immunohistochemical analysis of vasohibin-1, is increased in cases that clinically respond to neoadjuvant AI therapy. We also found that changes in the ratio of vasohibin-1-positive cells were inversely correlated with the post-AI Ki-67 index, which supports former findings [49].

A summary of biomarkers of neoadjuvant AI therapy is shown in Table 14.1. A primary aim of neoadjuvant ET is to shrink the tumor prior to surgery and to validate predictive factors of response at the time of surgery, which could facilitate the selection of an appropriate adjuvant therapy. At present, immunohistochemical analysis of Ki-67 expression is the most appropriate method to predict response to AI therapy. However, a more accurate biomarker to predict short-term, as well as long-term, responses and acquired resistance to AIs has not yet been established. The goal of effective personalized medicine is the ability to identify cancer patients who will respond to anticancer therapies. Also, it is desirable to identify at which point the cancer cells acquire resistance to ongoing therapy. Clinically, some patients relapse while receiving AI therapy, whereas others relapse after treatment completion. ET is an effective AI to potently suppress cancer growth via inhibition of estrogen activity. Unfortunately, no current biomarker is suitable to distinguish such cases from the outset. Therefore, new biomarkers to predict AI resistance are urgently needed. Since relevant miRNAs can be detected in the circulation of cancer patients, these circulating miRNAs may be a new promising class of potential biomarkers that can be readily measured in real time in serum to facilitate

Table 14.1 Summary of biomarkers of neoadjuvant AI therapy

Biomarkers	Altered by AI treatment	Predict response	Predict resistance	Reference
Clinical factors		Menopausal status		[2]
Tumor size	Yes	No	No	[6]
Pathological features				
Mitosis	Yes	Yes	No	[7]
Nuclear pleomorphism	No	No	No	[8]
Immunohistochemistry				
ER	No	Yes	No	[10–12]
PR	Yes	No	No	[14]
HER2	No	No	Yes	[14, 16]
Ki-67	Yes	Yes	No	[14, 15, 20, 21]
Tissue concentration of sex steroid				
E2	Yes	No	No	[24]
Androgen	Yes	No	No	[27]
RNA	Yes	No	No	[28–30]
MicroRNAs	Yes	Hopeful	Hopeful	[33–43]
Tumor-infiltrating lymphocytes	Yes	Yes	No	[48]
Angiogenesis	Yes	Yes	No	[49]

the choice of the most beneficial and effective treatment. Until then, immunohistochemical analysis is one of the most effective methods available, and neoadjuvant therapy compared to adjuvant therapy allows for disease assessment both pre- and post-AI therapy.

References

1. Bradley KL, Tyldesley S, Speers CH, Woods R, Villa D (2014) Contemporary systemic therapy for male breast cancer. Clin Breast Cancer 14(1):31–39. doi:10.1016/j.clbc.2013.09.001
2. Montagna E, Cancello G, Colleoni M (2013) The aromatase inhibitors (plus ovarian function suppression) in premenopausal breast cancer patients: ready for prime time? Cancer Treat Rev 39(8):886–890. doi:10.1016/j.ctrv.2013.04.007
3. Lonning PE, Haynes BP, Dowsett M (2014) Relationship of body mass index with aromatisation and plasma and tissue oestrogen levels in postmenopausal breast cancer patients treated with aromatase inhibitors. Eur J Cancer 50(6):1055–1064. doi:10.1016/j.ejca.2014.01.007
4. Noruzinia M, Coupier I, Pujol P (2005) Is BRCA1/BRCA2-related breast carcinogenesis estrogen dependent? Cancer 104(8):1567–1574. doi:10.1002/Cncr.21367

5. Gorski JJ, Kennedy RD, Hosey AM, Harkin DP (2009) The complex relationship between BRCA1 and ER alpha in hereditary breast cancer. Clin Cancer Res 15(5):1514–1518. doi:10.1158/1078-0432.Ccr-08-0640
6. Eiermann W, Paepke S, Appfelstaedt J, Llombart-Cussac A, Eremin J, Vinholes J, Mauriac L, Ellis M, Lassus M, Chaudri-Ross HA, Dugan M, Borgs M (2001) Preoperative treatment of postmenopausal breast cancer patients with letrozole: a randomized double-blind multicenter study. Ann Oncol: Off J Eur Soc Med Oncol/ESMO 12(11):1527–1532
7. Miller WR, Dixon JM, Macfarlane L, Cameron D, Anderson TJ (2003) Pathological features of breast cancer response following neoadjuvant treatment with either letrozole or tamoxifen. Eur J Cancer 39(4):462–468
8. Rakha EA, El-Sayed ME, Lee AH, Elston CW, Grainge MJ, Hodi Z, Blamey RW, Ellis IO (2008) Prognostic significance of Nottingham histologic grade in invasive breast carcinoma. J Clin Oncol: Off J Am Soc Clin Oncol 26(19):3153–3158. doi:10.1200/JCO.2007.15.5986
9. Thomas JS, Julian HS, Green RV, Cameron DA, Dixon MJ (2007) Histopathology of breast carcinoma following neoadjuvant systemic therapy: a common association between letrozole therapy and central scarring. Histopathology 51(2):219–226. doi:10.1111/j.1365-2559.2007.02752.x
10. Burstein HJ, Griggs JJ, Prestrud AA, Temin S (2010) American society of clinical oncology clinical practice guideline update on adjuvant endocrine therapy for women with hormone receptor-positive breast cancer. J Oncol Pract/Am Soc Clin Oncol 6(5):243–246. doi:10.1200/JOP.000082
11. Patani N, Martin LA (2014) Understanding response and resistance to oestrogen deprivation in ER-positive breast cancer. Mol Cell Endocrinol 382(1):683–694. doi:10.1016/j.mce.2013.09.038
12. Goldhirsch A, Ingle JN, Gelber RD, Coates AS, Thurlimann B, Senn HJ (2009) Thresholds for therapies: highlights of the St Gallen International Expert Consensus on the primary therapy of early breast cancer 2009. Ann Oncol: Off J Eur Soc Med Oncol/ESMO 20(8):1319–1329. doi:10.1093/annonc/mdp322
13. Chanplakorn N, Chanplakorn P, Suzuki T, Ono K, Chan MS, Miki Y, Saji S, Ueno T, Toi M, Sasano H (2010) Increased estrogen sulfatase (STS) and 17beta-hydroxysteroid dehydrogenase type 1(17beta-HSD1) following neoadjuvant aromatase inhibitor therapy in breast cancer patients. Breast Cancer Res Treat 120(3):639–648. doi:10.1007/s10549-010-0785-3
14. Yamashita H, Takahashi S, Ito Y, Yamashita T, Ando Y, Toyama T, Sugiura H, Yoshimoto N, Kobayashi S, Fujii Y, Iwase H (2009) Predictors of response to exemestane as primary endocrine therapy in estrogen receptor-positive breast cancer. Cancer Sci 100(11):2028–2033. doi:10.1111/j.1349-7006.2009.01274.x
15. Ellis MJ, Coop A, Singh B, Tao Y, Llombart-Cussac A, Janicke F, Mauriac L, Quebe-Fehling E, Chaudri-Ross HA, Evans DB, Miller WR (2003) Letrozole inhibits tumor proliferation more effectively than tamoxifen independent of HER1/2 expression status. Cancer Res 63(19):6523–6531
16. Dowsett M, Ebbs SR, Dixon JM, Skene A, Griffith C, Boeddinghaus I, Salter J, Detre S, Hills M, Ashley S, Francis S, Walsh G, Smith IE (2005) Biomarker changes during neoadjuvant anastrozole, tamoxifen, or the combination: influence of hormonal status and HER-2 in breast cancer – a study from the IMPACT trialists. J Clin Oncol: Off J Am Soc Clin Oncol 23(11):2477–2492. doi:10.1200/JCO.2005.07.559
17. Ellis MJ, Tao Y, Young O, White S, Proia AD, Murray J, Renshaw L, Faratian D, Thomas J, Dowsett M, Krause A, Evans DB, Miller WR, Dixon JM (2006) Estrogen-independent proliferation is present in estrogen-receptor HER2-positive primary breast cancer after neoadjuvant letrozole. J Clin Oncol: Off J Am Soc Clin Oncol 24(19):3019–3025. doi:10.1200/JCO.2005.04.3034
18. Gong P, Wang YX, Liu GV, Zhang J, Wang ZY (2013) New insight into Ki67 expression at the invasive front in breast cancer. PLoS One 8(1). doi:ARTN e54912. doi:10.1371/journal.pone.0054912

19. Cheang MC, Chia SK, Voduc D, Gao D, Leung S, Snider J, Watson M, Davies S, Bernard PS, Parker JS, Perou CM, Ellis MJ, Nielsen TO (2009) Ki67 index, HER2 status, and prognosis of patients with luminal B breast cancer. J Natl Cancer Inst 101(10):736–750. doi:10.1093/jnci/djp082
20. Miller WR, Dixon JM (2002) Endocrine and clinical endpoints of exemestane as neoadjuvant therapy. Cancer Control: J Moffitt Cancer Cent 9(2 Suppl):9–15
21. Dowsett M, Smith IE, Ebbs SR, Dixon JM, Skene A, Griffith C, Boeddinghaus I, Salter J, Detre S, Hills M, Ashley S, Francis S, Walsh G (2005) Short-term changes in Ki-67 during neoadjuvant treatment of primary breast cancer with anastrozole or tamoxifen alone or combined correlate with recurrence-free survival. Clin Cancer Res 11(2):951s–958s
22. Dowsett M, Smith IE, Ebbs SR, Dixon JM, Skene A, A'Hern R, Salter J, Detre S, Hills M, Walsh G (2007) Prognostic value of Ki67 expression after short-term presurgical endocrine therapy for primary breast cancer. J Natl Cancer Inst 99(2):167–170. doi:10.1093/jnci/djk020
23. Geisler H (2003) Breast cancer tissue estrogens and their manipulation with aromatase inhibitors and inactivators. J Steroid Biochem 86(3–5):245–253. doi:10.1016/S0960-0760(03)00364-9
24. Lonning PE, Geisler J (2010) Evaluation of plasma and tissue estrogen suppression with third-generation aromatase inhibitors: of relevance to clinical understanding? J Steroid Biochem Mol Biol 118(4–5):288–293. doi:10.1016/j.jsbmb.2009.09.013
25. Geisler J, Detre S, Berntsen H, Ottestad L, Lindtjorn B, Dowsett M, Einstein Lonning P (2001) Influence of neoadjuvant anastrozole (Arimidex) on intratumoral estrogen levels and proliferation markers in patients with locally advanced breast cancer. Clin Cancer Res: Off J Am Assoc Cancer Res 7(5):1230–1236
26. Geisler J, Helle H, Ekse D, Duong NK, Evans DB, Nordbo Y, Aas T, Lonning PE (2008) Letrozole is superior to anastrozole in suppressing breast cancer tissue and plasma estrogen levels. Clin Cancer Res: Off J Am Assoc Cancer Res 14(19):6330–6335. doi:10.1158/1078-0432.CCR-07-5221
27. Takagi K, Miki Y, Nagasaki S, Hirakawa H, Onodera Y, Akahira J, Ishida T, Watanabe M, Kimijima I, Hayashi S, Sasano H, Suzuki T (2010) Increased intratumoral androgens in human breast carcinoma following aromatase inhibitor exemestane treatment. Endocr Relat Cancer 17(2):415–430. doi:10.1677/ERC-09-0257
28. Miller WR, Anderson TJ, White S, Larionov A, Murray J, Evans D, Krause A, Dixon JM (2005) Aromatase inhibitors: cellular and molecular effects. J Steroid Biochem Mol Biol 95(1–5):83–89. doi:10.1016/j.jsbmb.2005.04.010
29. Miller WR, Larionov A (2010) Changes in expression of oestrogen regulated and proliferation genes with neoadjuvant treatment highlight heterogeneity of clinical resistance to the aromatase inhibitor, letrozole. Breast Cancer Res: BCR 12(4):R52. doi:10.1186/bcr2611
30. Mackay A, Urruticoechea A, Dixon JM, Dexter T, Fenwick K, Ashworth A, Drury S, Larionov A, Young O, White S, Miller WR, Evans DB, Dowsett M (2007) Molecular response to aromatase inhibitor treatment in primary breast cancer. Breast Cancer Res: BCR 9(3):R37. doi:10.1186/bcr1732
31. Filipowicz W, Bhattacharyya SN, Sonenberg N (2008) Mechanisms of post-transcriptional regulation by microRNAs: are the answers in sight? Nat Rev Genet 9(2):102–114. doi:10.1038/nrg2290
32. Kosaka N, Iguchi H, Ochiya T (2010) Circulating microRNA in body fluid: a new potential biomarker for cancer diagnosis and prognosis. Cancer Sci 101(10):2087–2092. doi:10.1111/j.1349-7006.2010.01650.x
33. Maillot G, Lacroix-Triki M, Pierredon S, Gratadou L, Schmidt S, Benes V, Roche H, Dalenc F, Auboeuf D, Millevoi S, Vagner S (2009) Widespread estrogen-dependent repression of micrornas involved in breast tumor cell growth. Cancer Res 69(21):8332–8340. doi:10.1158/0008-5472.CAN-09-2206

34. Masri S, Liu Z, Phung S, Wang E, Yuan YC, Chen S (2010) The role of microRNA-128a in regulating TGFbeta signaling in letrozole-resistant breast cancer cells. Breast Cancer Res Treat 124(1):89–99. doi:10.1007/s10549-009-0716-3
35. Wang X, Cao L, Wang Y, Liu N, You Y (2012) Regulation of let-7 and its target oncogenes (review). Oncol Lett 3(5):955–960. doi:10.3892/ol.2012.609
36. Shibahara Y, Miki Y, Onodera Y, Hata S, Chan MS, Yiu CC, Loo TY, Nakamura Y, Akahira J, Ishida T, Abe K, Hirakawa H, Chow LW, Suzuki T, Ouchi N, Sasano H (2012) Aromatase inhibitor treatment of breast cancer cells increases the expression of let-7f, a microRNA targeting CYP19A1. J Pathol 227(3):357–366. doi:10.1002/path.4019
37. Manavalan TT, Teng Y, Appana SN, Datta S, Kalbfleisch TS, Li Y, Klinge CM (2011) Differential expression of microRNA expression in tamoxifen-sensitive MCF-7 versus tamoxifen-resistant LY2 human breast cancer cells. Cancer Lett 313(1):26–43. doi:10.1016/j.canlet.2011.08.018
38. Miller TE, Ghoshal K, Ramaswamy B, Roy S, Datta J, Shapiro CL, Jacob S, Majumder S (2008) MicroRNA-221/222 confers tamoxifen resistance in breast cancer by targeting p27Kip1. J Biol Chem 283(44):29897–29903. doi:10.1074/jbc.M804612200
39. Zhao JJ, Lin J, Yang H, Kong W, He L, Ma X, Coppola D, Cheng JQ (2008) MicroRNA-221/222 negatively regulates estrogen receptor alpha and is associated with tamoxifen resistance in breast cancer. J Biol Chem 283(45):31079–31086. doi:10.1074/jbc.M806041200
40. Rao X, Di Leva G, Li M, Fang F, Devlin C, Hartman-Frey C, Burow ME, Ivan M, Croce CM, Nephew KP (2011) MicroRNA-221/222 confers breast cancer fulvestrant resistance by regulating multiple signaling pathways. Oncogene 30(9):1082–1097. doi:10.1038/onc.2010.487
41. Cittelly DM, Das PM, Salvo VA, Fonseca JP, Burow ME, Jones FE (2010) Oncogenic HER2 {delta}16 suppresses miR-15a/16 and deregulates BCL-2 to promote endocrine resistance of breast tumors. Carcinogenesis 31(12):2049–2057. doi:10.1093/carcin/bgq192
42. Cittelly DM, Das PM, Spoelstra NS, Edgerton SM, Richer JK, Thor AD, Jones FE (2010) Downregulation of miR-342 is associated with tamoxifen resistant breast tumors. Mol Cancer 9:317. doi:10.1186/1476-4598-9-317
43. Garcia-Becerra R, Santos N, Diaz L, Camacho J (2012) Mechanisms of resistance to endocrine therapy in breast cancer: focus on signaling pathways, miRNAs and genetically based resistance. Int J Mol Sci 14(1):108–145. doi:10.3390/ijms14010108
44. Soares J, Pinto AE, Cunha CV, Andre S, Barao I, Sousa JM, Cravo M (1999) Global DNA hypomethylation in breast carcinoma: correlation with prognostic factors and tumor progression. Cancer 85(1):112–118
45. Widschwendter M, Jones PA (2002) DNA methylation and breast carcinogenesis. Oncogene 21(35):5462–5482. doi:10.1038/sj.onc.1205606
46. Connolly R, Stearns V (2012) Epigenetics as a therapeutic target in breast cancer. J Mammary Gland Biol Neoplasia 17(3–4):191–204. doi:10.1007/s10911-012-9263-3
47. Lujambio A, Esteller M (2007) CpG island hypermethylation of tumor suppressor microRNAs in human cancer. Cell Cycle 6(12):1455–1459
48. Dunn GP, Old LJ, Schreiber RD (2004) The immunobiology of cancer immunosurveillance and immunoediting. Immunity 21(2):137–148. doi:10.1016/j.immuni.2004.07.017
49. Chan MS, Wang L, Chanplakorn N, Tamaki K, Ueno T, Toi M, Loo WT, Chow LW, Suzuki T, Sasano H (2012) Effects of estrogen depletion on angiogenesis in estrogen-receptor-positive breast carcinoma – an immunohistochemical study of vasohibin-1 and CD31 with correlation to pathobiological response of the patients in neoadjuvant aromatase inhibitor therapy. Expert Opin Ther Targets 16(Suppl 1):S69–S78. doi:10.1517/14728222.2011.628938

Part V
Preoperative Chemotherapy

Chapter 15
Essence of Neoadjuvant Therapy

Jenny Furlanetto and Gunter von Minckwitz

Abstract The neoadjuvant approach is widely used because it offers several clinical advantages. Importantly, it allows to monitor treatment response and to discontinue ineffective therapy in the event of disease progression, thus sparing the patients of potentially toxic and inadequate drugs. Moreover, the preoperative setting provides an in vivo model to explore the efficacy of new drugs and to investigate biomarkers that could help to identify patients with a higher chance of treatment benefit.

This chapter addresses the following topics: differences between adjuvant and neoadjuvant chemotherapy, aims of neoadjuvant chemotherapy, recommended treatment options in the preoperative setting, differences between pCR (pathological complete response) definitions and their associations with outcome, and prognosis in patients with residual disease. Moreover, the hot topic of surrogacy of pCR will be discussed.

Keywords Breast cancer • Neoadjuvant chemotherapy • Pathological complete response • Surrogate endpoint

15.1 Introduction

Neoadjuvant chemotherapy was originally used to allow for operability of a tumor initially not amenable to surgery. However, in recent years it has become a new standard of care in patients with locally advanced breast cancer and an important option for patients with operable tumors. The extensive use of this approach is mainly due to the unique opportunity to monitor tumor chemosensitivity and to adjust the therapeutic plan according to the response. Moreover, the neoadjuvant setting allows testing of new drugs and identification of biomarkers predicting response and outcome. In this chapter, we will discuss the major concepts applicable in the neoadjuvant setting.

J. Furlanetto • G. von Minckwitz (✉)
German Breast Group, c/o GBG Forschungs GmbH, Neu-Isenburg, Martin-Behaim-Straße 12, 63263 Neu-Isenburg, Germany
e-mail: Gunter.vonMinckwitz@germanbreastgroup.de

M. Toi et al. (eds.), *Personalized Treatment of Breast Cancer*,
DOI 10.1007/978-4-431-55552-0_15

15.2 Basic Concepts

15.2.1 Definition

Neoadjuvant treatment is the standard therapy for locally advanced breast cancer and is an option for primary operable disease. Three different terms are currently used to define this approach. The term *primary systemic therapy* focuses on the position of this treatment modality within the entire treatment course; *preoperative therapy* underlines the timing in regard to surgery; and the term *neoadjuvant therapy* refers more to the aim of the treatment, the healing of the patient, similar to the adjuvant approach. Although the first two terms give a more accurate description of the treatment itself, the latter is the more frequently used.

15.2.2 Neoadjuvant vs Adjuvant

A meta-analysis of nine randomized trials, including a total of 3946 patients, found no statistically or clinically significant differences between neoadjuvant and adjuvant treatment arms in relation to death (risk ratio [RR] 1.00, 95 % confidence interval [CI] 0.90–1.12), disease progression (RR 0.99, 95 % CI 0.91–1.07), and distant disease recurrence (RR 0.99, 95 % CI 0.94, 95 % CI 0.83–1.06). However, neoadjuvant therapy was significantly associated with an increased risk of locoregional disease recurrence compared to adjuvant chemotherapy (RR 1.22, 95 % CI 1.04–1.43). The increased risk in the preoperative arm largely reflected the use of radiotherapy without any surgery for patients who had a complete clinical response [1].

In the NSABP B-18 study, patients were randomly assigned to either surgery followed by four cycles of AC chemotherapy (doxorubicin 60 mg/m^2 and cyclophosphamide 600 mg/m^2) every 21 days or the same regimen followed by surgery. The results from this protocol show no statistically significant differences in disease-free survival (DFS) and overall survival (OS) between the two groups. Only a trend in favor of preoperative chemotherapy for DFS and OS in women younger than 50 years was observed (DFS HR = 0.85, $p = 0.09$; OS HR = 0.81, $p = 0.06$). In the NSABP B-27 study, all patients were assigned to receive four cycles of AC every 21 days before surgery. Patients in group 1 did not receive further preoperative chemotherapy; patients in group 2 received four cycles of docetaxel 100 mg/m^2 preoperatively after completion of AC, whereas in group 3 docetaxel was given after surgery. No significant differences were seen for OS and DFS between the treatment groups [2].

Taken together, these trials demonstrate the equivalence of neoadjuvant and adjuvant treatments for breast cancer in terms of survival, disease progression, and distant recurrence.

15.2.3 Aims of Neoadjuvant Chemotherapy (NACT)

Three main reasons for choosing neoadjuvant therapy can be identified: to improve the surgical option, to determine the response to preoperative treatment, and to obtain long-term disease-free survival. As stated by a panel of experts, the relative importance of these three objectives differs in different breast cancer settings. In locally advanced breast cancer, the major goal is to improve the surgical option and secondly to obtain freedom from disease; in operable breast cancer patients that are candidates for adjuvant chemotherapy, to obtain freedom from disease; and in operable breast cancer patients that are candidates for adjuvant endocrine treatment alone, to improve the surgical option and secondly to gain information on tumor response [3].

As shown in several randomized trials the breast-conserving surgery (BCS) rate is increased by neoadjuvant chemotherapy without an increased risk of local relapse [4–6]. Recently the prospective multicentric ACOSOG Z1071 trial shows that the incidence of BCS correlates with tumor biology, triple-negative breast cancer (TNBC), and HER2-positive breast cancers having the highest rates of BCS (TNBC 46.8 %; HER2+ 43.0 %; HER2− 34.5 %; $p = 0.019$) and pCR (TNBC 38.2 %; HER2+ 45.4 %; HER2− 11.4 %; $p < 0.0001$); after neoadjuvant chemotherapy patients with these subtypes are possible candidates for less invasive surgical approaches after chemotherapy [7].

Other potential benefits may include the opportunity to monitor response during treatment with the possibility of an adjustment in systemic therapy, an improvement in cosmetic outcome and a decrease in the extent of axillary surgery [8]. Moreover, the neoadjuvant approach has become a valuable research approach, allowing the investigation of new drugs or of new combinations of old drugs in smaller trials and in less time if compared to the adjuvant setting. The possibility to perform multiple biopsies during treatment and the direct observation of tumor response permit identification of biomarkers to predict response and safety and to understand how tumor biology is modified by the treatment itself.

15.2.4 Neoadjuvant Treatment

Since the goals of treatment in terms of ultimate systemic control are the same, the selection of regimen for neoadjuvant chemotherapy generally follows the guidelines applying to the conventional adjuvant setting. Some important advices should be followed:

- The addition of taxanes to anthracycline-based NACT improves pCR and DFS and decreases the incidence of local recurrence [16].
- The full course of chemotherapy should be completed before surgery to increase the chance of pCR [15].

- The optimal duration of NACT has not been clearly defined. At least six cycles of chemotherapy should be administered [9, 10].
- Dose-dense NACT has been shown to improve pCR [11]; notably a recent meta-analysis found a potential surrogate value of pCR for survival in trials comparing dose-dense regimens versus standard regimens [32]. Among patients who did not respond to standard initial NACT, switching to a non-cross-resistant regimen did not show additional benefit [12, 13].
- In patients with HER2-positive disease, anti-HER2 therapy should be included, because increased rates of response could be obtained [14, 19, 20].
- Endocrine treatment should be started after surgery and NACT. In fact, the concurrent use of chemotherapy and tamoxifen may be detrimental in terms of both survival and toxicity [14].
- No additional postoperative adjuvant chemotherapy following a full course of NACT is recommended, whether pCR was achieved or not [15, 16].

15.3 Pathological Complete Remission

15.3.1 Definitions

Several definitions of pathological complete remission are used by different international breast cancer groups. They vary according to the different acceptance for residual breast cancer in breast and nodes (Table 15.1). The more stringent definition is used by the German Breast Group (GBG) and by the Arbeitsgemeinschaft Gynäkologische Onkologie Breast Group (AGO-B), whereas the more tolerant is used by French groups.

Table 15.1 Definitions of pathological complete remission currently used by different international research groups

Classification	Definition	Currently used by
*yp*T0 *yp*N0	No invasive and no noninvasive residual in breast and nodes	GBG
		AGO-B [17]
*yp*T0/is *yp*N0	No invasive residual in breast and nodes	MD Anderson Cancer Center [18]
		Austrian Breast and Colorectal Cancer Study Group [19]
		Neo-Breast International Group [20]
*yp*T0/is *yp*N0/+	No invasive residual in breast. Noninvasive residual in breast and infiltrated lymph nodes are allowed	National Surgical Adjuvant Breast and Bowel Project [21]
*yp*T $\leq$1*mic* *yp*N0/+	No gross invasive residual in breast; focal invasive and noninvasive residuals in breast and infiltrated lymph nodes are allowed	French groups [22]

15.3.2 pCR as a Surrogate Marker for Outcome

Whether or not pCR can be considered a surrogate marker for outcome is under a lot of debate. Results are contradictory among studies and a clear consent has not yet been found. The main reason is the heterogeneity between the different trials according to selection criteria, baseline parameters, and pCR definition used and the different subgroups analyzed. Two big meta-analyses tried to address this issue in the last years. The German Breast Group investigated the association between pCR according to the different definitions available and outcome in 6.377 patients with primary breast cancer receiving neoadjuvant anthracycline-taxane-based chemotherapy in seven randomized trials. The impact of subgroups and of residual disease in breast and nodes has been clearly shown. Patients with no residual disease in breast and nodes (*yp*T0 *yp*N0) experienced a better DFS and OS. This was particularly true when compared with *yp*T0/is *yp*N+ (DFS HR 3.18; 95 % CI 2.31–4.38; $p < 0.001$; OS HR 4.05; 95 % CI 2.63–6.24: $p < 0.001$), but also if only in situ residual disease in breast was present (DFS HR 1.74; 95 % CI 1.28–2.36; $p < 0.001$; OS HR 1.41; 95 % CI 0.87–2.29; $p = 0166$). Moreover, in less aggressive tumor (low proliferation, lobular, grade 1, hormone receptor positive), pCR was not predictive for OS and DFS. In patients with grade 2–3 tumors, hormone receptor negative, and ductal histology, the achievement of a pCR was associated with a better outcome. When considering the different breast cancer subgroups, no impact of pCR on prognosis was seen for luminal A-like (ER and/or PgR positive, HER2 negative, grade 1 or 2) and in luminal B/HER2-positive tumors, whereas a great impact was seen for HER2 positive, TNBC, and luminal B/HER2-negative tumors. Given these results it seems that pCR could only be a good surrogate endpoint in this latter group [23]. Considering the importance of the availability of new drugs for breast cancer patients and the great advantages that neoadjuvant trials offer in comparison to adjuvant studies (smaller sample sizes, short drug exposure, response monitoring within a short time frame, shorter follow-up), the FDA (Food and Drug Administration) initiated the CTNeoBC meta-analysis, in order to better understand pCR correlation with long-term outcome. The main goal was to define if pCR could be used as an endpoint to support accelerated approval of cancer drugs in high-risk early breast cancer patients. A total of 12 trials including 11,955 patients and almost all studies included in the German meta-analysis were analyzed. The strongest definition of pCR (ypT0 ypN0) was associated with a better outcome (event-free survival [EFS] HR 0.24, 95 % CI 0.39–0.51; OS HR 0.36 95 % CI 0.30–0.44), and the effect was greater in aggressive subtypes (TNBC, HER2 positive, HER2 negative). No difference in outcome was observed when patients with ypT0 ypN0 and widely overlapping group of patients with ypT0/is ypN0 were compared [24]. The study failed to define what magnitude of pCR improvement was needed to predict long-term clinical benefit. In fact when odds ratio for pCR was plotted against hazard ratios of event-free survival, no correlation was found. Two possible explanations could be identified: in the trials analyzed all BC subtypes were included, even if it is known that they could respond differently to the same treatment and an imprecise assessment of subgroups was done (mainly locally, no quality control, PAM50 test was not performed). Moreover, only small differences in terms of pCR between the compared CT regimens were identified. After the completion of the CTNeoBC trial, FDA recognized ypT0/is ypN0 as the preferred definition for pCR as a regulatory endpoint. Two main reasons underline this decision. First of all the use of the more stringent definition could lead to a lower rate of pCR, affecting the real benefit of the drug. Even if an association between pCR and outcome has not yet been proven for all patients affected by breast cancer, several studies showed that this association might exist for HER2-positive tumors. The NOAH study demonstrated a 20 % increased pCR rate for the combination of chemotherapy with an anti-HER2 agent as well as an improvement in event-free survival [25]. This trial therefore led to the approval of trastuzumab in the neoadjuvant setting by the European Medical Agency. Moreover, the NOAH study was the only trial included in the Cortazar meta-analysis to demonstrate a good surrogacy, probably due to the use of a targeted therapy for a specific subpopulation of patients. This results were confirmed by the NeoSphere study that clearly showed that a double anti-HER2 blockade with trastuzumab and pertuzumab can lead to a greater chance of pCR and consequently to a better outcome [26].

Confirmatory trials that should already be started at the time of the decision are mandatory for the accelerated approval of a drug [27]. Indeed the demonstration of an improvement in DFS and OS will be required until a formal validation of the surrogacy of pCR is obtained. Moreover, late and cumulative toxicities need to be accurately investigated.

For the first time in September 30, 2013, the FDA granted accelerated approval to pertuzumab for use in combination with trastuzumab and docetaxel as neoadjuvant treatment of patients with HER2-positive, locally advanced, inflammatory or early stage breast cancer, based on a significant improvement of pCR [28].

Controversy about the value of pCR as a surrogate endpoint has been reconfirmed by the results of the ALTTO trial that investigated the use of trastuzumab and/or lapatinib in the adjuvant setting. The NeoALTTO trial previously showed that dual anti-HER2 blockade with trastuzumab and lapatinib resulted in a near doubling of the pathological complete response, corresponding to a 62 % reduction in events as compared with no pathological response [20]. After a median follow-up of 4.5 years, the ALTTO results showed that dual targeting was associated with a slight numerical reduction in disease recurrences, but the difference was not statistically significant [29]. Unexpectedly, the outstanding results in terms of pCR obtained in the neoadjuvant setting did not translate in a survival advantage in the adjuvant setting. Several reasons can explain this finding. First of all the predefined level of significance alpha was split (≤ 0.025) in order to test both the concurrent and the sequential treatments of lapatinib with trastuzumab.

Secondly the relative dose intensity was much lower in the adjuvant regimen compared to the neoadjuvant setting. Furthermore other neoadjuvant trials did not confirm the results of NeoALTTO study. In the NSABP B-41 and in the CALGB 40601, the combined anti-HER2-targeted therapy produced only an insignificantly higher pCR than single-agent HER2-directed therapy [30, 31]. Correlative analysis of tissue sample is ongoing in order to identify subgroups of patients that could derive a benefit from the adjuvant combination.

A recent meta-regression analysis of 29 studies based on literature extracted data also failed to support the use of pCR as surrogate endpoint for DFS and OS. Interestingly the analysis found a correlation between pCR and outcome for trials comparing conventional doses with intensified/dose-dense regimens [32].

15.4 Prognosis of Patients Without a pCR

15.4.1 How to Define Prognosis of Patients Without a pCR After Neoadjuvant Chemotherapy

The identification of patients at high risk after neoadjuvant chemotherapy is essential in order to develop new strategies to improve their outcome. The classic TNM system can also be applied to residual disease after primary chemotherapy in order to define the prognostic impact. As previously described, data from the German meta-database clearly showed the correlation between outcome and this staging system [15]. Currently the most used classification systems are the following:

- CPS-EG (clinicopathological stage and biological markers) score: the integration of estrogen receptor status and tumor grading in the CPS score allowed the identification of seven distinct patients groups having different metastasis-free survival and disease-specific survival and provide a useful tool to stratify patients eligible for clinical trials with novel therapeutics. In particular ER-negative disease and G3 tumors were additional independent risk factors [33, 34]. The CPS-EG score was developed and validated by the MD Anderson group. The GBG also found that the system provides valuable prognostic information especially in patients with HR-positive, HER2-negative disease.
- RCB (residual cancer burden) score: the score is calculated as a continuous index combining pathological measurements of primary tumor (size and cellularity) and nodal metastases (number and size) to predict distant relapse-free survival. In particular the presence of an extensive residual disease is associated with poor prognosis, irrespective of the type of neoadjuvant chemotherapy administered, adjuvant hormone therapy, or the pathological stage of the residual disease. All data can be obtained from pathologic reports and entered in a freely available online calculator [35].

- RPCB (integrated score of RCB and Ki67) score: high post-treatment Ki67 value measured on the surgical excision specimen was independently associated with poorer DFS and OS. Moreover, post-treatment Ki67 was found to be more predictive of long-term outcome than the pretreatment value or the change from pre- to post-treatment [36]. The integration of post-treatment Ki67 with RCB provides more prognostic information than the two variables alone [37].

Several studies are ongoing to define if new agents could improve the prognosis of patients with residual disease after a preoperative chemotherapy. The only published phase III trial in this setting, the NaTaN study, failed to demonstrate an improvement in terms of DFS in patients treated with zoledronate as postneoadjuvant therapy after standard anthracycline-taxane-based NACT for early BC [38]. Therefore, even if residual invasive disease predicts high risk of relapse, given the lack of data on the efficacy of alternative agents in this setting, the current standard in patients with residual disease after NACT is no further therapy beyond endocrine and anti-HER2 treatment.

15.4.2 Ongoing Trials in Patients with Residual Disease

Several studies are ongoing to assess the efficacy of new drugs in patients not achieving a pCR after NACT:

- PENELOPE (NCT01864746): based on a randomized phase II trial in HR-positive metastatic breast cancer showing an improvement of progression-free survival [39], the study investigates the role of palbociclib, a cyclin D kinase 4/6 inhibitor, in addition to standard endocrine therapy in patients with a CPS-EG score $\geq$3 or 2 but with metastatic lymph nodes after NACT.
- KATHERINE (NCT01772472): based on data from the phase III EMILIA study, which showed that trastuzumab emtansine (TDM-1) significantly improved survival of women with HER2-positive metastatic breast cancer [40], the study randomly compares the use of trastuzumab vs TDM-1 as adjuvant therapy in patients with HER2-positive breast cancer who have residual tumor in the breast.
- OLYMPIA (NCT02032823): based on two phase II trials assessing safety and efficacy of olaparib in advanced breast cancer patients [41, 42], the study investigates the role of olaparib as adjuvant therapy in TNBC patients harboring germline BRCA1/2 mutations. Patients having had neoadjuvant chemotherapy are eligible in case they do not show a pCR.

15.5 Conclusion

The neoadjuvant setting provides the unique opportunity to directly observe the effect of the therapy on the tumor and to tailor the treatment according to the response. Moreover, the investigation of biomarkers correlated with response allows a better selection of patients for subsequent treatment. Further research is warranted to spare those patients unlikely to derive treatment benefit from toxicities and to maximize the overall cost-benefit rate.

References

1. Mauri D, Pavlidis N, Ioannidis JP (2005) Neoadjuvant versus adjuvant systemic treatment in breast cancer: a meta-analysis. J Natl Cancer Inst 97(3):188–194
2. Rastogi P, Anderson SJ, Bear HD, Geyer CE, Kahlenberg MS, Robidoux A et al (2008) Preoperative chemotherapy: updates of National Surgical Adjuvant Breast and Bowel Project Protocols B-18 and B-27. J Clin Oncol 26(5):778–785
3. Kaufmann M, Hortobagyi GN, Goldhirsch A, Scholl S, Makris A, Valagussa P et al (2006) Recommendations from an international expert panel on the use of neoadjuvant (primary) systemic treatment of operable breast cancer: an update. J Clin Oncol 24(12):1940–1949
4. Chen AM, Meric-Bernstam F, Hunt KK, Thames HD, Oswald MJ, Outlaw ED et al (2004) Breast conservation after neoadjuvant chemotherapy: the MD Anderson cancer center experience. J Clin Oncol 22(12):2303–2312
5. Lichter AS, Lippman ME, Danforth DN Jr, d'Angelo T, Steinberg SM, de Moss E et al (1992) Mastectomy versus breast-conserving therapy in the treatment of stage I and II carcinoma of the breast: a randomized trial at the National Cancer Institute. J Clin Oncol 10(6):976–983
6. Fisher B, Bryant J, Wolmark N, Mamounas E, Brown A, Fisher ER et al (1998) Effect of preoperative chemotherapy on the outcome of women with operable breast cancer. J Clin Oncol 16(8):2672–2685
7. Boughey JC, McCall LM, Ballman KV, Mittendorf EA, Ahrendt GM, Wilke LG et al (2014) Tumor biology correlates with rates of breast-conserving surgery and pathologic complete response after neoadjuvant chemotherapy for breast cancer: findings from the ACOSOG Z1071 (Alliance) Prospective Multicenter Clinical Trial. Ann Surg 260(4):608–614
8. Kaufmann M, von Minckwitz G, Mamounas EP, Cameron D, Carey LA, Cristofanilli M et al (2012) Recommendations from an international consensus conference on the current status and future of neoadjuvant systemic therapy in primary breast cancer. Ann Surg Oncol 19 (5):1508–1516
9. von Minckwitz G, Kümmel S, Vogel P, Hanusch C, Eidtmann H, Hilfrich J, German Breast Group et al (2008) Intensified neoadjuvant chemotherapy in early-responding breast cancer: phase III randomized GeparTrio study. J Natl Cancer Inst 100(8):552–562
10. Steger GG, Galid A, Gnant M, Mlineritsch B, Lang A, Tausch C et al (2007) ABCSG-14. Pathologic complete response with six compared with three cycles of neoadjuvant epirubicin plus docetaxel and granulocyte colony-stimulating factor in operable breast cancer: results of ABCSG-14. J Clin Oncol 25(15):2012–2018
11. Untch M, Möbus V, Kuhn W, Muck BR, Thomssen C, Bauerfeind I et al (2009) Intensive dose-dense compared with conventionally scheduled preoperative chemotherapy for high-risk primary breast cancer. J Clin Oncol 27(18):2938–2945
12. Huober J, Fasching PA, Hanusch C, Rezai M, Eidtmann H, Kittel K et al (2013) Neoadjuvant chemotherapy with paclitaxel and everolimus in breast cancer patients with non-responsive

tumours to epirubicin/cyclophosphamide (EC) ± bevacizumab -results of the randomised GeparQuinto study (GBG 44). Eur J Cancer 49(10):2284–2293
13. von Minckwitz G, Kümmel S, Vogel P, Hanusch C, Eidtmann H, Hilfrich J, German Breast Group et al (2008) Neoadjuvant vinorelbine-capecitabine versus docetaxel-doxorubicin-cyclophosphamide in early nonresponsive breast cancer: phase III randomized GeparTrio trial. J Natl Cancer Inst 100(8):542–551
14. von Minckwitz G, Costa SD, Raab G, Blohmer JU, Eidtmann H, Hilfrich J, German Preoperative Adriamycin-Docetaxel and German Adjuvant Breast Cancer Study Groups et al (2001) Dose-dense doxorubicin, docetaxel, and granulocyte colony-stimulating factor support with or without tamoxifen as preoperative therapy in patients with operable carcinoma of the breast: a randomized, controlled, open phase IIb study. J Clin Oncol 19(15):3506–3515
15. Goldhirsch A, Winer EP, Coates AS, Gelber RD, Piccart-Gebhart M, Thürlimann B et al (2013) Personalizing the treatment of women with early breast cancer: highlights of the St Gallen International Expert Consensus on the Primary Therapy of Early Breast Cancer 2013. Ann Oncol 24(9):2206–2223
16. NCCN guidelines http://www.nccn.org/professionals/physician_gls/f_guidelines.asp#site
17. Sinn HP, Schmid H, Junkermann H, Huober J, Leppien G, Kaufmann M et al (1994) Histologic regression of breast cancer after primary (neoadjuvant) chemotherapy. Geburtshilfe Frauenheilkd 54(10):552–558
18. Green MC, Buzdar AU, Smith T, Ibrahim NK, Valero V, Rosales MF et al (2005) Weekly paclitaxel improves pathologic complete remission in operable breast cancer when compared with paclitaxel once every 3 weeks. J Clin Oncol 23(25):5983–5992
19. Steger GG, Greil R, Lang A, Rudas M, Fitzal F, Mlineritsch B, Austrian Breast and Colorectal Study Group (ABCSG) et al (2014) Epirubicin and docetaxel with or without capecitabine as neoadjuvant treatment for early breast cancer: final results of a randomized phase III study (ABCSG-24). Ann Oncol 25(2):366–371
20. Baselga J, Bradbury I, Eidtmann H, Di Cosimo S, de Azambuja E, Aura C, NeoALTTO Study Team et al (2012) Lapatinib with trastuzumab for HER2-positive early breast cancer (NeoALTTO): a randomised, open-label, multicentre, phase 3 trial. Lancet 379 (9816):633–640
21. Bear HD, Anderson S, Brown A, Smith R, Mamounas EP, Fisher B, National Surgical Adjuvant Breast and Bowel Project Protocol B-27 et al (2003) The effect on tumor response of adding sequential preoperative docetaxel to preoperative doxorubicin and cyclophosphamide: preliminary results from National Surgical Adjuvant Breast and Bowel Project Protocol B-27. J Clin Oncol 21(22):4165–4174
22. Sataloff DM, Mason BA, Prestipino AJ, Seinige UL, Lieber CP, Baloch Z (1995) Pathologic response to induction chemotherapy in locally advanced carcinoma of the breast: a determinant of outcome. J Am Coll Surg 180(3):297–306
23. von Minckwitz G, Untch M, Blohmer JU, Costa SD, Eidtmann H, Fasching PA et al (2012) Definition and impact of pathologic complete response on prognosis after neoadjuvant chemotherapy in various intrinsic breast cancer subtypes. J Clin Oncol 30(15):1796–1804
24. Cortazar P, Zhang L, Untch M, Mehta K, Costantino JP, Wolmark N et al (2014) Pathological complete response and long-term clinical benefit in breast cancer: the CTNeoBC pooled analysis. Lancet 384(9938):164–172
25. Gianni L, Eiermann W, Semiglazov V, Manikhas A, Lluch A, Tjulandin S et al (2010) Neoadjuvant chemotherapy with trastuzumab followed by adjuvant trastuzumab versus neoadjuvant chemotherapy alone, in patients with HER2-positive locally advanced breast cancer (the NOAH trial): a randomised controlled superiority trial with a parallel HER2-negative cohort. Lancet 375(9712):377–384
26. Gianni L, Pienkowski T, Im YH, Roman L, Tseng LM, Liu MC et al (2012) Efficacy and safety of neoadjuvant pertuzumab and trastuzumab in women with locally advanced, inflammatory, or early HER2-positive breast cancer (NeoSphere): a randomised multicentre, open-label, phase 2 trial. Lancet Oncol 13(1):25–32

27. Prowell T, Cortazar P (2012) Guidance for industry pathological complete response in neoadjuvant treatment of high-risk early-stage breast cancer: use as an endpoint to support accelerated approval. Draft guidance for industry. Silver Spring (MD): FDA, Office of Hematology Oncology Group; 2012 May. Report No.:FDA-2012-D-0432. Available from: http://www.fda.gov/Drugs/ucm309182.htm
28. Amiri-Kordestani L, Wedam S, Zhang L, Tang S, Tilley A, Ibrahim A et al (2014) First FDA approval of neoadjuvant therapy for breast cancer: pertuzumab for the treatment of patients with HER2-positive breast cancer. Clin Cancer Res 20(21):5359–5364
29. Piccart-Gebhart MJ, Holmes AP, Baselga J, De Azambuja E, Dueck AC, Viale G et al (2014) First results from the phase III ALTTO trial (BIG 2-06; NCCTG [Alliance] N063D) comparing one year of anti-HER2 therapy with lapatinib alone (L), trastuzumab alone (T), their sequence (T→L), or their combination (T+L) in the adjuvant treatment of HER2-positive early breast cancer (EBC). J Clin Oncol 32:5s (suppl; abstr LBA4)
30. Robidoux A, Tang G, Rastogi P, Geyer CE Jr, Azar CA, Atkins JN et al (2013) Lapatinib as a component of neoadjuvant therapy for HER2-positive operable breast cancer (NSABP protocol B-41): an open-label, randomised phase 3 trial. Lancet Oncol 14(12):1183–1192
31. Carey LA, Berry DA, Ollila D, Harris L, Krop IE, Weckstein D et al (2013) Clinical and translational results of CALGB 40601: a neoadjuvant phase III trial of weekly paclitaxel and trastuzumab with or without lapatinib for HER2-positive breast cancer. J Clin Oncol 31:15s (suppl; abstr 500)
32. Berruti A, Amoroso V, Gallo F, Bertaglia V, Simoncini E, Pedersini R et al (2014) Pathologic complete response as a potential surrogate for the clinical outcome in patients with breast cancer after neoadjuvant therapy: a meta-regression of 29 randomized prospective studies. J Clin Oncol 32(34):3883–3891
33. Jeruss JS, Mittendorf EA, Tucker SL, Gonzalez-Angulo AM, Buchholz TA, Sahin AA et al (2008) Combined use of clinical and pathologic staging variables to define outcomes for breast cancer patients treated with neoadjuvant therapy. J Clin Oncol 26(2):246–252
34. Mittendorf EA, Jeruss JS, Tucker SL, Kolli A, Newman LA, Gonzalez-Angulo AM et al (2011) Validation of a novel staging system for disease-specific survival in patients with breast cancer treated with neoadjuvant chemotherapy. J Clin Oncol 29(15):1956–1962
35. Symmans WF, Peintinger F, Hatzis C, Rajan R, Kuerer H, Valero V et al (2007) Measurement of residual breast cancer burden to predict survival after neoadjuvant chemotherapy. J Clin Oncol 25(28):4414–4422
36. Jones RL, Salter J, A'Hern R, Nerurkar A, Parton M, Reis-Filho JS et al (2009) The prognostic significance of Ki67 before and after neoadjuvant chemotherapy in breast cancer. Breast Cancer Res Treat 116(1):53–68
37. Sheri A, Smith IE, Johnston SR, A'Hern R, Nerurkar A, Jones RL et al (2015) Residual proliferative cancer burden to predict long-term outcome following neoadjuvant chemotherapy. Ann Oncol 26(1):75–80
38. von Minckwitz G, Rezai M, Eidtmann H, Tesch H, Huober J, Gerber B et al. Zoledronate for patients with invasive residual disease after anthracyclines-taxane-based chemotherapy for early breast cancer –the Phase III NeoAdjuvant Trial Add-oN (NaTaN) study (GBG 36/ABCSG 29) San Antonio Breast Cancer Symposium. Abstract S5-05. Presented 13 Dec 2013
39. Finn RS, Crown JP, Lang I, Boer K, Bondarenko IM, Kulyk SO et al (2015) The cyclin-dependent kinase 4/6 inhibitor palbociclib in combination with letrozole versus letrozole alone as first-line treatment of oestrogen receptor-positive, HER2-negative, advanced breast cancer (PALOMA-1/TRIO-18): a randomised phase 2 study. Lancet Oncol 16(1):25–35
40. Verma S, Miles D, Gianni L, Krop IE, Welslau M, Baselga J, EMILIA Study Group et al (2012) Trastuzumab emtansine for HER2-positive advanced breast cancer. N Engl J Med 367(19):1783–1791

41. Tutt A, Robson M, Garber JE, Domchek SM, Audeh MW, Weitzel JN et al (2010) Oral poly (ADP-ribose) polymerase inhibitor olaparib in patients with BRCA1 or BRCA2 mutations and advanced breast cancer: a proof-of-concept trial. Lancet 376(9737):235–244
42. Gelmon KA, Tischkowitz M, Mackay H, Swenerton K, Robidoux A, Tonkin K et al (2011) Olaparib in patients with recurrent high-grade serous or poorly differentiated ovarian carcinoma or triple-negative breast cancer: a phase 2, multicentre, open-label, non-randomised study. Lancet Oncol 12(9):852–861

Chapter 16
The Challenge to Overcome Triple-Negative Breast Cancer Heterogeneity

Hiroko Masuda and Norikazu Masuda

Abstract Triple-negative breast cancer (TNBC) is not a simple unit but a collection of biologically heterogeneous groups. Gene profiling allows us to identify distinct tumor subtypes in TNBC that have the potential for exploring new optimal treatments based on their biological features. To date chemotherapy has been the only treatment option for TNBC, and cytotoxic chemotherapies are insufficient for treating this aggressive breast cancer. We need to find better treatment strategies that are less toxic, improve the risk of recurrence, and are more targeted to each of the homogeneous TNBC subtypes. This chapter focuses on the molecular stratification of TNBC and introduces potential treatment strategies and current clinical trials in order to address the problem of TNBC heterogeneity.

Keywords Gene expression analysis • Molecular subtype • TNBC heterogeneity • Targeted therapy • PARP inhibitors

16.1 Introduction: Triple-Negative Breast Cancer

Triple-negative breast cancer is estrogen receptor negative and progesterone receptor negative and lacks amplification of HER2. This means it is a collective unit that does not have any well-known target genes to identify it. Recent TNBC research has previously suggested TNBC's heterogeneity, and there is currently a consensus that TNBC is not a simple unit but a collection of biologically heterogeneous groups [1, 2].

TNBC represents approximately 15–20 % of all patients with breast cancer and is associated with high recurrence rate and short survival [2]. Neoadjuvant chemotherapy, followed by definitive local therapy (surgery, radiation therapy, or both), is part of the current standard strategy for newly diagnosed primary TNBC treatment. The use of neoadjuvant chemotherapy revealed TNBC heterogeneity and large differences in efficacy in patients; the discovery of heterogeneity guided subsequent individual treatment [3]. In TNBC, chemotherapy sensitivity of current

H. Masuda (✉) • N. Masuda
National Hospital Organization, Osaka National Hospital, 2-1-14 Hoenzaka, Chuo-ku, Osaka 540-0006, Japan
e-mail: hmasuda@med.showa-u.ac.jp

M. Toi et al. (eds.), *Personalized Treatment of Breast Cancer*,
DOI 10.1007/978-4-431-55552-0_16

anthracycline and/or taxane regimens is compatible with the other BC subtypes [3]. Approximately 20–30 % patients with TNBC achieved pathological complete response (pCR) by these chemotherapy regimens, and pCR is strongly associated with improved overall survival and event-free survival [4]. Liedtke et al. [3] reported that they analyzed 1118 patients who received neoadjuvant chemotherapy at MD Anderson Cancer Center for stage I–III breast cancer from 1985 to 2004 and compared clinical and pathological parameters, pathological complete response (pCR) rates, survival measurements, and organ-specific relapse rates for patients with TNBC and non-TNBC. They showed that TNBC patients had significantly higher pCR rates (22 % vs. 11 %, $p = 0.034$), but decreased 3-year progression-free survival rates ($p < 0.0001$) and 3-year overall survival (OS) rates ($p < 0.0001$). And if pCR was achieved, patients with TNBC and non-TNBC had similar survival rates ($p = 0.24$).

In most cases, patients who had a progression of disease (PD) during neoadjuvant chemotherapy also had TNBC. And at this moment, we do not have any alternative treatments for TNBC, and PD cases showed significantly poorer outcomes. This significant difference in treatment responses we assumed is caused by TNBC heterogeneity. For patients with TNBC, worse survival rates were caused by higher relapse rates among tumors not eradicated by chemotherapy. Because of an absence of well-defined molecular targets, patients with TNBC derive no benefit from molecularly targeted treatments such as endocrine therapy or combination therapy of HER2-targeted therapy. We therefore need to identify the subtypes of primary TNBC that are associated with high or low pCR rates and to provide individualized treatment for patients who do not show enough efficacy with current chemotherapy. This individualization by molecular profiling will help us develop the optimal targeting drugs for TNBC. In order to improve TNBC prognosis, we have to distinguish these heterogeneous groups and develop new treatment strategies for patients who have residual disease or PD under current chemotherapy regimens.

16.2 Classification of TNBC Subtypes

Though several targeted agents have been tested for treatment in TNBC, so far none have been successful [5–7]. Some have proposed that this might be due to the molecular heterogeneity of TNBC tumors. In order to overcome TNBC heterogeneity and find appropriate targeted therapies in each subtype, we have tried to identify the biologically homogeneous TNBC subtypes.

16.2.1 Genomic Profiling

To classify heterogeneous TNBC into several homogeneous subtypes, we often used gene expression analysis because of its value for investigating more than 20,000 gene expression patterns encyclopedically. And gene expression analyses have identified molecular subtypes of TNBC that are refining our understanding of breast cancer biology and our ability to develop targeting therapies.

16.2.1.1 Basal/Non-basal-Like Subtype

In 2000, Perou et al. reported that there is an intrinsic subtype in breast cancer [1]. They characterized variation in gene expression patterns in a set of 65 surgical specimens of human breast tumors from 42 different individuals, using complementary DNA microarrays representing 8102 human genes. These patterns provided a distinctive molecular portrait of each tumor, and they identified "intrinsic" subtypes that we now call luminal A, luminal B, HER2-enriched, basal-like, and normal-like subtype. In order to adapt the clinical setting, we have also tried to identify these subtypes using immunohistochemical (IHC) staining. We recognized that basal-like breast cancer was similar to TNBC, and TNBC and basal-like breast cancer definitions have been used interchangeably to identify breast cancers that lack expression of hormone receptors and overexpression and/or amplification of HER2. However, there are substantial discordance rates between these two groups and 60–80 % of TNBC conformed with basal-like breast cancer (Fig. 16.1). There have been some reports that chemotherapy sensitivity was different with basal and non-basal TNBC, and basal tumors may have higher rates of pCR to standard chemotherapy compared with other TNBC subtypes [8–11].

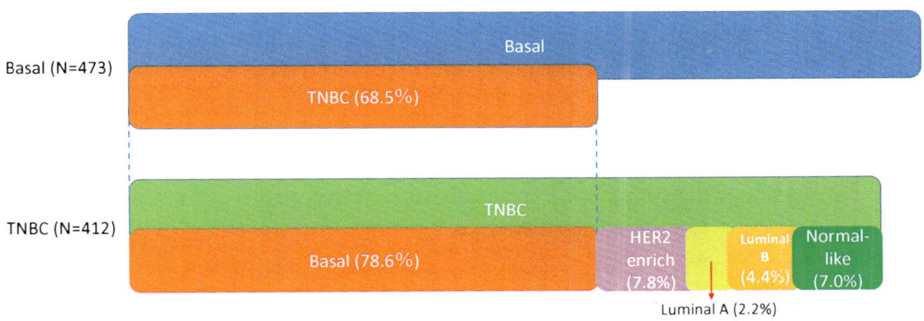

Fig. 16.1 Distribution of the intrinsic molecular and pathology-based subtypes within triple-negative and basal-like tumors [9]

16.2.1.2 Claudin-Low Subtype

Perou et al. used gene expression studies to identify a breast cancer subset having enriched EMT features and high expression of stem cell-like biological processes; they termed this subset "claudin low" because this group of tumors demonstrated low gene expression of the tight junction proteins claudin 3, 4, and 7 [12, 13]. Most claudin-low tumors are triple-receptor negative (61–71 %) and vimentin positive (55 %). This subtype was also associated with metaplastic and medullary histological differentiation, and lymphocytic infiltration was found in 37 % of cases. Its real frequency and clinical relevance are still under investigation.

16.2.1.3 Seven Molecular Subtypes

In 2011, Lehmann et al. [14] classified TNBC into seven subtypes, one of which is an unstable group. These TNBC subtypes were identified using 21 public breast cancer mRNA expression datasets and cluster analysis. These datasets included 587 TNBC tumor samples. To identify global differences in gene expression (GE) between TNBC subtypes, k-means clustering was performed on the most differentially expressed genes. Lehmann et al. were able to classify the TNBC samples into subtypes and then performed gene set enrichment analysis to determine the top canonical pathways associated with each TNBC subtype. The seven TNBC subtypes were characterized on the basis of gene ontologies and differential GE and labeled as basal-like 1 (BL1); cell cycle and DNA damage response gene expression signatures, basal-like 2 (BL2); similar with BL1 and the other enriched in growth factor signaling and myoepithelial markers, immunomodulatory (IM); enriched for gene ontologies in immune cell processes, mesenchymal (M); high expression of genes involved in differentiation and growth factor pathways, mesenchymal stem-like (MSL); and similar to M and enriched in gene expression of epithelial-mesenchymal transition and stem cell markers, luminal androgen receptor (LAR), a luminal subtype driven by androgen signaling and unstable (UNS). Lehmann et al. also classified breast cancer cell lines according to their subtypes. Xenograft tumors established from their TNBC subtypes display differential sensitivity to cisplatin, bicalutamide, and NVP-BEZ235. Lehmann et al. showed that their subtypes had a predictive effect on therapy selection. In a preclinical model, the BL1 and BL2 cell lines, for example, which were associated with the DNA damage response, were highly sensitive to cisplatin; the LAR cell line, which expresses high levels of AR mRNA, was highly sensitive to AR antagonist; and the MSL cell line that was associated with the PI3K pathway was highly sensitive to NVP-BEZ235 (PI3K/mTOR inhibitor). Masuda et al. [15] reproduced their seven TNBC molecular subtypes and analyzed 130 TNBC patients who received neoadjuvant chemotherapy mainly treated with anthracycline and taxane regimens and showed significantly correlated with six subtypes and pathological complete response rates. BL1 subtype showed the highest pCR rate (52 %), and BL2 and

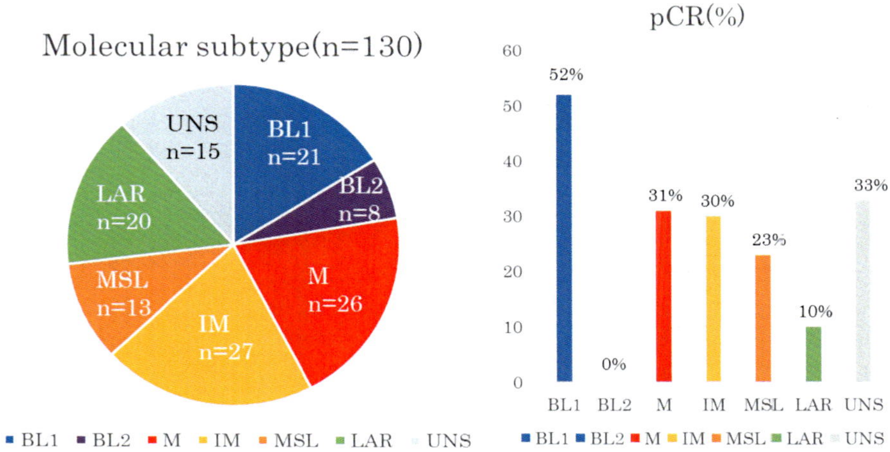

Fig. 16.2 Distribution of pCR status by seven molecular subtypes [15]

LAR showed the lowest pCR rates (0 % and 10 %, respectively). There was no significant association between TNBC subtype and OS, DFS. Masuda et al. commented that, interestingly, the LAR group had delayed recurrences compared with the other groups and did not have the lowest OS rate despite having the lowest pCR rate. The clinical course of the LAR group was thus more similar to that of the luminal intrinsic subtype. These results suggest that within TNBC we need to distinguish the LAR subtype and design a different treatment strategy for that group. Pathologically, AR expression in ER-negative tumors was associated with lower histological grade and apocrine histological differentiation. Of course further studies are needed to comprehend the TNBC subtypes and clinical relation (Fig. 16.2).

16.2.1.4 Relationship Between the Intrinsic Subtypes and Seven Molecular Subtypes

Some reports have compared the intrinsic subtypes and TNBC seven molecular subtypes [9, 15, 16].

Most TNBC seven molecular subtypes are classified as a basal-like intrinsic subtype; however, MSL and LAR subtypes also belonged to the non-basal subtypes. Abramson et al. [16, 17] reported that in MLS TNBCs approximately 50 % were basal-like, 27.8 % were normal-like, 13.9 % were luminal B, and the remaining approximately 8 % were HER2 and luminal A by intrinsic subtypes. In the LAR subtype, 74.3 % were HER2 and 14.4 % were luminal B by intrinsic subtypes (Fig. 16.3).

Prat et al. reported that when they explored the similarities and differences between six molecular subtypes and intrinsic subtypes, these entities largely

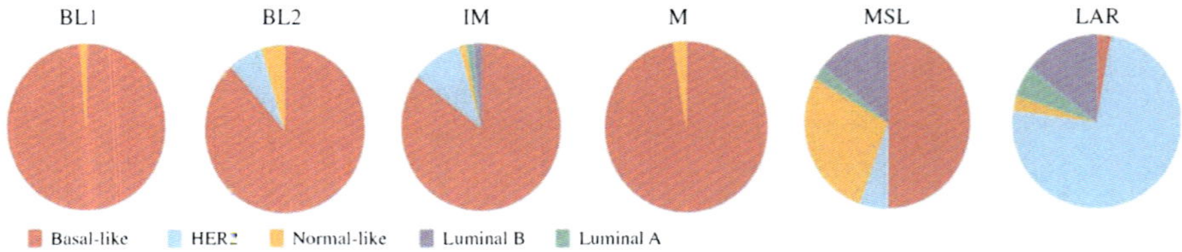

Fig. 16.3 Pie charts display the TNBC type composition of intrinsic subtype and seven molecular subtypes [17]

overlap with intrinsic and claudin-low subtypes. Six molecular subtypes were observed, and four main gene expression clusters were identified representing a stromal gene signature, a luminal signature, an immune signature, and a basal epithelial signature. They also showed HER2 and luminal tumors were highly expressing the LAR cluster; however, they suggested that IM and MSL subtypes are mostly defined by the high expression of genes likely coming from the microenvironment, not from the actual tumor cells, and mentioned the possibility that previously described TN heterogeneity in part reflects tumor heterogeneity plus microenvironmental heterogeneity. TN disease is thus a broad and diverse category for which additional subclassifications are needed.

Gene expression analyses still have some challenges for clinical use such as the difficulty of methods of analysis and the quality of reproducibility. Even among the well-known intrinsic subtypes, several types of gene signatures were derived in each study and none of the classification systems tested produced perfect agreement [18–21]. Prospective future studies are needed to establish the clinical relevancy of dividing the subtypes by gene profiling. In addition, prospective validation is needed to measure these findings and a new treatment strategy using targeted agents derived from molecular profiling. We also need to investigate whether mRNA overexpressed has a truly significant function and activation at the protein expression level by methods such as reverse-phase protein arrays (RPPA) or IHC staining. Then we have to develop methods to identify the TNBC subtypes that could be easily adapted to a clinical setting for developing optimal individual treatments.

16.2.2 Identify Mutations

The Cancer Genome Atlas (TCGA) research network analyzed primary breast cancers using beyond gene expression, including protein expression using RPPA, genomic DNA copy number arrays, DNA methylation, exome sequencing, messenger RNA arrays, and microRNA sequencing [22]. This study allowed integration of information across platforms, provided key insights into previously defined gene expression subtypes, and demonstrated the existence of four main breast cancer classes (luminal A, luminal B, HER2 enriched, and basal-like) when combining data from five platforms, each of which shows significant molecular heterogeneity.

There were numerous subtype-associated and novel gene mutations, and some of them have the potential to develop therapeutic targets. The overall mutation rate was highest in the basal-like and HER2-enriched subtypes. In the basal-like subtype, the most frequent loss of function alterations genes were associated with DNA damage repair, including *TP53*, *RB1*, and *BRCA1*, and gain of function alterations were phosphatidylinositol 3-kinase (*PI3K*) signaling pathways. Eighty percent of basal-like tumors showed *TP53* mutations, and the next most common gene mutation was *PIK3CA* (9 %). Aberrant activation of PI3K pathway occurs due to loss of negative regulators, such as phosphatase and tensin homolog (*PTEN*) and inositol polyphosphate 4-phosphatase type II (*INPP4B*) or activating mutations in PIK3 catalytic subunit (*PIK3CA*). Consistent with previous reports, this study also confirmed that germline BRCA1 mutations were strongly associated with basal-like breast cancer [19, 23].

About 20 % of basal-like tumors had germline and/or somatic *BRCA1* and *BRCA2* variants, and that means there is a possibility that PARP inhibitors and/or platinum compounds might have some benefit for these patients. Interestingly, comparison of basal-like breast tumors with high-grade serous ovarian tumors showed many molecular commonalities, indicating a related etiology and similar therapeutic opportunities such as platinum analogs and taxanes. Focused on the therapeutic targets derived from TCGA research network, gene amplification is also remarkable. In basal-like tumors, PI3K and RAS-RAF-MEK pathways were amplified, including *PIK3CA* (49 %), *KRAS* (32 %), *BRAF* (30 %), and *EGFR* (23 %). *FGFR1*, *FGFR2*, *IGFR1*, *c-KIT*, *MET*, and PDGFRA were also identified.

The TCGA network concluded that the biological finding of the four main breast cancer subtypes caused by different subsets of genetic and epigenetic abnormalities raises the possibility that much of the clinically observable plasticity and heterogeneity occurs within, and not across, these major biological subtypes of breast cancer.

16.3 Treatment Strategy to Overcome Triple-Negative Breast Cancer Heterogeneity

Because of the aforementioned new discoveries in subtype classifications, mutations, and amplified genes, the challenge of providing individualized treatment strategies in TNBC has begun (Fig. 16.4a, b) and is being investigated in currently ongoing TNBC neoadjuvant clinical trials.

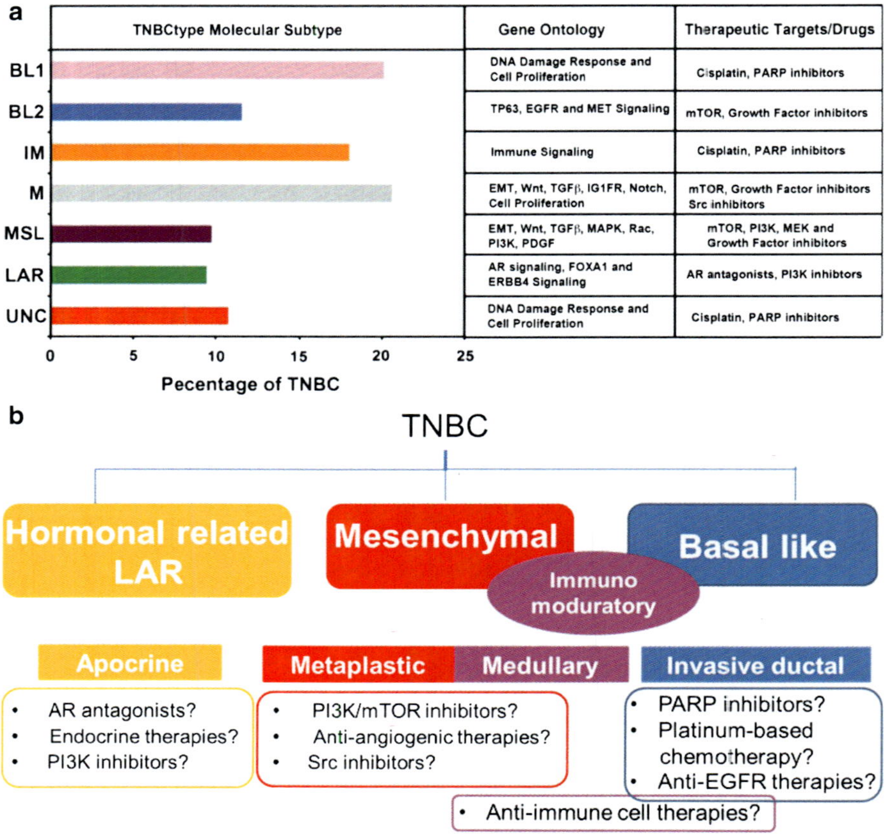

Fig. 16.4 (**a**) The distribution of triple-negative breast cancer (*TNBC*) subtypes from The Cancer Genome Atlas is illustrated with enriched gene ontology and potential therapeutic targets. Bar graphs display the subtype percentage relative to TNBC [16]. (**b**) Treatment strategies for TNBC regarding to the subtypes

16.3.1 Basal-Like Subtype/BRCA Mutation

In addition to or instead of anthracycline and/or taxane, which have been the standard chemotherapy regimens until now, the agent that is currently most assertively being tested in trials is the DNA-damaging agent platinum.

As we mentioned, 60–80 % of TNBC belong to the basal-like subtype. Its biological features showed overexpression of cell cycle and DNA damage response gene signatures, often have *TP53* and *BRCA1* mutation, and often have loss of function of *RB1*, which is a tumor suppressor protein that prevents excessive cell growth by inhibiting cell cycle progression. Because of dysfunction of these genes, these tumors are highly proliferative, on average, as illustrated by the proliferation index, regardless of whether proliferation is measured by Ki-67, proliferating cell nuclear antigen, immunohistochemistry, or gene expression proliferation. *TP53* loss, *RB* loss, and *BRCA1* pathway association are responsible for the high aneuploidy seen in these tumors, including a huge number of chromosomal changes, translocations, and losses [24]. So according to their biological features, platinum agents such as cisplatin and carboplatin, inter-strand cross-linking agents that damage the DNA, might have a potential to have efficacy for basal-like subtypes.

In fact there are some clinical trials that showed the efficacy of platinum agents for TNBC patients at neoadjuvant setting. CALGB 40603 is a randomized phase II neoadjuvant trial that tested the addition of carboplatin with or without bevacizumab to weekly paclitaxel followed by doxorubicin and cyclophosphamide (AC) for stage II–III TNBC patients. The result showed that addition of carboplatin (AUC 6 q3 week × 4) significantly increased pCR rate (60 % v 44 %, $p=0.0018$) [25]. GeparSixto is also a randomized phase II neoadjuvant trial for stage II–III triple-negative and HER2-positive breast cancer. In this trial, TNBC patients received weekly paclitaxel 80 mg/m^2 and non-pegylated liposomal doxorubicin 20 mg/m^2 and bevacizumab 15 mg/kg q3w with and without weekly carboplatin AUC 1.5. In TNBC patients, 84 (53.2 %, 54.4–60.9) of 158 patients achieved a pathological complete response with carboplatin, compared with 58 (36.9 %, 29.4–44.5) of 157 without ($p=0.005$) [26]. At the ASCO 2014 annual meeting, von Minckwitz et al. reported [27] the additional results of GeparSixto trial: the patients who have BRCA mutation and also have family history of breast cancer and/or ovarian cancer showed the highest pCR rate for this regimen (81.8 %). These randomized neoadjuvant studies have now established that inclusion of carboplatin increases pCR rate in TNBC, and this provides a valuable new treatment option for patients with high-risk TNBC. Patients in these studies also received bevacizumab, an antiangiogenesis agent that targets vascular endothelial growth factor (VEGF) and is attractive for TNBC.

There is a distinct neoadjuvant phase II trial named I-SPY2 aimed at investigating efficacy of investigational targeted agents and effective patient selection at the same time. This is done by employing "adaptive trial design"—an innovative automated algorithm that graduates a treatment in one or more biomarker types when there is an >85 % predicted likelihood that the experimental arm will produce higher pCR rate than weekly T + AC in a 300-patient randomized phase III study in that biomarker subset—that would accelerate drug approval with minimal resources. The first graduated regimen and population of this study was veliparib (50 mg po)/carboplatin (AUC 6, q3 week ×4) + weekly paclitaxel followed by AC for TNBC patients. Veliparib is a poly(ADP-ribose) polymerase (PARP) inhibitor that targets an alternate DNA repair pathway in BRCA-deficient cells, producing a synthetic lethal effect. The activity of veliparib was likely influenced by germline BRCA status and may also depend on the extent of homologous DNA recombination repair defect [28]. BRCA mutation carrier is a population that should be distinguished from other TNBC patients. It has been found to be associated with basal-like subtype and important therapeutic implications with PARP inhibitors. Significant single-agent activity was reported with the PARP inhibitor olaparib in patients with BRCA1 or BRCA2 mutations and advanced breast cancer [29]. PARP inhibitors are also actively being investigated at adjuvant and neoadjuvant setting with TNBC and/or BRCA mutation carriers.

Over half of basal-like breast cancers express EGFR, and expression of EGFR by IHC has been associated with a poor response to chemotherapy and decreased survival in patients with triple-negative breast cancer [30]. In preclinical models, inhibitors of EGFR induced apoptosis and enhanced response to chemotherapy. Two phase II clinical trials evaluated the efficacy of cetuximab alone or in combination with platinum-based chemotherapy for triple-negative breast cancer [5, 6] and found that addition of cetuximab to carboplatin did not improve outcome. These results so far have been disappointing. One of the reasons for these unexpected results is the lack of biomarkers for predicting which patients are most likely to respond to EGFR inhibitors. Molecular analysis using RT-PCR (PAM50) of paraffin-embedded tumor samples from triple-negative breast cancer patients enrolled in both trials ($n = 132$) revealed that 67 % of the triple-negative breast cancer patients treated displayed the basal phenotype. This benefit from cetuximab might be correlated with higher expression of PTEN or lack of amplification of KRAS. EGFR inhibitor also might have potential as a targeted drug for basal-like subtype.

16.3.2 Luminal Androgen Subtype

This subtype, which is driven by AR signaling and luminal signatures and is associated with a high rate of PI3K activation/mutation, may be uniquely sensitive to androgen blockers and PI3K-directed therapy [31]. A nonrandomized phase II trial evaluating treatment of patients with metastatic, AR+ (defined as 15 % or higher AR expression by IHC) TNBC with bicalutamide demonstrated no measurable responses by RECIST but demonstrated a 6-month clinical benefit rate of 19 % [32]. Another clinical trial that is evaluating enzalutamide is being conducted for patients with TNBC who express the AR (NCT01889238).

Preclinical data indicate that the combination of bicalutamide with a PI3K inhibitor produces an additive/synergistic effect in LAR cell lines. This is also a potential treatment strategy for this subtype [31].

16.3.3 Mesenchymal/Mesenchymal Stem Cell-Like/Claudin-Low Subtype

These subtypes shared similar molecular features including low expression of claudins 3, 4, and 7 as well as high expression of genes associated with EMT. Mesenchymal-like TNBCs carry a high rate of molecular aberrations that activate the PI3K/Akt/mTOR axis, suggesting that this subgroup may be responsive to therapeutic regimens targeting this pathway [14]. The cell lines that were classified as MSL have dedifferentiated morphologies observed in breast carcinosarcoma as well as metaplastic and anaplastic carcinomas, and the EMT core signature associates closely with the claudin-low and metaplastic breast cancer subtypes and correlates negatively with pathological complete response. Additionally, the expression level of FOXC1, another EMT inducer, correlates strongly with poor survival of breast cancer patients [17, 33]. Early data from a phase I clinical trial enriched with patients diagnosed with metaplastic breast cancer also suggest that PI3K inhibition may be a viable target for this subtype of TNBC. Moulder et al. [34] treated the metaplastic breast cancer patients with liposomal doxorubicin, bevacizumab, and temsirolimus (DAT) according to their biological features that display high levels of angiogenesis and commonly express VEGF and HIF-1. Temsirolimus inhibits mammalian target of rapamycin (mTOR), and preclinical data have implicated the PI3K/mTOR pathway in breast CSC survival and tumorigenicity, which can be reversed by treating with rapamycin. Overall, this combination regimen achieved 1 CR, 1 PR, 1 SD, 2 PD and they continued to recruit the patients and planning a phase II trial in multicenter. These results further emphasize the need to characterize TNBC tumors molecularly to enrich for response in targeted therapy.

16.3.4 Immunomodulatory Subtype

Immunotherapy and tumor immunity of TNBC is now being aggressively investigated because it also may be a drug target for TNBC. Several studies have emphasized the prognostic and predictive impact of tumor-infiltrating lymphocytes (TILs) in TNBC [35, 36]. High baseline TILs can predict high pCR, and increasing lymphocytic infiltration was associated with improved outcomes for patients with TNBC. These findings could be useful in providing the rationale for evaluating immunotherapeutic approaches and selecting the patient's population.

At the 2014 ASCO annual meeting, Vinayak et al. [37] reported that they evaluated the patients who enrolled the PrECOG 0105, a neoadjuvant trial of carboplatin, gemcitabine, and iniparib, and investigated the association of pre-therapy TILs in PrECOG 0105 with pathologic response, germline BRCA1/2 genotype, and gene expression profiles, including TNBC subtypes. They determined the density of stromal (sTILs) and intratumoral (iTILs) lymphocytes. Seventy patients were included in this analysis. Of those, 20 % of patients had BRCA1/2 mutant and 76 % of tumors had at least 10 % sTILs (range 10–80 %) and 31 % at least 10 % iTILs (range 10–40 %). Lymphocyte-predominant BC (LPBC), defined as ≥50 % sTILs, was seen in 13 %. pCR rate was highest (56 %) in LPBC, though not significantly different from the non-LPBC group (38 %, $p = 0.47$). sTILs were significantly associated with TNBC subtype: median sTIL = 40 % in the IM subtype, 15 % in BL1, 20 % in BL2, 10 % in LAR, 0 % in M, and 10 % in MSL ($p = 0.0005$). iTILs were also significantly associated with TNBC subtypes

($p = 0.0003$): iTIL >0 for 10/14 (71 %) in IM subtype, 1/7 (14 %) in BL1, and 0 in others. Association with BRCA1/2 mutation status was not significant. In a multivariate model, each 10 % increase in iTILs (OR 2.62 [95 % CI 1.08–6.35]; $p = 0.03$) but not sTILs (OR 1.17 [95 % CI 0.87–1.58]; $p = 0.28$) was independently associated with pCR (RCB = 0). Both sTILs and iTILs are predictive of response to platinum-based neoadjuvant therapy and are significantly associated with TNBC subtypes, with the highest frequency in the IM subtype [37].

The expression of immune regulatory targets in the TNBC population suggests that immune-targeted therapies may be effective in subset of TNBC. Among the most promising approaches to activating therapeutic antitumor immunity is the blockade of immune checkpoints, and cytotoxic T lymphocyte-associated antigen 4 (CTLA4) antibodies were the first of this class of immunotherapeutics to achieve US Food and Drug Administration (FDA) approval. Preliminary clinical findings with blockers of additional immune-checkpoint proteins, such as programmed cell death protein 1 (PD1) and its receptor ligand, programmed death ligand-1 (PDL-1), indicate broad and diverse opportunities to enhance antitumor immunity with the potential to produce durable clinical responses [38]. There are anticipated targeted agents for TNBC that await further studies.

16.4 Summary

The prospects for overcoming TNBC heterogeneity and improving this refractory and complex breast cancer's outcome are now developing dramatically. Gene profiling, which allows identification of TNBC subtypes and classification of them into homogenous subtypes reflecting their biological features, has the potential to derive the targeted agents for each group. However, we still have several challenges to address before using these methods in clinical settings. For instance, new technology such as next-generation sequencing gave us more information, and so this technology must be combined with new findings in order to create optimal treatment strategies for TNBC. Preclinical, translational research and hypothesis-driven clinical trials are needed to make TNBC as a controllable disease.

References

1. Perou CM, Sorlie T, Eisen MB, van de Rijn M, Jeffrey SS, Rees CA, Pollack JR, Ross DT, Johnsen H, Akslen LA, Fluge O, Pergamenschikov A, Williams C, Zhu SX, Lonning PE, Borresen-Dale AL, Brown PO, Botstein D (2000) Molecular portraits of human breast tumours. Nature 406(6797):747–752. doi:10.1038/35021093
2. Gluz O, Liedtke C, Gottschalk N, Pusztai L, Nitz U, Harbeck N (2009) Triple-negative breast cancer – current status and future directions. Ann Oncol 20(12):1913–1927, doi:mdp492 [pii]
3. Liedtke C, Mazouni C, Hess KR, Andre F, Tordai A, Mejia JA, Symmans WF, Gonzalez-Angulo AM, Hennessy B, Green M, Cristofanilli M, Hortobagyi GN, Pusztai L (2008)

Response to neoadjuvant therapy and long-term survival in patients with triple-negative breast cancer. J Clin Oncol: Off J Am Soc Clin Oncol 26(8):1275–1281. doi:10.1200/JCO.2007.14.4147

4. Rastogi P, Anderson SJ, Bear HD, Geyer CE, Kahlenberg MS, Robidoux A, Margolese RG, Hoehn JL, Vogel VG, Dakhil SR, Tamkus D, King KM, Pajon ER, Wright MJ, Robert J, Paik S, Mamounas EP, Wolmark N (2008) Preoperative chemotherapy: updates of National Surgical Adjuvant Breast and Bowel Project Protocols B-18 and B-27. J Clin Oncol 26 (5):778–785. doi:10.1200/JCO.2007.15.0235
5. Carey LA, Rugo HS, Marcom PK, Mayer EL, Esteva FJ, Ma CX, Liu MC, Storniolo AM, Rimawi MF, Forero-Torres A, Wolff AC, Hobday TJ, Ivanova A, Chiu WK, Ferraro M, Burrows E, Bernard PS, Hoadley KA, Perou CM, Winer EP (2012) TBCRC 001: randomized phase II study of cetuximab in combination with carboplatin in stage IV triple-negative breast cancer. J Clin Oncol: Off J Am Soc Clin Oncol 30(21):2615–2623. doi:10.1200/JCO.2010.34.5579
6. Khambata-Ford S, O'Shaughnessy J, Brickman D, et al (2010) Candidate predictive biomarkers of cetuximab benefit in triple-negative breast cancer. J Clin Oncol 28(suppl): abstr 1056
7. O'Shaughnessy J, et al (2010) Meta-analysis of patients with triple-negative breast cancer (TNBC) from three randomized trials of first-line bevacizumab (BV) and chemotherapy treatment for metastatic breast cancer (MBC). Cancer Res 70(Suppl 24):452s.[15]
8. Carey LA, Dees EC, Sawyer L, Gatti L, Moore DT, Collichio F, Ollila DW, Sartor CI, Graham ML, Perou CM (2007) The triple negative paradox: primary tumor chemosensitivity of breast cancer subtypes. Clin Cancer Res 13(8):2329–2334. doi:13/8/2329 [pii], 10.1158/1078-0432.CCR-06-1109
9. Prat A, Adamo B, Cheang MC, Anders CK, Carey LA, Perou CM (2013) Molecular characterization of basal-like and non-basal-like triple-negative breast cancer. Oncologist 18 (2):123–133. doi:10.1634/theoncologist.2012-0397
10. Nielsen TO, Hsu FD, Jensen K, Cheang M, Karaca G, Hu Z, Hernandez-Boussard T, Livasy C, Cowan D, Dressler L, Akslen LA, Ragaz J, Gown AM, Gilks CB, van de Rijn M, Perou CM (2004) Immunohistochemical and clinical characterization of the basal-like subtype of invasive breast carcinoma. Clin Cancer Res 10(16):5367–5374. doi:10.1158/1078-0432.CCR-04-0220, 10/16/5367 [pii]
11. Rouzier R, Perou CM, Symmans WF, Ibrahim N, Cristofanilli M, Anderson K, Hess KR, Stec J, Ayers M, Wagner P, Morandi P, Fan C, Rabiul I, Ross JS, Hortobagyi GN, Pusztai L (2005) Breast cancer molecular subtypes respond differently to preoperative chemotherapy. Clin Cancer Res 11(16):5678–5685. doi:11/16/5678 [pii], 10.1158/1078-0432.CCR-04-2421
12. Prat A, Parker JS, Karginova O, Fan C, Livasy C, Herschkowitz JI, He X, Perou CM (2010) Phenotypic and molecular characterization of the claudin-low intrinsic subtype of breast cancer. Breast Cancer Res 12(5):R68. doi:bcr2635 [pii], 10.1186/bcr2635
13. Herschkowitz JI, Simin K, Weigman VJ, Mikaelian I, Usary J, Hu Z, Rasmussen KE, Jones LP, Assefnia S, Chandrasekharan S, Backlund MG, Yin Y, Khramtsov AI, Bastein R, Quackenbush J, Glazer RI, Brown PH, Green JE, Kopelovich L, Furth PA, Palazzo JP, Olopade OI, Bernard PS, Churchill GA, Van Dyke T, Perou CM (2007) Identification of conserved gene expression features between murine mammary carcinoma models and human breast tumors. Genome Biol 8(5):R76. doi:gb-2007-8-5-r76 [pii], 10.1186/gb-2007-8-5-r76
14. Lehmann BD, Bauer JA, Chen X, Sanders ME, Chakravarthy AB, Shyr Y, Pietenpol JA (2011) Identification of human triple-negative breast cancer subtypes and preclinical models for selection of targeted therapies. J Clin Invest 121(7):2750–2767. doi:10.1172/JCI45014, 45014 [pii]
15. Masuda H, Baggerly KA, Wang Y, Zhang Y, Gonzalez-Angulo AM, Meric-Bernstam F, Valero V, Lehmann BD, Pietenpol JA, Hortobagyi GN, Symmans WF, Ueno NT (2013) Differential response to neoadjuvant chemotherapy among 7 triple-negative breast cancer

molecular subtypes. Clin Cancer Res: Off J Am Assoc Cancer Res 19(19):5533–5540. doi:10.1158/1078-0432.CCR-13-0799

16. Abramson VG, Lehmann BD, Ballinger TJ, Pietenpol JA (2014) Subtyping of triple-negative breast cancer: implications for therapy. Cancer. doi:10.1002/cncr.28914
17. Lehmann BD, Pietenpol JA (2014) Identification and use of biomarkers in treatment strategies for triple-negative breast cancer subtypes. J Pathol 232(2):142–150. doi:10.1002/path.4280
18. Sorlie T, Perou CM, Tibshirani R, Aas T, Geisler S, Johnsen H, Hastie T, Eisen MB, van de Rijn M, Jeffrey SS, Thorsen T, Quist H, Matese JC, Brown PO, Botstein D, Lonning PE, Borresen-Dale AL (2001) Gene expression patterns of breast carcinomas distinguish tumor subclasses with clinical implications. Proc Natl Acad Sci U S A 98(19):10869–10874. doi:10.1073/pnas.191367098, 98/19/10869 [pii]
19. Sorlie T, Tibshirani R, Parker J, Hastie T, Marron JS, Nobel A, Deng S, Johnsen H, Pesich R, Geisler S, Demeter J, Perou CM, Lonning PE, Brown PO, Borresen-Dale AL, Botstein D (2003) Repeated observation of breast tumor subtypes in independent gene expression data sets. Proc Natl Acad Sci U S A 100(14):8418–8423. doi:10.1073/pnas.0932692100, 0932692100 [pii]
20. Hu Z, Fan C, Oh DS, Marron JS, He X, Qaqish BF, Livasy C, Carey LA, Reynolds E, Dressler L, Nobel A, Parker J, Ewend MG, Sawyer LR, Wu J, Liu Y, Nanda R, Tretiakova M, Ruiz Orrico A, Dreher D, Palazzo JP, Perreard L, Nelson E, Mone M, Hansen H, Mullins M, Quackenbush JF, Ellis MJ, Olopade OI, Bernard PS, Perou CM (2006) The molecular portraits of breast tumors are conserved across microarray platforms. BMC Genomics 7:96. doi:1471-2164-7-96 [pii], 10.1186/1471-2164-7-96
21. Parker JS, Mullins M, Cheang MC, Leung S, Voduc D, Vickery T, Davies S, Fauron C, He X, Hu Z, Quackenbush JF, Stijleman IJ, Palazzo J, Marron JS, Nobel AB, Mardis E, Nielsen TO, Ellis MJ, Perou CM, Bernard PS (2009) Supervised risk predictor of breast cancer based on intrinsic subtypes. J Clin Oncol 27(8):1160–1167. doi:10.1200/JCO.2008.18.1370, JCO.2008.18.1370 [pii]
22. The Cancer Genome Atlas Network (2012) Comprehensive molecular portraits of human breast tumours. Nature 490 (7418):61–70. doi:10.1038/nature11412, nature11412 [pii]
23. Foulkes WD, Stefansson IM, Chappuis PO, Begin LR, Goffin JR, Wong N, Trudel M, Akslen LA (2003) Germline BRCA1 mutations and a basal epithelial phenotype in breast cancer. J Natl Cancer Inst 95(19):1482–1485
24. Perou CM (2011) Molecular stratification of triple-negative breast cancers. Oncologist 16 (Suppl 1):61–70. doi:10.1634/theoncologist.2011-S1-61
25. Sikov WM, Berry DA, Perou CM, Singh B, Cirrincione CT, Tolaney SM, Kuzma CS, Pluard TJ, Somlo G, Port ER, Golshan M, Bellon JR, Collyar D, Hahn OM, Carey LA, Hudis CA, Winer EP (2014) Impact of the addition of carboplatin and/or bevacizumab to neoadjuvant once-per-week paclitaxel followed by dose-dense doxorubicin and cyclophosphamide on pathologic complete response rates in stage II to III triple-negative breast cancer: CALGB 40603 (Alliance). J Clin Oncol. doi:JCO.2014.57.0572 [pii], 10.1200/JCO.2014.57.0572
26. von Minckwitz G, Schneeweiss A, Loibl S, Salat C, Denkert C, Rezai M, Blohmer JU, Jackisch C, Paepke S, Gerber B, Zahm DM, Kummel S, Eidtmann H, Klare P, Huober J, Costa S, Tesch H, Hanusch C, Hilfrich J, Khandan F, Fasching PA, Sinn BV, Engels K, Mehta K, Nekljudova V, Untch M (2014) Neoadjuvant carboplatin in patients with triple-negative and HER2-positive early breast cancer (GeparSixto; GBG 66): a randomised phase 2 trial. Lancet Oncol 15(7):747–756. doi:10.1016/S1470-2045(14)70160-3, S1470-2045(14)70160-3 [pii]
27. von Minckwitz G, Hahnen E, Fasching PA et al (2014) Pathological complete response (pCR) rates after carboplatin-containing neoadjuvant chemotherapy in patients with germline BRCA (gBRCA) mutation and triple-negative breast cancer (TNBC): results from GeparSixto. ASCO annual meeting. Abstract 1005. Presented 2 Jun 2014. J Clin Oncol 32:5s (suppl; abstr 1005)

28. Rugo HS, Olopade O, DeMichele A et al (2013) Veliparib/carboplatin plus standard neoadjuvant therapy for high-risk breast cancer: first efficacy results from the I-SPY2 trial. 2013 San Antonio Breast Cancer Symposium. Abstract S5-02. Presented 13 Dec 2013
29. Tutt A, Robson M, Garber JE, Domchek SM, Audeh MW, Weitzel JN, Friedlander M, Arun B, Loman N, Schmutzler RK, Wardley A, Mitchell G, Earl H, Wickens M, Carmichael J (2010) Oral poly(ADP-ribose) polymerase inhibitor olaparib in patients with BRCA1 or BRCA2 mutations and advanced breast cancer: a proof-of-concept trial. Lancet 376(9737):235–244. doi:10.1016/S0140-6736(10)60892-6, S0140-6736(10)60892-6 [pii]
30. Corkery B, Crown J, Clynes M, O'Donovan N (2009) Epidermal growth factor receptor as a potential therapeutic target in triple-negative breast cancer. Ann Oncol: Off J Eur Soc Med Oncol/ESMO 20(5):862–867. doi:10.1093/annonc/mdn710
31. Lehmann BD, Bauer JA, Schafer JM, Pendleton CS, Tang L, Johnson KC, Chen X, Balko JM, Gomez H, Arteaga CL, Mills GB, Sanders ME, Pietenpol JA (2014) PIK3CA mutations in androgen receptor-positive triple negative breast cancer confer sensitivity to the combination of PI3K and androgen receptor inhibitors. Breast Cancer Res: BCR 16(4):406. doi:10.1186/s13058-014-0406-x
32. Gucalp A, Tolaney S, Isakoff SJ, Ingle JN, Liu MC, Carey LA, Blackwell K, Rugo H, Nabell L, Forero A, Stearns V, Doane AS, Danso M, Moynahan ME, Momen LF, Gonzalez JM, Akhtar A, Giri DD, Patil S, Feigin KN, Hudis CA, Traina TA (2013) Phase II trial of bicalutamide in patients with androgen receptor-positive, estrogen receptor-negative metastatic Breast Cancer. Clin Cancer Res 19(19):5505–5512. doi:10.1158/1078-0432.CCR-12-3327, 1078-0432.CCR-12-3327 [pii]
33. Taube JH, Herschkowitz JI, Komurov K, Zhou AY, Gupta S, Yang J, Hartwell K, Onder TT, Gupta PB, Evans KW, Hollier BG, Ram PT, Lander ES, Rosen JM, Weinberg RA, Mani SA (2010) Core epithelial-to-mesenchymal transition interactome gene-expression signature is associated with claudin-low and metaplastic breast cancer subtypes. Proc Natl Acad Sci U S A 107(35):15449–15454. doi:10.1073/pnas.1004900107
34. Moulder S, Moroney J, Helgason T, Wheler J, Booser D, Albarracin C, Morrow PK, Koenig K, Kurzrock R (2011) Responses to liposomal doxorubicin, bevacizumab, and temsirolimus in metaplastic carcinoma of the breast: biologic rationale and implications for stem-cell research in breast cancer. J Clin Oncol: Off J Am Soc Clin Oncol 29(19):e572–e575. doi:10.1200/JCO.2010.34.0604
35. Loi S, Michiels S, Salgado R, Sirtaine N, Jose V, Fumagalli D, Kellokumpu-Lehtinen PL, Bono P, Kataja V, Desmedt C, Piccart MJ, Loibl S, Denkert C, Smyth MJ, Joensuu H, Sotiriou C (2014) Ann Oncol: Off J Eur Soc Med Oncol/ESMO 25(8):1544–1550. doi:10.1093/annonc/mdu112
36. Loi S, Sirtaine N, Piette F, Salgado R, Viale G, Van Eenoo F, Rouas G, Francis P, Crown JP, Hitre E, de Azambuja E, Quinaux E, Di Leo A, Michiels S, Piccart MJ, Sotiriou C (2013) Prognostic and predictive value of tumor-infiltrating lymphocytes in a phase III randomized adjuvant breast cancer trial in node-positive breast cancer comparing the addition of docetaxel to doxorubicin with doxorubicin-based chemotherapy: BIG 02-98. J Clin Oncol: Off J Am Soc Clin Oncol 31(7):860–867. doi:10.1200/JCO.2011.41.0902
37. Vinayak S, Gray RJ, Adams S et al (2014) Association of increased tumor-infiltrating lymphocytes (TILs) with immunomodulatory (IM) triple-negative breast cancer (TNBC) subtype and response to neoadjuvant platinum-based therapy in PrECOG0105. J Clin Oncol 32:5s (suppl; abstr 1000^)
38. Pardoll DM (2012) The blockade of immune checkpoints in cancer immunotherapy. Nat Rev Cancer 12(4):252–264. doi:10.1038/nrc3239, nrc3239 [pii]

Chapter 17
Surgical Management of Breast Cancer After Preoperative Systemic Treatment

John Mathew, Carol-Ann Courtney, Kelly K. Hunt, and John F. Robertson

Abstract Surgery following neoadjuvant systemic therapy involves complex decision making within the entire multidisciplinary team. The selection of which systemic therapy to use (i.e. endocrine therapy, chemotherapy, anti-HER2 agents) and the role of radiotherapy therapy must be carefully considered on a case-by-case basis. Tumour size before, during and after the systemic therapy needs to be carefully and accurately measured by the most appropriate imaging technique(s), before deciding on the final surgical approach. For the small percentage of patients whose tumour progresses during treatment or where there is no volume reduction and the tumour remains unsuitable for breast-conserving surgery, mastectomy with or without reconstruction remains an option. For the remaining patients, there are various surgical options available from standard breast-conserving surgery to oncoplastic breast-conserving surgery. The choice will be determined by a number of factors including the size of the tumour, surgical decision making regarding the need to remove the entire initial tumour volume or residual tumour volume, the size of the breast, the location of the tumour, the radiologic appearance after neoadjuvant therapy and the tumour subtype and patient's concerns.

Keywords Preoperative systemic treatment • Neoadjuvant treatment • Oncoplastic surgery

17.1 Introduction

The terms preoperative therapy and neoadjuvant therapy are used to describe systemic therapy as an initial treatment before surgery. Neoadjuvant therapy was introduced in the 1970s with one of the initial reports involving 110 patients with locally advanced breast cancer treated with doxorubicin and vincristine showing an

J. Mathew • C.-A. Courtney • J.F. Robertson (✉)
Royal Derby Hospital Centre, University of Nottingham, Uttoxeter Road, Derby DE22 3DT, UK
e-mail: john.robertson@nottingham.ac.uk

K.K. Hunt
The University of Texas MD Anderson Cancer Center, Houston, TX, USA

M. Toi et al. (eds.), *Personalized Treatment of Breast Cancer*,
DOI 10.1007/978-4-431-55552-0_17

objective response rate of 89 % [1]. This led to further studies evaluating the efficacy of neoadjuvant systemic therapy for those presenting with inoperable breast cancer [2–4]. Neoadjuvant systemic treatment has the potential to improve outcome as most patients with locally advanced primary breast cancer have micrometastases at the time of presentation and benefit from systemic treatment. To date there has been no evidence from randomised trials to show an overall survival (OS) benefit from neoadjuvant chemotherapy compared to adjuvant therapy [5, 6].

For those presenting with operable cancers, neoadjuvant systemic therapy has been shown to improve the rate of breast-conserving surgery. However, this has been reported to be associated with an increased risk of local recurrence in the conserved breast [6].

NSABP B-18 [5] was the first large prospective randomised trial to investigate the role of neoadjuvant chemotherapy in women presenting with primary operable breast cancer [5]. In this study, 1523 women were randomised to receive four cycles of doxorubicin and cyclophosphamide (AC) chemotherapy either preoperatively or postoperatively. There were no significant differences between arms with regard to the primary end points of OS, disease-free survival (DFS) and recurrence-free survival (RFS) after 16 years. The study included patients with tumours which were suitable for conservation surgery from the outset as well as patients with tumours for which mastectomy was initially advised. In the latter group, the reported local recurrence rate for patients who were initially advised and went on to have mastectomy was 6.9 % versus 14.5 % for those patients initially advised mastectomy but after neoadjuvant chemotherapy had breast-conserving surgery. Furthermore, the rate of breast-conserving surgery in B-18 only increased from 60 % with adjuvant chemotherapy to 68 % with neoadjuvant chemotherapy, although this difference was statistically significant.

The B-18 trial was followed by the NSABP B-27 study, which had three arms [6]. Here patients were randomised to four cycles of preoperative AC followed by surgery or four cycles of preoperative AC followed by four cycles of docetaxel and then surgery or four cycles of preoperative AC followed by surgery and adjuvant therapy consisting of four cycles of docetaxel. No significant difference in OS, DFS or RFS between the three arms was demonstrated; however, the addition of docetaxel sequential to AC preoperatively did increase the pCR rate versus AC alone, although it did not increase the breast conservation rate.

Other than improving the rate of breast-conserving surgery, neoadjuvant treatment would appear to have little advantage compared to adjuvant treatment for patients with primary operable breast cancer. The neoadjuvant approach does allow for assessment of response to chemotherapy which has been reported to be a surrogate marker of outcome [7]. Pathological complete response has been reported to be a marker of improved survival as shown in the B-18 trial. Women who had a pCR had superior outcomes compared with women who did not (OS HR = 0.32, $P < .0001$; DFS HR = 0.47, $P < .0001$) [5]. The B-27 trial also showed improved OS (HR = 0.36, $P < .0001$) and DFS (HR = 0.49, $P < .0001$) in patients who experienced a pCR [6]. With the opportunity to assess response to therapy, there is the potential to change drug treatment during neoadjuvant therapy or postoperatively in the adjuvant setting if no clinical response or progression is noted with the conventional agents. However, progression during chemotherapy is rare, and in the absence of progression (i.e. stable disease or partial response), it is not clear whether changing treatment will affect the outcome. A recent pooled analysis of neoadjuvant trials has reported on the relationship between response (including pathological response) and outcome [8]. For a trial to be included in this analysis, several criteria had to be met: it had to include at least 200 patients with primary breast cancer; patients had to be treated with neoadjuvant chemotherapy followed by surgery; pCR, EFS and OS data had to be available; and median follow-up had to be at least 3 years. There were 12 trials included; however, the analysis could not validate pathological complete response as a surrogate end point for improved OS [8].

One advantage of neoadjuvant therapy is the ability to study the effects of drugs on the biological and histological features of a tumour in vivo by means of sequential tumour biopsies [9]. This approach can potentially predict the response of different breast cancers to different therapies based on molecular profiles and thus may be one way to progress towards a more individualised therapy and develop novel agents.

In this chapter we discuss the various controversies of neoadjuvant systemic treatment with chemotherapy or endocrine agents as well as the evidence behind the surgical choices available following neoadjuvant treatment of breast cancer.

17.2 Indications for Neoadjuvant Systemic Treatment

Patients who are confirmed to be candidates for adjuvant chemotherapy (e.g. high-grade tumour, node positive, HER2-positive, triple negative) can be considered for neoadjuvant chemotherapy [10]. It may be the preferred option for those patients in whom breast conservation is either not possible or would result in suboptimal cosmesis [10]. Although conventionally used for locally advanced breast cancers, neoadjuvant chemotherapy has more recently been used in some centres for smaller T2 (2–5 cm) tumours [11]. It would be reasonable to offer neoadjuvant chemotherapy in these patients especially if adverse prognostic factors have been identified, such as high nuclear grade [10] or triple-negative tumours [12]. Young age is an independent risk factor for recurrence and survival, and it has been suggested that these patients would be potential candidates for neoadjuvant treatment [13]: the biological or clinical rationale for this suggestion is not clear to the authors.

In the B-18 trial, women under the age of 50 appeared to have the greatest benefit from neoadjuvant chemotherapy. A retrospective analysis of this study shows OS in women under the age of 50 was slightly better in the preoperative chemotherapy group (61 % vs. 55 %, $P = 0.06$) although this was not statistically significant [5]. This trend was also seen in DFS for this group (44 % v 38 %, $P = 0.09$).

There are tumour subtypes which may have a much lower rate of response to neoadjuvant chemotherapy and therefore may not achieve the same benefits as with other tumour types. For example, Guarneri and colleagues published a single centre study that reported the pCR rate of hormone receptor-negative tumours was 24 % versus 8 % for hormone receptor-positive tumours [14]. Cristofanilli et al. found that in invasive lobular cancers, a subgroup of hormone receptor-positive tumours, the pCR rate was only 3 % [15].

17.3 Endocrine Therapy Versus Chemotherapy

Neoadjuvant endocrine therapy is increasingly utilised to achieve tumour shrinkage before surgery in postmenopausal women with oestrogen receptor (ER)-positive tumours [16]. Although there is a lack of randomised data on the use of neoadjuvant endocrine therapy versus adjuvant endocrine therapy, reviews of the available literature have shown clinical response rates ranging from 13.5 to 100 % with treatment periods between 3 and 24 months [16, 17]. These reviews have also demonstrated the superiority of aromatase inhibitors compared to tamoxifen in terms of tumour response and rates of breast-conserving surgery in postmenopausal patients. However, there are few studies of neoadjuvant endocrine therapy which link initial tumour size, response rates, resulting breast conservation rates and outcome (i.e. local recurrence or overall survival). Studies of neoadjuvant (and primary) endocrine therapy show not only continued response with treatment durations longer than 3 months but that tumour response rate increases with increased duration of treatment. Therefore, longer durations of neoadjuvant endocrine therapy are feasible and should be considered in selected patients.

The majority of neoadjuvant trials have utilised chemotherapy with or without biologic agents, with only a few randomised clinical trials comparing the clinical effectiveness of neoadjuvant chemotherapy versus neoadjuvant endocrine therapy [18, 19]. Semiglazov et al. in a phase 2 randomised trial examined the clinical effectiveness of these two forms of treatment in patients with ER-positive disease who were not eligible for breast-conserving surgery at presentation [18]. There were 121 patients who received neoadjuvant endocrine therapy (anastrozole (61 patients) or exemestane (60 patients)) and 118 patients who received neoadjuvant chemotherapy. There were no statistically significant differences in the overall response rate between the groups after 3 months of treatment (anastrozole 62 %, exemestane 67 %, chemotherapy 63 %; $P > 0.05$). More patients in the endocrine therapy group (33 %) were eligible for breast conservation surgery compared to the chemotherapy group (23 %) although this did not reach statistical significance. After a median follow-up of 36 months, there was no significant difference in the incidence of local recurrence between the two groups (endocrine therapy 3.3 % versus chemotherapy 3.4 %). Patients in this study were older (median age of 67 and 68 years in the endocrine therapy and chemotherapy groups, respectively), and this may have had an impact on response and outcome.

It is recognised that the incidence of hormone receptor-positive breast cancer increases with age as does the extent of ER positivity [20]. It has also been shown that the benefits of chemotherapy in primary breast cancer are reduced in an older population [21]. Furthermore, there is evidence that neoadjuvant chemotherapy in ER-positive tumours, particularly invasive lobular breast cancer, produces significantly fewer pCRs [14, 15]. In a randomised trial reported by Alba et al., 95 patients with luminal type breast cancer were randomised to neoadjuvant chemotherapy (epirubicin plus cyclophosphamide × four cycles followed by docetaxel × four cycles) or neoadjuvant endocrine therapy (exemestane 25 mg daily × 24 weeks) [19]. The primary end point was response measured by magnetic resonance imaging (MRI), and it did not show a statistical difference in the response rate measured by MRI (66 % for neoadjuvant chemotherapy versus 48 % for neoadjuvant endocrine therapy; $P = 0.075$). The grade 3/4 toxicity was more frequent with chemotherapy.

Pathological complete response to neoadjuvant chemotherapy has come to be accepted as a surrogate marker of outcome. A single centre publication reported that pCR was associated with better outcomes regardless of hormone receptor status in breast cancer patients [14], and a further review reports a range of pCR from 4 to 29.2 % with chemotherapy [22]. However, a recent pooled analysis of 12 studies where response criteria, including pCR, were compared to clinical outcome measures reported no link between pCR and clinical outcome, although in certain more aggressive subtypes, the prognostic value of pCR was greater than in other less aggressive subtypes [8].

Few neoadjuvant endocrine therapy studies have reported on pathological complete response rates. In those already mentioned [14, 15, 18, 19], the pCR rate ranged from 0 to 8 % for hormone receptor-positive tumours. Milla-Santos and colleagues reported on 112 postmenopausal women with stage 3 locally advanced breast cancers receiving neoadjuvant endocrine therapy for 3 months followed by surgery in responders with a pCR rate of 12 % [23].

Thomas et al. evaluated pathologic response in 50 patients receiving neoadjuvant chemotherapy for 3 months and 53 patients receiving neoadjuvant endocrine therapy (letrozole) for 3 months [24]. Excised tumours were compared with preoperative core biopsy specimens. Neoadjuvant chemotherapy produced more pathologic complete responses; however, a pattern of scattered residual cells in the tumour bed was also seen more frequently ($P = 0.035$) with neoadjuvant chemotherapy. Letrozole produced substantially more central scars (31 patients with neoadjuvant endocrine therapy versus 2 patients with neoadjuvant chemotherapy; $P = 0.0001$). There was also a statistically significant correlation with central scarring and clinical tumour volume reduction ($P = 0.034$). It was proposed that differences in the type of response and correlation with tumour volume reduction may have an impact on the amount of tissue removed following neoadjuvant treatment. However, this was not a randomised trial, and analysis of the pretreatment characteristics of the two groups showed them to be different in terms of age, tumour stage, nodal status and ER status. It is therefore not clear if the different histological pattern is due to the different treatments, the different types of tumours or a combination of both. However, the point raised by the authors that central tumour shrinkage, which was less frequent with chemotherapy, may be an important factor in downsizing tumours and enabling subsequent conservation surgery requires consideration given the meta-analyses which report an increased rate of local recurrence in patients undergoing breast conservation following neoadjuvant chemotherapy. The ACOSOG Z1031 trial also has shown that in a population of 352 patients with stage 2 or 3 primary hormone receptor-positive breast cancer (Allred score 6–8), the third-generation aromatase inhibitors (i.e. using exemestane, anastrozole or letrozole) resulted in breast-conserving surgery in the following subgroups of patients: 83 % (157/189) of patients who were deemed borderline for breast conservation at presentation, 51 % (81/159) deemed suitable by standard mastectomy and 75 % (3/4) deemed inoperable by standard mastectomy. The authors reported that this 'low toxicity approach is therefore a reasonable standard of care for selected patients with ER-rich, HER2-negative breast cancer who desire breast conservation despite clinical stage 2 or 3 disease' [25].

17.4 Tumour Imaging and Localisation and Margin of Excision in Patients Receiving Neoadjuvant Systemic Treatment

All patients should have mammography at diagnosis and again prior to surgery on completion of systemic therapy. Other imaging modalities include ultrasound and MRI, and MRI may be more accurate in measuring tumour size although not everyone uses it. In a study by Segara et al., the accuracy of physical examination and ultrasound in assessing tumour size was compared to MRI at the time of diagnosis and prior to surgery; these measurements were then compared to the final pathologic tumour size. MRI scan predicted the size within a centimetre in 76 % of patients compared with 66 % for ultrasound and 54 % with physical examination (not statistically significant) [26].

There is some controversy regarding how much tissue should be resected at the time of breast-conserving surgery following neoadjuvant therapy. Some will make the argument that the entire footprint of the original tumour should be resected along with a margin of normal tissue. This may be feasible in small volume tumours or when there is a relatively small tumour volume to breast volume ratio. Oncoplastic breast-conserving techniques such as mammoplasty or volume replacement procedures such as LICAP flaps may permit larger resections whilst maintaining a cosmetically acceptable outcome.

Many surgeons take the view that only the residual tumour burden, along with a margin of normal tissue, needs to be resected, and removing the original footprint of the tumour would preclude the opportunity for breast-conserving surgery.

It is usual practice to place a radiological marker in the centre of the tumour at the time of initial presentation. This allows the residual radiological abnormality to be targeted with wires even in the presence of complete clinical or radiological response. In a retrospective review of 373 patients (145 had radio-opaque markers placed and 228 did not), those with markers had an improved rate of local control when compared to those who did not (98.6 % vs. 91.7 %, $P = 0.02$) after a follow-up of approximately 4 years [27]. In this study patients usually only had one clip placed in the centre of the tumour, and the surgeons did not try to excise the full extent of the original tumour footprint. Likewise, in a study by Boughey and colleagues, a smaller volume of tissue was excised in patients treated with neoadjuvant chemotherapy (i.e. not including the original tumour footprint with a cuff of normal tissue), but there was similar local recurrence rates compared to patients treated with surgery followed by adjuvant chemotherapy [28]. Regardless of opinion on the optimal extent of resection, it is clear that a multidisciplinary approach is essential in these complex cases, and careful discussion between patients, surgeons, radiologists, pathologists and oncologists should take place prior to the patient starting neoadjuvant treatment and again at the end of neoadjuvant therapy prior to deciding on the final surgical approach. The question of how much tissue should be resected for particular tumour subtypes and/or particular neoadjuvant therapies is an important area for future research.

17.5 Management of the Axilla with Neoadjuvant Systemic Treatment

Management of the axilla in patients undergoing primary surgery for breast cancer is controversial, and this is also the case for neoadjuvant treatment with no consensus as to what is the best approach. For those in whom positive nodes are identified at the time of initial diagnosis, approximately 50 % [29], axillary clearance after neoadjuvant treatment remains standard practice. In those with a clinically and radiologically negative axilla at presentation, the timing of sentinel lymph node biopsy (SLNB) in the neoadjuvant setting is controversial. Initial studies regarding the efficacy of SNLB following neoadjuvant chemotherapy showed an unacceptably high false-negative rate with one small study showing a 30 % false-negative rate in patients undergoing SLNB after chemotherapy [30]. There have not been any randomised controlled trials evaluating the reliability (identification rate and false-negative rate) of sentinel node biopsy following neoadjuvant chemotherapy. In the NSABP-B27 trial, many participating surgeons performed SLNB followed by axillary dissection [31]. There were 428 patients in whom the surgeon attempted SLNB following neoadjuvant chemotherapy. In this group, 15 women had a negative sentinel lymph node but were found to have metastatic disease in at least one non-sentinel lymph node, giving a false-negative rate of 10.7 %. Of the total, 343 had at least one sentinel node identified followed by a completion axillary dissection with an overall success rate of 84.8 % in identifying the sentinel node. More recently, a multicentre prospective cohort study was designed to evaluate a specific algorithm for timing of a standardised sentinel lymph node biopsy procedure in patients who undergo neoadjuvant chemotherapy [32]. The primary end point was to assess the false-negative rate of SLNB after NAC for patients who converted from clinically node-positive disease before chemotherapy (cN1) to node-negative disease (cN0) following chemotherapy. In this group there was a false-negative rate (FNR) of 14.2 % and an identification rate (IR) of 80.1 %. This study and the results from the B-27 trial above report a less than optimal identification rate of SLNs following NAC and higher FNRs compared to sentinel node trials performed in the upfront surgery setting. In the NSABP B-32 trial, the false-negative rate was 9.8 % with an overall success rate of 97.2 % [33]. Results of the ALMANAC validation study involving 842 patients reported a success rate of 96.1 % using combined technique of blue dye and radioisotope and a false-negative rate of 6.7 % [34]. In both the NSABP B-32 and ALMANAC trials, these were randomised trials which required training and proctoring of the surgeons before they could enrol patients on the trial.

No randomised trials have been conducted to evaluate the reliability of SLNB after NAC. We know from cohort studies of SLNB after NAC that the axillary recurrence rates are low and such an RCT is unlikely to occur as the number needed to recruit into the trial will be too high to make it feasible. Recent cohort studies have reported better identification rates and lower false-negative rates with SLNB following NAC. There have been five meta-analyses combining these cohort studies which report an identification rate between 89 and 95 % and false-negative rate between 8 and 14 % [35–39]. The first three meta-analyses had broader inclusion criteria including patients with both clinically positive and clinically negative axillary nodes. They reported an identification rate between 88 and 90.9 % and FNR between 8.4 and 12 % [35–37]. Tan et al. in 2011 in their meta-analysis looked into the feasibility and accuracy of SLNB in a population of patients who were clinically node negative following NAC [38]. They reported an identification rate of 94.3 % and FNR of 9.4 %. The most recent meta-analysis includes 15 studies of clinically node-positive breast cancer patients who underwent SLNB after NAC followed by axillary node dissection [39]. They report a pooled identification rate of 89 % and an FNR of 14 %. In the recent Z1071 trial, 649 patients with node-positive breast cancer underwent NAC followed by SLNB and ALND. They reported an identification rate of 93.9 % and FNR of 12.6 % [40]. Another recent prospective multicentre cohort study in patients with biopsy-proven node-positive breast cancer who underwent SLNB after NAC included 153 patients and reported an identification rate of 87.6 % and an FNR of 8.4 % [41].

Proponents of SLNB prior to initiating chemotherapy argue that because of its high accuracy, it could potentially avoid an axillary node clearance if the sentinel node is negative. Conversely, it follows that a positive sentinel node in this scenario would mean the patient undergoes axillary node clearance as their definitive axillary procedure after chemotherapy. However, up to 40 % of patients receiving neoadjuvant chemotherapy will have downstaging of their axilla; thus, axillary clearance may be unnecessary and could be associated with significant morbidity [40–45]. Although there are no data from randomised clinical trials to support the approach of omitting axillary dissection post-chemotherapy in patients, the meta-analysis of cohort studies has shown the feasibility and to some extent the reliability of SLNB following NAC.

17.6 Oncological Safety of Breast Conservation Surgery Following Neoadjuvant Systemic Treatment

There is consensus that neoadjuvant chemotherapy can increase the breast conservation rate, as shown in the NSABP B-18 trial, EORTC 10902 trial and a subsequent meta-analysis [5, 7, 46]. Data from the NSABP B-18 trial suggested a trend towards increased local recurrence (13 % vs. 10 %, $P = 0.21$) in patients undergoing breast conservation following neoadjuvant chemotherapy, although this did not reach statistical significance. In the EORTC 10902 phase III RCT, 698 patients were enrolled to receive four cycles of neoadjuvant FEC or four cycles of adjuvant FEC [46]. More patients were eligible to be treated by breast conservation surgery with NAC (23 % downstaged) compared to adjuvant treatment with no significant differences in overall survival, progression-free survival and locoregional control.

Subsequently, a meta-analysis suggested an increase in local recurrence in those having breast conservation following neoadjuvant chemotherapy [7]. However, proponents of neoadjuvant treatment argue that increase in local recurrence largely reflects the use of radiotherapy without surgery in patients with complete clinical response, and thus local recurrence is not increased as long as surgery remains part of the treatment even after complete clinical response (HR, 1.12; 95 % CI, 0.92–1.37; p, 0.25).

Chemotherapy can result in different patterns of tumour shrinkage. This can be a concentric shrinkage or a 'honeycomb' or 'Swiss cheese' regression of the tumour leaving microscopic islands of disease within the original footprint of the primary tumour [24]. This 'honeycomb' type regression, which can be seen in up to 40 % of tumours, could be hypothesised to be the cause of the trend towards increased rates of local recurrence following neoadjuvant chemotherapy. Although results from B-18 suggested a trend towards increased local recurrence in the conserved breast, there are other studies that show neoadjuvant chemotherapy may in fact have a positive impact on clear excision margins and reoperation rates. For example, Christy et al. showed neoadjuvant chemotherapy significantly reduced the rate of reoperation for positive margins in patients whose tumours measured between 2 and 4 cm [11]. There was also a significantly decreased number of positive margins in those patients who received neoadjuvant chemotherapy compared to post-operative chemotherapy (10 % vs. 32 %, $P = <0.01$). This led to decreased rates of reoperation (3 % vs. 35 %, $P = <0.01$) and mastectomy (3 % vs. 19 %, $P = <0.01$). In a retrospective review of data from patients involved in trials of neoadjuvant versus adjuvant chemotherapy, patients with tumours more than 2 cm had significantly smaller volumes of breast tissue excised when treated with neoadjuvant chemotherapy compared to those who had surgery first followed by adjuvant chemotherapy, and the re-excision rates did not significantly differ between groups [28]. Clough et al. reported on 175 patients with a median tumour size of 25 mm (range 4–90 mm) treated by breast-conserving surgery with various quadrant-specific oncoplastic techniques described later in the chapter. There were 136 (77.7 %) patients who had surgery as their initial treatment and 39 (22.3 %) patients received neoadjuvant therapy. Of these, 13.1 % of patients had involved margins, and only 3 (1.7 %) developed local recurrence after a median follow-up of 49 (23–96) months [47].

17.7 Oncoplastic Procedures Following Neoadjuvant Systemic Treatment

Breast reconstruction following neoadjuvant chemotherapy and mastectomy is beyond the scope of this chapter. This section will focus on partial breast reconstruction using oncoplastic techniques of volume displacement and volume replacement where simple wide local excision alone would leave a significant cosmetic defect.

The aim of oncoplastic breast conservation surgery is to allow potentially large areas of breast tissue to be excised with a margin whilst preserving a natural-looking shape to the conserved breast. This can be achieved by a number of different surgical approaches. The oncological safety in terms of margin status and recurrence has been reported to compare favourably with traditional breast conservation surgery (BCS) [48–52]. As noted above, Clough's series of 175 patients undergoing mammoplasty at the time of BCS reported low rates of margin involvement and local recurrence. That series also assessed the cosmetic outcome rated on a 5-point scale (excellent, 5; good, 4; fair, 3; poor, 2; bad, 1). Of the 80 patients (45.7 %) assessed, the mean cosmetic score was 4.6 with 85 % of that group scoring 4 or 5. Caution should be exercised in interpreting these results as over half the patients in the series did not have assessment of their cosmetic outcome, and the 39 patients who had neoadjuvant chemotherapy had a median tumour size of only 25 mm. Indeed, Schaverien and colleagues reported on the quality of information reporting in studies of standard and oncoplastic breast-conserving surgery [53], and they carried out a systematic review to establish the completeness of reporting of key patient, tumour, treatment and outcome information. They compared standard breast-conserving surgery considered to be the 'gold standard' with the reporting of the same key criteria for all published studies of oncoplastic breast-conserving surgery. They included six randomised controlled trials of standard BCS ($n = 11{,}767$ patients) and 53 studies for oncoplastic BCS ($n = 3236$ patients), none of which were randomised trials. The oncoplastic studies reported a mean of 54 % of key criteria (range 10–85 %). The authors proposed standards by which to judge future studies of BCS reporting key information and outcomes, and the collection of robust, validated data and randomised controlled trials on the long-term safety of oncoplastic techniques are needed.

We know from previous studies that once approximately 20 % of the breast volume is excised with conventional breast conservation, there is a risk of cosmetic deformity [54, 55]. With oncoplastic techniques, up to 50 % of the breast volume can be excised whilst preserving a natural breast shape [48]. With these techniques an average 200 g of tissue is removed; however, up to 1000 g or even more can be excised in patients with large breasts with no significant adverse cosmetic outcome [56]. Preservation of an acceptable breast shape and volume may be achieved with techniques that rely primarily on reshaping the breast tissue, such as reduction or therapeutic mammoplasty, or introducing autologous tissue from elsewhere to maintain breast volume such as local perforator flaps. For those patients undergoing mammoplasty, the volume of the conserved breast may be considerably smaller than the preoperative size. This volume deficit may be further exacerbated by post-operative radiotherapy. It is common that patients undergoing these procedures require adjustment to the contralateral breast in order to maintain symmetry, and careful discussion and planning of this with the patient are an essential part of the treatment pathway. These techniques will now be outlined.

17.8 Mammoplasty Techniques for Patients Undergoing Breast Conservation

The wise pattern or inverted T mammoplasty has long been used for cosmetic breast reduction and is well established as a safe and reliable procedure. Many authors have described using this technique or modifications thereof to excise tumours from the breast, essentially combining a wide excision with a breast reduction in what has become known as a therapeutic mammoplasty. It is a highly adaptable technique allowing excision of tumours from any quadrant of the breast [57, 58] and has become established as a key procedure in oncoplastic breast conservation surgery.

However, Clough et al. believe that it cannot be adapted in all situations especially in patients with large breasts and describe a quadrant-per-quadrant atlas of mammoplasty technique for large breast cancers [47].

Alternative approaches such as vertical or round block mammoplasty are also useful, and careful patient selection is the key to successful oncological and cosmetic outcomes.

For clarity, tumour position within the breast will be categorised as central, upper pole, lower pole or by quadrant (superolateral, inferolateral, superomedial, inferomedial) and the choices of surgical approach to each of these locations discussed.

17.9 Tumours of the Upper Pole

For these tumours a classical inverted T approach is a good option especially for large breasts. For small or moderately sized breasts, this technique can be used, but a vertical pattern mammoplasty or round block technique may be more appropriate.

17.9.1 Wise Pattern or Inverted T Mammoplasty

This approach opens up the whole breast from medial to lateral, enabling wide excision of the tumour with a margin and then filling up the defect with the surrounding tissue and the mobilised pedicle. An inferior pedicle is classically used for upper pole tumours; however, superior-based pedicles are also an option.

The surgeon marks the midline from the suprasternal notch to the umbilicus. A line is drawn from the mid-clavicular point towards the nipple and down through the inferior pole of the breast – this marks the breast meridian. The new nipple position is marked on this line. A finger can be placed in the inframammary fold, and the position of the tip of the finger is marked anteriorly on the breast. The distance from the suprasternal notch to the new nipple should be between 18 and 22 cm, and the distance from the midline to the new nipple should be 9–11 cm [54]. The breast is rotated medially and laterally against the meridian to mark the medial and lateral pillars and plot the area to be excised, which may be within the wise 'keyhole' pattern or around it. Within this keyhole the inferior pedicle incorporating the nipple areola complex is marked. Wide excision of the tumour is then carried out. The de-epithelialised pedicle is then advanced into the defect, and the pillars are stitched together as shown in Fig. 17.1a. The appearance of the final scar is shown in Fig. 17.1b. When marking the inferior pedicle, aim for a width of approximately 8–10 cm and extend the pedicle 1.5 cm superiorly from the areola [54]. The thickness of pedicle should be 4–10 cm at the base and 3–5 cm at the

Fig. 17.1a Wise pattern inferior pedicle mammoplasty for superior pole tumours

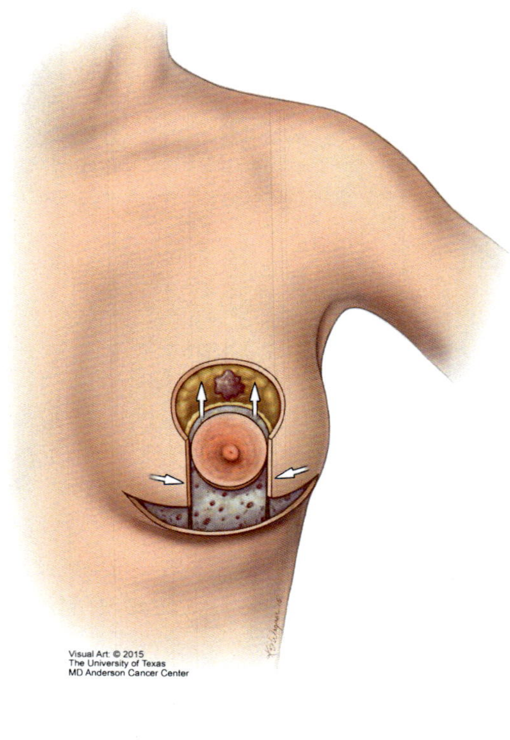

Fig. 17.1b Final appearance of scar after wise pattern mammoplasty

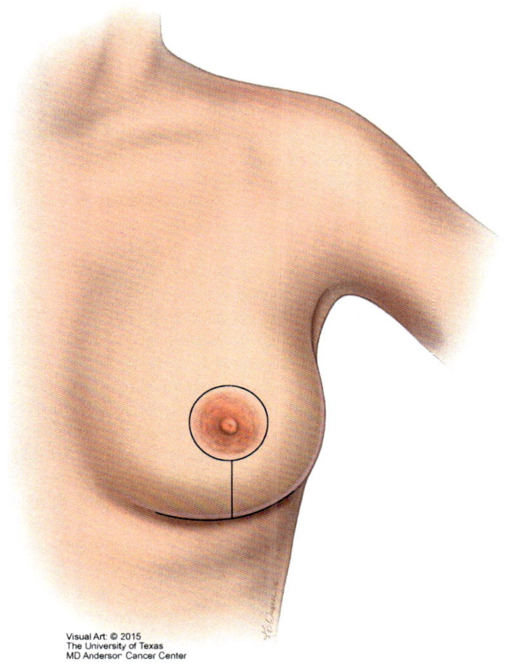

nipple areola complex [54]. For superior-based flaps, the keyhole pattern remains the same; however, a de-epithelialised superior-based flap is rotated into the defect as shown in Fig. 17.2a. If the wide excision defect is large, a secondary pedicle can be fashioned and advanced into the defect to create volume in the upper pole. This can be achieved, for example, by using the tissue that would have been used for an inferior pedicle. This can be de-epithelialised and mobilised into the defect.

17.9.2 Vertical Pattern Mammoplasty

Vertical reduction mammoplasty has been championed by a number of authors including Le Jour and Hall-Finlay and can be easily adapted for therapeutic mammoplasty. This approach reduces the scarring on the breast and relies on a superior-based pedicle. The initial post-operative result gives a very puckered looking appearance to the breast, and it is important to warn patients of this and give reassurance that a natural-looking breast appearance will be achieved within the coming weeks.

Fig. 17.2a Wise pattern superior medial pedicle for upper pole tumours

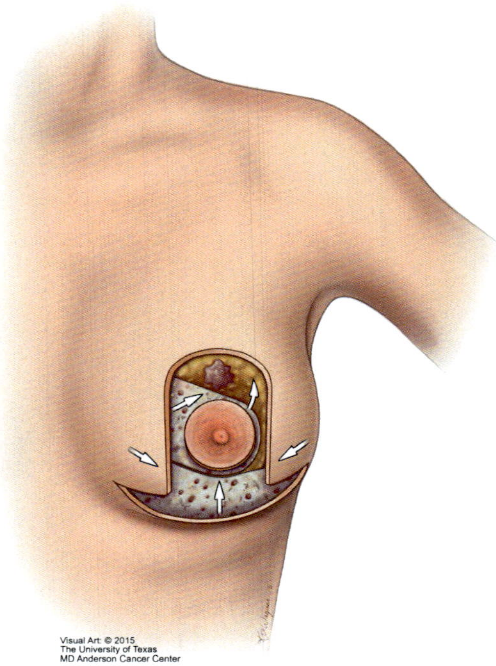

The preoperative markings have some common elements with the inverted T mammoplasty. The breast meridian and new nipple position are marked as before. The new superior border of the areola is marked approximately 2 cm above the new nipple position, and then a dome shape is drawn to define the new areolar border. The vertical markings, like the inverted T, are defined by rotating the breast medially and laterally in continuity with the breast meridian and joining these lines in a U shape approximately 2 cm proximal to the inframammary fold. This plots the area to be excised. A superomedial pedicle is then fashioned and can be rotated into the defect left by the wide local excision as shown in Fig. 17.2b. The medial and lateral pillars are plicated and the skin closed.

17.9.3 The Round Block Mammoplasty

This technique is useful in patients with small or moderately sized breasts and offers the advantage of minimal scarring. It was first described by Benelli [59]. The breast meridian is marked along with the inframammary fold and the position of the

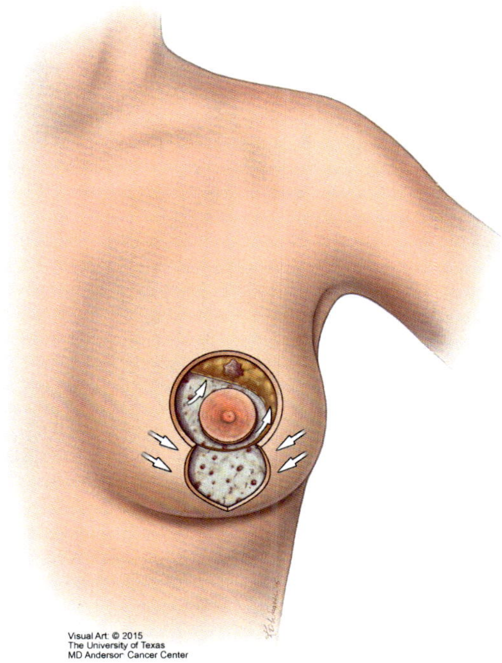

Fig. 17.2b Vertical pattern superior medial pedicle for upper pole tumours

new superior border of the areola. A periareolar ellipse is drawn, the size of which varies depending on tumour size, nipple position and the degree of ptosis. The skin is de-epithelialised as shown in Fig. 17.3. Skin flaps are raised around the tumour, and tumour excised with a margin and the surrounding breast tissue undergoes undermining and approximation for glandular reshaping. The skin incision is closed using a running suture technique to minimise the risk of stretching and distortion of the areola. Although used mainly for upper pole tumours, it can be adapted for tumours of any location of the breast [48]. A similar technique can be used on the opposite side for symmetry.

17.10 Tumours of the Lower Pole

A classical inverted T approach is a good option for lower pole tumours which can be resected with a wide margin without the need for a secondary pedicle to fill the defect as the area being resected falls within the 'keyhole' area. For these a superior-based pedicle is required. Figure 17.4a shows an inverted T mammoplasty

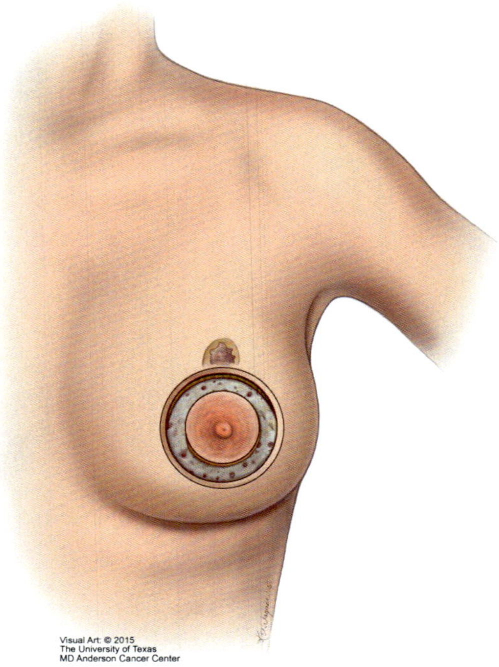

Fig. 17.3 Round block mammoplasty showing de-epithelialised area

with a superior-based pedicle. Vertical mammoplasty lends itself well to central lower pole tumours in moderately sized breasts as again the tumour falls within the area that would normally be resected as shown in Fig. 17.4b.

17.11 Tumours of the Upper Outer Quadrant

Here a lateral mammoplasty technique is a useful option [47]. Two oblique incisions are extended from the nipple areola complex towards the axilla. A small crescent of skin is de-epithelialised around the medial aspect of the nipple areola complex to restore a medial position of the nipple-areolar complex at the end of the procedure as shown in Fig. 17.5a. The oblique incision is deepened to excise the tumour with a wide margin along with the overlying skin. By undermining the surrounding glandular tissue from the pectoral fascia whilst maintaining attachment to overlying skin (thus maintaining the blood supply), glandular tissue is sutured together to obliterate the defect and achieve a good cosmetic result. At the end of

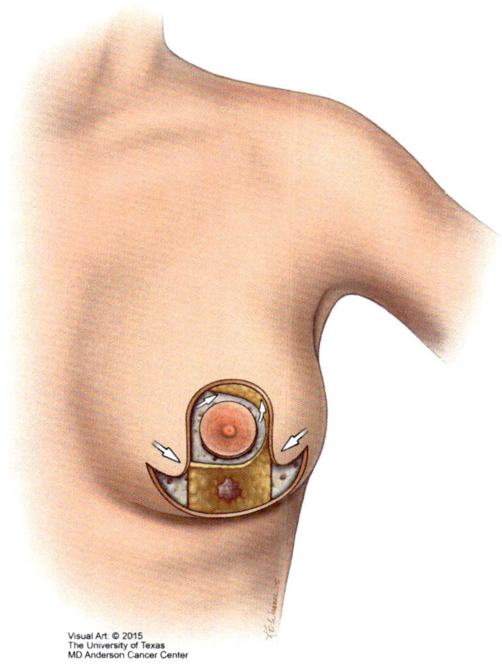

Fig. 17.4a Wise superior pedicle for inferior pole tumours

the procedure, there will be a scar surrounding the areola and extending laterally towards the axilla as shown in Fig. 17.5b.

For women who have large breasts in proportion to their body, inverted T approach is also a good option. The advantage here is that even if there are large defects following the excision of the tumour, an additional de-epithelialised secondary pedicle can be fashioned and mobilised into the defect [58]. For patients with fatty-replaced breasts, the blood supply to the pedicle will be through the subdermal plexus or through the pectoral muscles; therefore, dual undermining of the breast tissue should be avoided to prevent fat necrosis.

17.12 Tumours of the Lower Outer Quadrant of the Breast

In this area the J mammoplasty is a simple option [60]. This approach is similar to lateral mammoplasty for upper outer quadrant tumours except that the first incision starts at the medial edge of the de-epithelialised periareolar area as shown in Fig. 17.6a and extends towards the inframammary fold in a J fashion for right-

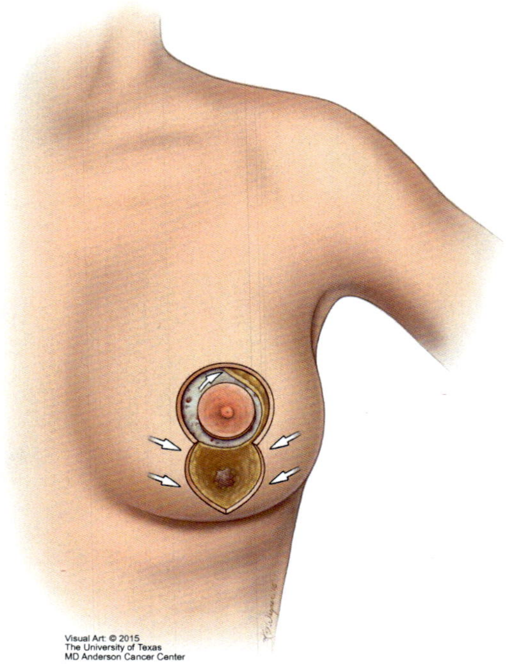

Fig. 17.4b Vertical pattern superior medial pedicle for lower pole tumours

sided tumours and reversed J shaped for left-sided tumours. The second incision starts at the lateral edge of the de-epithelialised periareolar area and follows a similar pattern. After excision of the tumour with the skin, the retroareolar gland is released from the nipple-areolar complex, and the three glandular pillars (central, medial and lateral) are mobilised into the excision cavity. Alternatively, the tip of the J can be extended upwards along the inframammary fold as shown in Fig. 17.6b, and the flap is pulled down to fill the defect.

Once again an inverted T incision or a vertical mammoplasty incision based on a superior-based pedicle can be used with excellent cosmetic results. If the tumour falls within the keyhole area for excision, the procedure is carried out as for a breast reduction. If a vertical approach is adopted, Fig. 17.7 demonstrates how a wide excision can be taken and the de-epithelialised lower pole tissue can be rotated into the defect as a secondary pedicle.

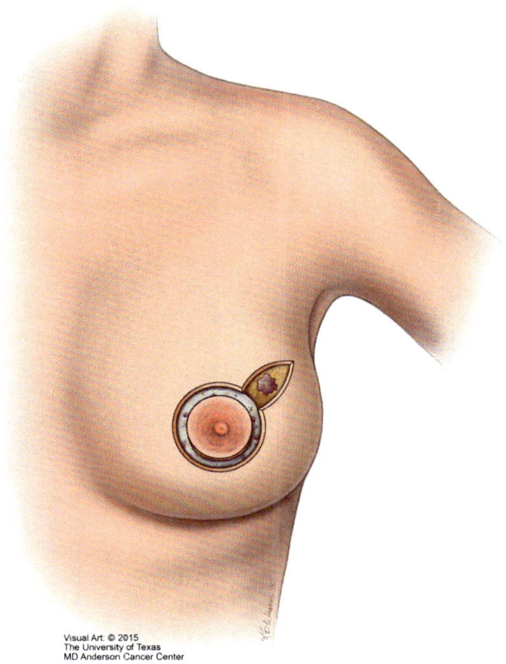

Fig. 17.5a Lateral mammoplasty incision and de-epithelialised periareolar part for upper outer quadrant tumours

17.13 Tumours of the Lower Inner Quadrant

The inverted T mammoplasty or vertical mammoplasty can be used in this location, and the approach is more or less a mirror image of the one described above for tumours of the lower outer quadrant. An alternative is a V mammoplasty, where a pyramidal section of the gland with its base located in the inframammary fold and apex at the border of the areola is excised along with the skin [47]. The submammary fold is then incised internally from the resection site to the anterior axillary line to allow adequate rotation of the remaining gland into the defect. The lower pole of the breast is undermined from the pectoral muscle and transferred medially to fill the defect. The nipple-areolar complex is then re-centralised on a de-epithelialised superior-based pedicle.

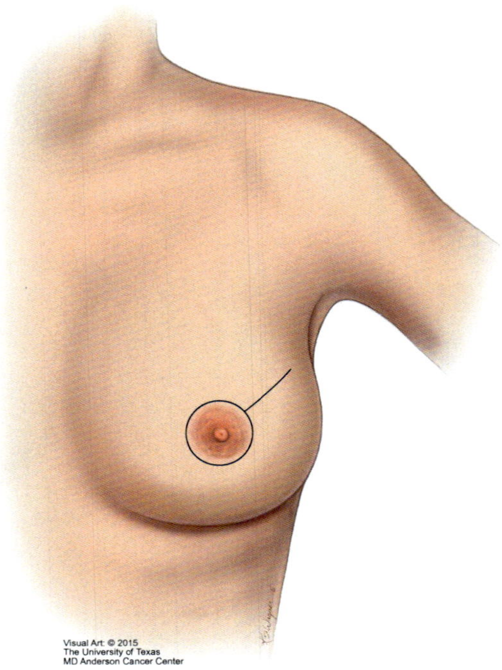

Fig. 17.5b Final scar following lateral mammoplasty

17.14 Tumours of the Upper Inner Quadrant

This is one of the most challenging areas in the breast to achieve a good cosmetic outcome following conservation due to the paucity of breast tissue in this area in many patients. The round block mammoplasty described earlier may be suitable for tumours at this location. A batwing technique of mammoplasty has also been described for tumours in this area [61]. For this technique a wing-like pattern is marked on the breast superior to the nipple-areolar complex as shown in Fig. 17.8a. The lesion is removed and the final pattern of scarring is illustrated in Fig. 17.8b. This approach should be used with caution for resections of more than 20 % of the volume of breast tissue.

As with other tumour locations discussed above, the inverted T or vertical mammoplasty can be adapted with the use of a secondary pedicle to fill the wide excision defect.

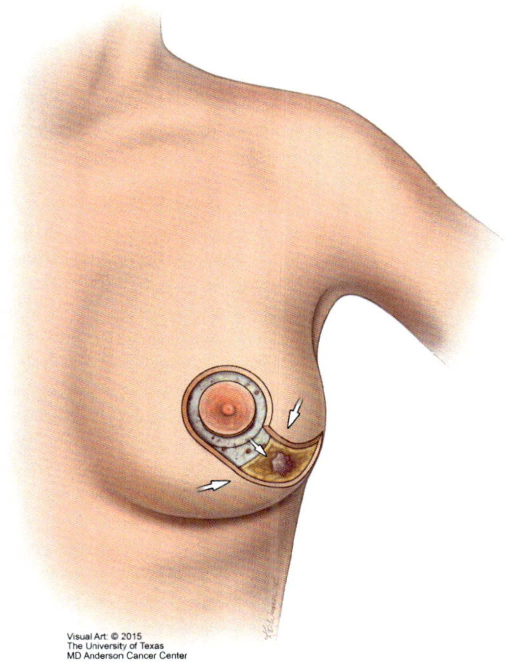

Fig. 17.6a J mammoplasty for lower outer quadrant tumours

17.15 Central Tumours

Central tumours will generally require excision of the nipple-areolar complex. Here the most straightforward option is an inverted T mammoplasty approach incorporating the nipple-areolar complex within the keyhole area if the breast is large enough to accommodate this. This can be closed directly, or a de-epithelialised inferior pedicle can be fashioned to fill the defect and improve projection. A nipple reconstruction can be fashioned at a later date if the patient wishes.

A simpler option for these central tumours is a 'melon slice' wedge mammoplasty [62] which lends itself well to women with larger breasts in proportion to their body and where there may be concerns regarding wound healing (smokers) and fat necrosis as there is no need for a pedicle.

For those women with a very central tumour in a smaller breast, there are still breast-conserving options. One would be the so-called starfish approach where a five-limbed starfish is drawn with the nipple-areolar complex at its centre. Each arm

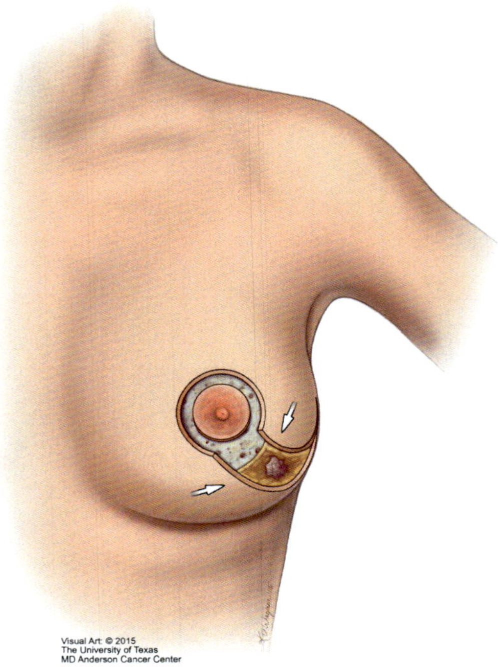

Fig. 17.6b Modified J mammoplasty where tip of the J is extended upwards along the inframammary fold

of the starfish is de-epithelialised. A circumareolar incision is made, and a full thickness cylinder of breast tissue is excised incorporating the tumour. The defect can then be obliterated with a series of purse-string sutures from bottom to top to bring the breast parenchyma together. The skin is then closed leaving a five-pointed star appearance. This approach maintains a nicely projected breast shape.

An alternative is the Grisotti flap. The nipple-areolar complex border is marked circumferentially and a similar sized circle marked below this. Medial and lateral lines extend from the margins of these circles inferiorly to the inframammary fold and incised down to the pectoral fascia. The skin inferior to the lower circle is de-epithelialised. Once the central tumour incorporating the nipple-areolar complex is excised, the flap can be mobilised into the defect with the remaining circle of skin acting as the new areola.

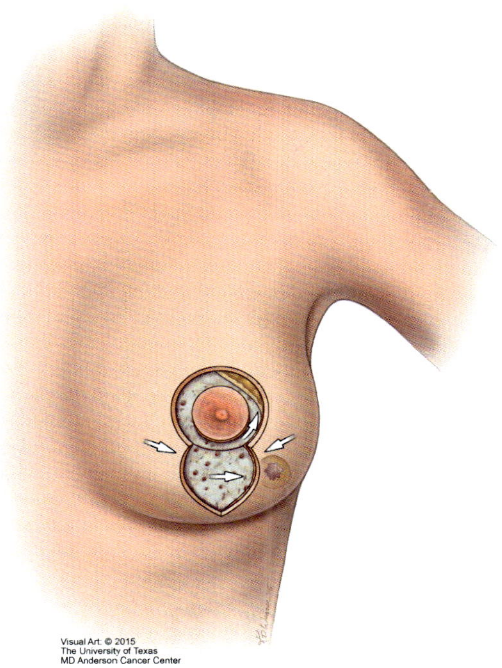

Fig. 17.7 Vertical mammoplasty with de-epithelialised secondary pedicle (infra areolar part) mobilised into the wide local excision site

17.16 Partial Breast Reconstruction Using Perforator Flaps for Volume Replacement

One of the downsides of mammoplasty is that, although breast shape is maintained, the volume of the conserved breast is reduced, often dramatically so. Therefore, many patients undergoing such surgery require a contralateral breast reduction in order to achieve symmetry. This necessitates further surgical procedures and scarring on an otherwise healthy breast. Women with large, pendulous breasts may welcome the opportunity to achieve an overall smaller breast size; however, for those women with smaller breasts, the loss of volume may be problematic. Options exist in the form of perforator flaps to maintain breast volume following wide excision. Such flaps are most suited to correct defects in the lateral aspect of the breast and have largely replaced the traditional myocutaneous latissimus dorsi (LD) 'mini-flap' as a means of oncoplastic volume replacement.

Two main types of perforator flaps have been described utilising either the lateral intercostal artery perforator (LICAP) or the thoracodorsal artery perforator (TDAP). These flaps rely on mobilising large areas of skin and subcutaneous tissue

Fig. 17.8a Batwing mammoplasty incision

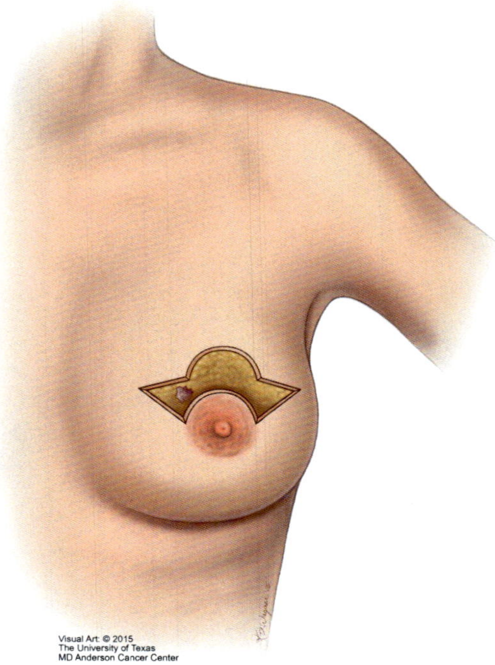

on perforators. They are initially more difficult to perform than the mini-LD flap but offer the advantage of sparing the LD muscle and hence reducing the morbidity associated with this procedure. Seroma formation is less, and the scars are generally well concealed, and patients report reduced pain as compared to the pedicled LD flap [63]. Another important consideration with perforator flaps is that they allow preservation of the LD muscle which is available for future use should the patient develop local recurrence and require mastectomy and reconstruction.

17.17 LICAP

The flap is drawn out lateral to the breast over the axilla and lateral chest wall. The anterior border of the flap should include the junction of the inframammary fold (IMF) with the anterior axillary line [64]. Lateral intercostal perforators are often present here. The perforators are localised and marked with a handheld Doppler and the flap marked incorporating the perforator as shown in Fig. 17.9a. The closest perforator to the breast, the most anterior one, is the ideal one to include within the

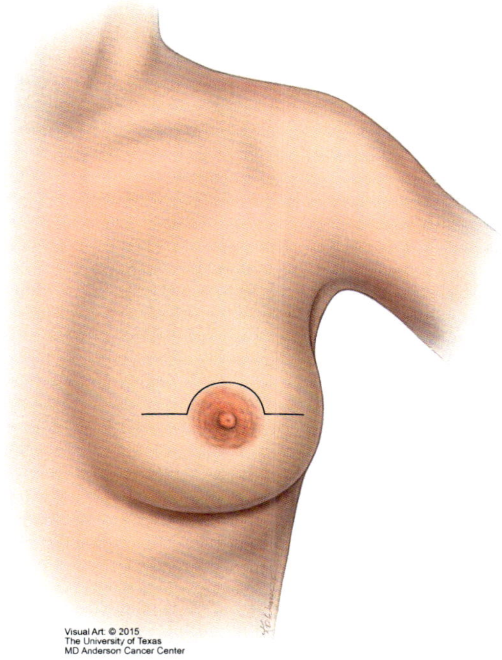

Fig. 17.8b Final scar following batwing mammoplasty

flap as this maximises the arc of rotation of the flap. A posterior approach is made first and the incision is developed to expose LD muscle; the dissection plane is above the muscle fascia. An anterior extension at the inferior border of the flap is used to expose the perforators and allow easy elevation of the flap and rotation into the defect. Several intercostal perforators may be encountered between the LD and pectoral major muscle. No large perforators should be sacrificed until a similar or larger one is found closer to the pectoral major muscle. Once the largest perforator is found, surrounding tissue is freed and allowed to fill the lateral defect in the breast. The donor site is closed primarily as shown in Fig. 17.9b.

17.18 TDAP

The precise perforator location is identified preoperatively with a handheld Doppler. The skin island is centred on the perforators that are typically located 8 cm below the posterior axillary fold and 2 cm behind the anterior border of the LD muscle where the proximal skin perforator exits the muscle into the subcutaneous tissue [65]. Once designed, the flap is elevated from posterior to anterior just above

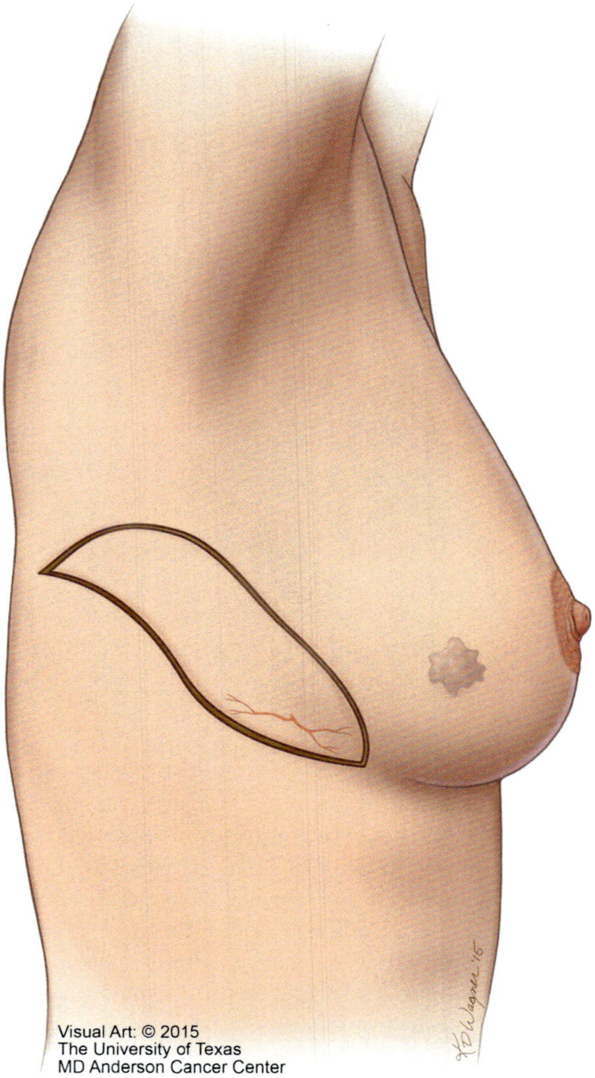

Fig. 17.9a Incision for LICAP flap with marked perforator

the LD muscle fascia, and care is taken to capture the maximal amount of soft tissue. The vascular pedicle is dissected to allow placement of the flap without tension. If a large-diameter (greater than 1 mm) pulsating perforator is identified, a TDAP or a muscle-sparing latissimus dorsi (MSLD) type 1 flap is performed. For a TDAP flap, the LD muscle is split, and the perforator is dissected proximally until the origin from the subscapular vessels is identified. Once dissection of the vessels

Fig. 17.9b Final scar following LICAP flap

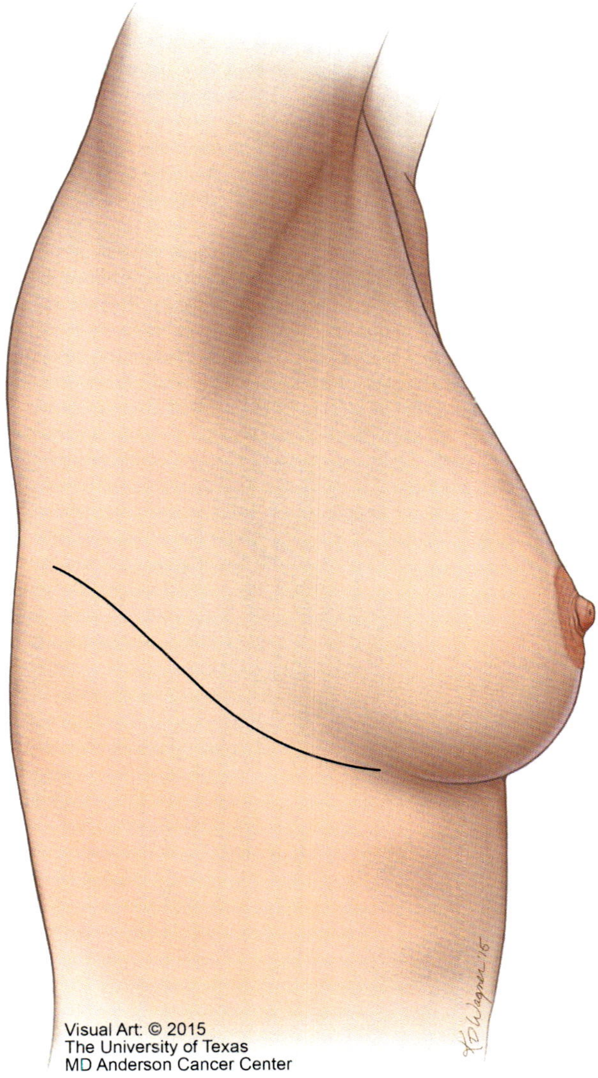

is complete, the skin paddle is carefully passed through the split LD muscle and then subcutaneously through the axillary region into the breast defect.

Alternatively, for an MSLD type 1 flap, a very small cuff of muscle is maintained around the perforators to prevent injuring the pedicle as it enters the flap [65]. If there were multiple small, nonpulsatile perforators, then an MSLD type 2 flap is performed, and here up to 5 cm of muscle is harvested.

References

1. De Lena M, Zucali R, Viganotti G, Valagussa P, Bonadonna G (1978) Combined chemotherapy radiotherapy approach in locally advanced breast cancer. Cancer Chemother Pharmacol 1 (1):53–59
2. Schick P, Goodstein J, Moor J, Butler J, Senter KL (1983) Preoperative chemotherapy followed by mastectomy for locally advanced breast cancer. J Surg Oncol 22(4):278–282
3. Perloff M, Lesnick GJ (1982) Chemotherapy before and after mastectomy in stage III breast cancer. Arch Surg 117(7):879–881
4. Swain SM, Sorace RA, Bagley CS, Danforth DN Jr, Bader J, Wesley MN, Steinberg SM, Lippman ME (1987) Neoadjuvant chemotherapy in the combined modality approach of locally advanced nonmetastatic breast cancer. Cancer Res 47(14):3889–3894
5. Fisher BBA, Mamounas E, Wieand S, Robidoux A, Margolese RG, Cruz AB Jr, Fisher ER WD, Wolmark N et al (1997) Effect of preoperative chemotherapy on local-regional disease in women with operable breast cancer: findings from National Surgical Adjuvant Breast and Bowel Project B-18. J Clin Oncol 15(7):2483–2493
6. Mamounas EP (1997) NSABP Protocol B-27. Preoperative doxorubicin plus cyclophosphamide followed by preoperative or postoperative docetaxel. Oncology (Williston Park) 11 (6 Suppl 6):37–40
7. Mieog JS, van der Hage JH, van de Velde CJ (2007) Preoperative chemotherapy for women with operable breast cancer. Cochrane Database Syst Rev 2(18):CD005002
8. Cortazar PZL, Untch M et al (2014) Pathological complete response and long-term benefit in breast cancer: the CT NeoBC pooled analysis. Lancet 384:164–172
9. Mathew J, Asgeirsson KS, Cheung KL, Chan S, Dahda A, Robertson JF (2009) Neoadjuvant chemotherapy for locally advanced breast cancer: a review of the literature and future directions. Eur J Surg Oncol 35(2):113–122
10. Kaufmann M, von Minchkwitz G, Bear HD et al (2007) Recommendations from an international expert panel on the use of neoadjuvant (primary) systemic treatment of operable breast cancer: new perspectives 2006. Ann Oncol 18:1927–1934
11. Christy CJ, Thorsteinsson D, Grube BJ, Black D, Abu-Khalaf M, Chung GG, DiGiovanna MP, Miller K, Higgins SA, Weidhaas J et al (2009) Preoperative chemotherapy decreases the need for re-excision of breast cancers between 2 and 4 cm diameter. Ann Surg Oncol 16(3):697–702
12. Kümmel SHJ, Loibl S (2014) Surgical treatment of primary breast cancer in the neoadjuvant setting. Br J Surg 101(8):912–924
13. Freedman RA, Partridge A (2013) Management of breast cancer in very young women. Breast 22(Suppl 2):S:176–S:179
14. Guarneri VBK, Kau SW et al (2006) Prognostic value of pathologic complete response after primary chemotherapy in relation to hormone status and other factors. J Clin Oncol 24 (7):1037–1044
15. Cristofanilli M, Cristofanilli M, Gonzalez-Angulo A, Sneige N et al (2005) Invasive lobular carcinoma classic type: response to primary chemotherapy and survival outcomes. J Clin Oncol 23(1):41–48
16. Mathew JAK, Jackson LR, Cheung KL, Robertson JF (2009) Neoadjuvant endocrine treatment in primary breast cancer – review of literature. Breast 6(18):339–344
17. Charehbili A, Fontein D, Kroep JR, Liefers GJ, Mieog JS, Nortier JW, van de Velde CJ (2014) Neoadjuvant hormonal therapy for endocrine sensitive breast cancer: a systematic review. Cancer Treat Rev 1(40):86–92
18. Semiglazov VF, Semiglazov V, Dashyan GA et al (2007) Phase 2 randomized trial of primary endocrine therapy versus chemotherapy in postmenopausal patients with estrogen receptor-positive breast cancer. Cancer 2(110):244–254
19. Alba E, Calvo L, Albanell J, De la Haba JR, Arcusa Lanza A, Chacon JI, Sanchez-Rovira P, Plazaola A, Lopez Garcia-Asenjo JA, Bermejo B, Carrasco E, Lluch A, GEICAM (2012) Chemotherapy (CT) and hormonotherapy (HT) as neoadjuvant treatment in luminal breast

cancer patients: results from the GEICAM/2006-03, a multicenter, randomized, phase-II study. Ann Oncol 12(23):3069–3074

20. MCcCarty KS Jr, Silva J, Cox EB et al (1983) Relationship of age and menopausal status to estrogen receptor content in primary carcinoma of the breast. Ann Surg 197:123–127
21. Early breast cancer trialists collaborative group. 2000 analysis overview results. Fifth meeting of early breast cancer trialists collaborative group. Oxford, September 2000, pp 21–23
22. Mieog JS, van der Hage J, van de Velde CJ (2007) Neoadjuvant chemotherapy for operable breast cancer. Br J Surg 10(94):1189–1200
23. Milla-Santos A, Milla L, Calvo N, Portella J, Rallo L, Casanovas JM, Pons M, Rodes J (2004) Anastrozole as neoadjuvant therapy for patients with hormone-dependent, locally-advanced breast cancer. Anticancer Res 2C(24):1315–1318
24. Thomas JS, Julian H, Green RV, Cameron DA, Dixon MJ (2007) Histopathology of breast carcinoma following neoadjuvant systemic therapy: a common association between letrozole therapy and central scarring. Histopathology 2(51):219–226
25. Ellis MJ, Suman VJ, Hoog J, Lin L, Snider J, Prat A, Parker S, Luo J, DeSchryver K, Allred DC, Esserman LJ, Unzeitig GW, Margenthaler J, Babiera GV, Marcom PK, Guenther JM, Watson MA, Leitch M, Hunt K, Olson JA (2011) Randomized phase II neoadjuvant comparison between letrozole, anastrozole, and exemestane for postmenopausal women with estrogen receptor rich stage 2 to 3 breast cancer: clinical and biomarker outcomes and predictive value of the baseline PAM50-based intrinsic subtype—ACOSOG Z1031. J Clin Oncol 29(17):2342–2349
26. Segara DKI, Garber JE, Winer E, Harris L, Bellon JR, Birdwell R, Lester S, Lipsitz S, Iglehart J et al (2007) Does MRI predict pathologic tumor response in women with breast cancer undergoing preoperative chemotherapy? J Surg Oncol 96(6):474–480
27. Oh JL, Nguyen G, Whitman GJ, Hunt KK, Yu TK, Woodward WA, Tereffe W, Strom EA, Perkins GHBT (2007) Placement of radiopaque clips for tumor localization in patients undergoing neoadjuvant chemotherapy and breast conservation therapy. Cancer 110 (11):2420–2427
28. Boughey JC, Florentia Peintinger M M.D., Meric-Bernstam F M.D., Perry AC P.A-.C., Hunt KK M.D., Babiera V M.D., Singletary SE M.D., Bedrosian I M.D., Lucci A M.D., Buzdar AU M.D., Pusztai L M.D., Ph.D., Kuerer HM M., Ph.D. (2006) Impact of preoperative versus postoperative chemotherapy on the extent and number of surgical procedures in patients treated in randomized clinical trials for breast cancer. Ann Surg 244:464–470
29. Damera A, Evans A, Cornford EJ et al (2003) Diagnosis if axillary nodal metastasis by ultrasound guided core biopsy in primary operable breast cancer. Br J Cancer 89:1310–1313
30. Nason KS, Anderson B, Byrd DR, Dunnwald LK, Eary JF, Mankoff DA, Livingston R, Schmidt RA, Jewell K, Yeung RS et al (2000) Increased false negative sentinel node biopsy rates after preoperative chemotherapy for invasive breast carcinoma. Cancer 89 (11):2187–2194
31. Mamounas EP, Brown A, Anderson S, Smith R, Julian T, Miller B, Bear HD, Caldwell CB, Walker A, Mikkelson WM et al (2005) Sentinel node biopsy after neoadjuvant chemotherapy in breast cancer: results from National Surgical Adjuvant Breast and Bowel Project Protocol B-27. J Clin Oncol 23(12):2694–2702
32. Kuehn T, Bauerfeind I, Fehm T, Fleige B, Hausschild M, Helms G, Lebeau A, Liedtke C, von Minckwitz G, Nekljudova V, Schmatloch S, Schrenk P, Staebler A, Untch M (2013) Sentinel-lymph node biopsy in patients with breast cancer before and after neoadjuvant chemotherapy (SENTINA): a prospective, multicentre cohort study. Lancet Oncol 7:609–618
33. Krag DN, Anderson S, Julian TB, Brown AM, Harlow SP, Ashikaga T, Weaver DL, Miller BJJL, Frazier TG et al (2007) Technical outcomes of sentinel-lymph-node resection and conventional axillary-lymph-node dissection in patients with clinically node-negative breast cancer: results from the NSABP B-32 randomised phase III trial. Lancet Oncol 8(10):881–888
34. Goyal A, Newcombe R, Chhabra A, Mansel RE, ALMANAC Trialists Group (2006) Factors affecting failed localisation and false-negative rates of sentinel node biopsy in breast cancer – results of the ALMANAC validation phase. Breast Cancer Res Treat 99(2):203–208

35. Xing Y, Foy M, Cox DD, Kuerer HM, Hunt KK, Cormier JN (2006) Meta-analysis of sentinel lymph node biopsy after preoperative chemotherapy in patients with breast cancer. Br J Surg 5:539–543
36. van Deurzen CH, Vriens B, Tjan-Heijnen VC, van der Wall E, Albregts M, van Hilligersberg R, Monninkhof EM, van Diest PJ (2009) Accuracy of sentinel node biopsy after neoadjuvant chemotherapy in breast cancer patients: a systematic review. Eur J Cancer 18:3124–3130
37. Kelly AM, Dwamena B, Cronin P, Carlos RC (2009) Breast cancer sentinel node identification and classification after neoadjuvant chemotherapy-systematic review and meta-analysis. Acad Radiol 16:551–563
38. Tan VK, Goh B, Fook-Chong S, Khin LW, Wong WK, Yong WS (2011) The feasibility and accuracy of sentinel lymph node biopsy in clinically node-negative patients after neoadjuvant chemotherapy for breast cancer – a systematic review and meta-analysis. J Surg Oncol 1:97–103
39. Fu J-F, Chen H-L, Yang J, Yi C-H, Zheng S (2014) Feasibility and accuracy of sentinel lymph node biopsy in clinically node-positive breast cancer after neoadjuvant chemotherapy: a meta-analysis. PLoS One 9:e105316
40. Boughey JC M.D., Suman J Ph.D., Mittendorf EA M.D., Ph.D., Ahrendt GM M.D., Wilke LG M.D., Taback B M.D., Leitch AM M.D., Kuerer HM M.D., Ph.D., Bowling M M.D., Flippo-Morton TS M.D., Byrd R M.D., Ollila DW M.D., Julian TB M.D., McLaughlin SA M.D., McCall L M.S., Symmans WF M.D., Le-Petross HT M.D., Haffty BG M.D., Buchholz TA M. D., Nelson H Md., Hunt KK M.D., for the Alliance for Clinical, Oncology Ti (2013) Sentinel lymph node surgery after neoadjuvant chemotherapy in patients with node-positive breast cancer the ACOSOG Z1071 (alliance) clinical trial. JAMA 14:1455–1461
41. Boileau JF, Poirier B, Basik M, Holloway CM, Gaboury L, Sideris L, Meterissian S, Arnaout A, Brackstone M, McCready DR, Karp SE, Trop I, Lisbona A, Wright FC, Younan RJ, Provencher L, Patocskai E, Omeroglu A, Robidoux A (2015) Sentinel node biopsy after neoadjuvant chemotherapy in biopsy-proven node-positive breast cancer: the SNFNAC study. J Clin Oncol 3:258–264
42. Kang SHKJ, Choi EA, Lee ES (2004) Sentinel lymph node biopsy after neoadjuvant chemotherapy. Breast Cancer 11(3):233–241
43. Veronesi PGO, Fernandez JR, Magnoni F (2009) Breast conservation and sentinel lymph node biopsy after neoadjuvant systemic therapy. Breast 18(3):S90–S92
44. Alvarado R et al (2012) The role for sentinel lymph node dissection after neoadjuvant chemotherapy in patients who present with node-positive breast cancer. Ann Surg Oncol 19:3177–3184
45. Dominici S et al (2010) Cytologically proven axillary lymph node metastases are eradicated in patients receiving preoperative chemotherapy with concurrent trastuzumab for HER2-positive breast cancer. Cancer 116:284–289
46. van der Hage JA, van de Velde C, Julien JP, Tubiana-Hulin M, Vandervelden C, Duchateau L (2001) Preoperative chemotherapy in primary operable breast cancer: results from the European Organization for Research and Treatment of Cancer trial 10902. J Clin Oncol 22:4224–4237
47. Clough KB, Ihrai T, Oden S, Kaufman G, Massey E, Nos C (2012) Oncoplastic surgery for breast cancer based on tumour location and a quadrant-per-quadrant atlas. Br J Surg 99 (10):1389–1395
48. Clough KB, Soussaline M, Campana F, Salmon RJ (1990) Mammoplasty combined with irradiation: conservative treatment of cancers located in the lower quadrants. Ann Chir Plast Esthet 35(2):117–122
49. Spear SL, Pelletiere C, Wolfe AJ et al (2002) Experience with reduction mammoplasty combined with breast conservation therapy in the treatment of breast cancer. Plast Reconstr Surg 111(3):1102–1109

50. Petit JY, Rietjens M, Garusi C et al (1998) Integration of plastic surgery in the course of breast-conserving surgery for cancer to improve results and radicality of tumor excision. Recent Results Cancer Res 152:202–211
51. Cothier-Savey I, Otmezguine Y, Calitchi E et al (1996) Value of reduction mammoplasty in the conservative treatment of breast neoplasm. A propos of 70 cases. Ann Chir Plast Esthet 41 (4):346–353
52. Mazouni C, Naveau A, Kane A, Dunant A, Garbay JR, Leymarie N, Sarfati B, Delaloge S, Rimareix F (2013) The role of oncoplastic breast surgery in the management of breast cancer treated with primary chemotherapy. Breast 22(6):1189–1193
53. Schaverien MV, Doughty J, Stallard S (2014) Quality of information reporting in studies of standard and oncoplastic breast conserving surgery. Breast 23(2):104–111
54. Yang JD, Lee JW, Cho YK, Kim WW, Hwang SO, Jung JH, Park HY (2012) Surgical techniques for personalized oncoplastic surgery in breast cancer patients with small- to moderate-sized breasts (part 1): volume displacement. J Breast Cancer 15(1):1–6
55. Bulstrode NW, Shrotria S (2001) Prediction of cosmetic outcome following breast conservation surgery using breast volume measurements. Breast 10:124–126
56. Kaur N, Petit J, Rietjens M et al (2005) Comparative study of surgical margins in oncoplastic surgery and quadrantectomy in breast cancer. Ann Surg Oncol 12(7):539–545
57. McCulley SJ, Macmillan R (2005) Therapeutic mammaplasty: analysis of 50 consecutive cases. Br J Plast Surg 58(7):902–907
58. McCulley SJ, Macmillan RD (2005) Planning and use of therapeutic mammoplasty – Nottingham approach. Br J Plast Surg 58:889–901
59. Benelli L (1990) A new periareolar mammaplasty: the "round block" technique. Aesthet Plast Surg 14(2):93–100
60. Gasperoni C, Salgarello M, Gasperoni P (2002) A personal technique: mammaplasty with J scar. Ann Plast Surg 48(2):124–130
61. Anderson BO, Masetti R, Silverstein MJ (2005) Oncoplastic approaches to partial mastectomy: an overview of volume-displacement techniques. Lancet Oncol 6:145–157
62. McCulley SJ, Durani P, Macmillan RD (2006) Therapeutic mammoplasty for centrally located breast tumours. Plast Reconstr Surg 117(2):366–373
63. Hamdi M, Van Landuyt K, Monstrey S et al (2004) Pedicled perforator flaps in breast reconstruction: a new concept. Br J Plast Surg 57:531–539
64. Hamdi M, Van Landuyt K, Blondeel P, Hijjawi B, Roche N, Monstrey S (2009) Autologous breast augmentation with the lateral intercostal artery perforator flap in massive weight loss patients. J Plast Reconstr Aesthet Surg 62:65–70
65. Bank J, Ledbetter K, Song DH (2014) Use of thoracodorsal artery perforator flaps to enhance outcomes in alloplastic breast reconstruction. Plast Reconstr Surg Glob Open 2(5):e140

Chapter 18
Imaging of Tumor Response by Preoperative Systemic Treatment

Shotaro Kanao and Masako Kataoka

Abstract In this chapter, imaging in evaluating treatment response of breast cancer by PST is reviewed. The advantage and disadvantage of imaging modalities including MMG, US, and MRI are compared. The main focus is the role of MRI in evaluating residual tumor and identifying pCR after NAC, since MRI is the most reliable and objective imaging tool. Technical aspect of MR scanner and DCE-MRI protocol is mentioned. RECIST-based measurement is the standard method of evaluation but is of limited value influenced by different morphology and different shrinkage pattern (concentric or dendritic). MR volumetry can be used as a more objective and accurate measurement tool. Variation of tumor response pattern with different therapeutic agents (e.g., taxane containing) may need to be considered in evaluating tumor response. Other emerging MRI techniques include DW-MRI as a non-contrast-enhanced imaging. Finally, FDG-PET is attracting attention as a functional imaging due to its promising results in response prediction.

Keywords FDG-PET • DCE-MRI • Neoadjuvant chemotherapy • MR volumetry • pCR

18.1 Tumor Response of Preoperative Systemic Treatment (PST) by Clinical Examination and Imaging Modalities

The aim of the preoperative systemic treatment (PST) is to evaluate treatment response of the primary tumor and potentially increase the chance of breast-conserving surgery. Preoperative systemic treatment (PST) was defined as a systemic therapy initiated before the locoregional treatment such as chemotherapy (NAC) or hormonal therapy (NAE). Initially, the treatment was offered to inoperable patients for reducing the tumor size and achieving secondary conserving surgery. Then, in the late 1990s, evidences came from NSABP B-18 trial showing

S. Kanao • M. Kataoka (✉)
Department of Radiology, Kyoto University Hospital, 54 Shogoin-kawaharacho, Sakyo-ku, Kyoto 606-8507, Japan
e-mail: makok@kuhp.kyoto-u.ac.jp

M. Toi et al. (eds.), *Personalized Treatment of Breast Cancer*,
DOI 10.1007/978-4-431-55552-0_18

that preoperative therapy is equivalent to adjuvant therapy [1–3]. Since then, preoperative neoadjuvant chemotherapy (NAC) has gradually become a treatment of choice for many more patients with locally advanced breast cancer, particularly for those who have tumors too large for breast-conserving surgery. Another potential advantage of preoperative systemic treatment is that pathological response of primary breast cancers to the neoadjuvant chemotherapy is a surrogate marker for patient outcome [2, 4].

Response evaluation criteria in solid tumors (RECIST) are the guideline of clinical evaluation of cancer therapeutics and first published in 2000. The principle of RECIST is simple: first, define the measurable target lesion at baseline; second, follow the sum of longest diameter (in case of lymph node, short axes); and third, evaluate the overall response of treatment by change of the diameter and additional findings. Complete response (CR) is complete vanishing of the tumor. Partial response (PR) is decrease of the sum of the longest diameter by more than 30 %. Stable disease (SD) is the sum of the longest diameter between −30 % and +20 %. Progressive disease (PD) is an increase of this sum by more than 20 %. Development of a new lesion is also regarded as PD [5]. The evaluation using RECIST plays an important role in treatment planning, particularly in response-guided approach [6].

Clinical (physical) examination is the basic and the most convenient method for assessing tumor response to PST. This simple method, however, is often unsatisfactory for the assessment of the tumor response. Nowadays, tumor response after PST is evaluated using various imaging modalities including mammography (MMG), ultrasonography (US), and magnetic resonance imaging (MRI) because these methods are more objective, accurate, and with better agreement with pathological assessment of the residual tumor after surgery. MMG, US, and MRI are morphology-based imaging modalities used for monitoring treatment response. In evaluating tumor response using these morphology-based methods, RECIST can be used as in clinical evaluation; the longest diameter of the target lesions is measured and summed up to assess the changes after treatment. There are advantages and disadvantages for each modality. MMG is the standard imaging for diagnosing breast disease and most easily available, yet it tended to underestimate residual tumor [7]. US is more accurate than MMG in assessing pathological response and easily performed in a ward or clinic. Drawbacks of US include operator dependency. Despite relatively higher cost and limited accessibility, MRI with the use of dynamic contrast enhancement (DCE-MRI) is becoming more popular in clinical setting. This modality demonstrated best correlation with pathology [7]. Objectiveness is another advantage of using MRI. Additional advantage of DCE-MRI includes obtaining anatomical information and vascular (functional) information together. Currently, DCE-MRI is becoming the standard imaging modality of choice in evaluating PST [8, 9], and many more clinical trials adopt DCE-MRI as a part of their protocol. On the other hand, nuclear imaging, particularly FDG-PET, is actively investigated as a potential tool in monitoring tumor response to PST in addition to response prediction at an early stage of the treatment [10, 11]. In RECIST 1.1 (the latest version), FDG-PET findings can be used as an evidence of new lesion (PD) [5] [Table 18.1].

Table 18.1 Comparison of clinical examination and imaging modalities in evaluating tumor response by PST

	Accuracy (size)	Vascularity evaluation	Cost	Accessibility
Clinical examination	△	x	Low	Easy
MMG	△	x	Medium	Easy
US	○	△	Medium	Easy
MRI	○	○	High	Limited
FDG-PET	–*	x	High	Limited

*metabolic activity is evaluated.

In this chapter, conventional morphology-based imaging including MMG and US is summarized. In the main part of the chapter, the role of MRI in monitoring tumor response is discussed. Problems and challenges in the current DCE-MRI techniques and emerging issues by new treatment regimen [12] are also mentioned. Recent evidences from major trials including ACRIN-6657/I-SPY trial [3, 13, 14] are reviewed.

18.2 Evaluation of Tumor Response by MMG and US

Measurement of tumor size using MMG may be difficult if (1) the lesion has ill-defined margin, (2) the lesion is not mass forming, or (3) the breast is composed of dense tissues. Measurement of the tumor diameter itself can be difficult if associated with ill-defined or spiculated margin. In addition, interpretation of calcification becomes more complicated; microcalcification may remain even with complete response [15], and new calcification may emerge during treatment. The reliability of mammography in evaluating tumor response depends on the degree of delineation from the surrounding breast tissue. If the margin of the tumor is definable in more than 50 % of the lesion, then the diameter of the tumor on mammography will show relatively good correlations ($r = 0.77$) with that on histopathology [16].

Compared to mammography, ultrasonography is more accurate in evaluating treatment response of breast cancer. Keune et al. retrospectively reviewed 104 primary breast cancers with neoadjuvant chemotherapy (NAC) and compared residual tumor size measured by ultrasound and mammography, using size on surgical pathology as a reference. Tumor size measured on ultrasound was accurate (within 1 cm) in 60 % of cases, while that measured on mammography was accurate in only 32 % of cases [17]. After NAC, nearly half (50/104) of the tumor became unable to be sized on mammography. A recent study on triple-negative breast cancer (TNBC) demonstrated that ultrasonography was more accurate than mammography and equivalent to MRI in evaluating residual tumor size following NAC. Accuracy to within 1 cm was the higher in US (83 %) and MRI (78 %) than in MMG (56 %) [18]. Breast tumors are often easier to delineate on US than on MMG. In a meta-analysis, US showed comparable degree of agreement to that of MRI [9]. Another potential advantage of US is evaluation of vascularity using Doppler function, although it is not quantitative. Practical benefit of US as evaluation of treatment response is that US examination can be combined with US-guided biopsy, if midcourse tissue sampling is necessary. Weaknesses of US as a tool in evaluating treatment response are operator dependency and reproducibility of measurement.

18.3 Evaluation of Tumor Response by MRI

18.3.1 Background

As stated in introduction, The primary aim of imaging during and after neoadjuvant therapy is to document and quantify tumor response, based on RECIST. The second and more interesting aim is to predict the pathological response early after the initiation of treatment, before the final morphological changes become evident. Dynamic contrast-enhanced MRI (DCE-MRI) has been shown to be superior to evaluate tumor diameter after PST compared to clinical examination and mammography, when pathological residual tumor was used as a reference standard. Ultrasound may be as accurate as DCE-MRI in assessing tumor response [18, 19]. However, MRI consistently demonstrated good agreement with pathological response evaluations [7] and is regarded as a more objective and reproducible imaging tool. As a result, DCE-MRI is often the imaging investigation of choice. If PST is given to a patient, the first breast MRI should be performed before the start of chemotherapy. A second MRI, for the evaluation of the effect of chemotherapy on the tumor, should be performed when approximately half of the course of chemotherapy has been administered. A third MRI investigation should be performed after the final course of chemotherapy to evaluate the residual disease. In clinical or trial setting, it would be recommended to schedule tissue sampling after MRI; incidental post-biopsy changes such as local hemorrhage may cause artifactual enhancement or mass effect and thus prevent accurate assessment of tumor response.

18.3.2 Technical Aspect of MRI

Technical advances in MRI in the last 10 years had an impact of the use of breast MRI. Introduction of a high-field magnet scanner into clinical practice, and shifting toward 1.5 tesla or even to 3.0 tesla, led to the improvement in signal-to-noise ratio. Development of a multichannel coil dedicated to breast MRI helped in shortening of image acquisition time and better image quality. In our institution, for example, hardware was renewed from a 1.5 tesla scanner with a two-channel dedicated breast coil in 2008 to a 3.0 tesla scanner with an 18-channel coil today. High-field-strength scanners have potential advantages related to the increased spatial and temporal resolution such as an increase in the signal-to-noise ratio by doubling of SNR at 3.0 T compared with 1.5 T.

Table 18.2 Breast MRI patient handling and sequences recommended by EUSOBI guidelines

	Comments
Coil	Dedicated bilateral breast coil
Position	Prone
T2-weighted image	For evaluating water-containing lesions, cysts/edema
T1-weighted image	Pre-contrast image
Post-contrast DCE early phase	Obtained within the first 2 min to capture peak enhancement of cancer
Post-contrast DCE delayed phase	At least one in delayed phase (three time points) to evaluate whether the lesion continues or enhances or shows a plateau or early washout
Pixel size	At least 1×1 mm (in plane resolution ≤ 1 mm), slice thickness <2.5 mm, in order to detect all lesions equal or over 5 mm

Significant improvement was reported in differential diagnosis of enhancing breast lesions at 3.0 T compared with 1.5 T in the same patients. In the context of tumor response evaluation, these technical advancements contributed to more accurate delineation of tumor, identification of small malignant lesion, small residual lesions that might have been missed with lower spatial resolution, discrimination with nonspecific background, or benign enhancing lesions. Update of softwares was also valuable in tumor evaluation. The technique of fat suppression becomes sophisticated. Parallel imaging technique also helps to speed up the image acquisition process. Breast MRI protocol should follow the EUSOBI guidelines in order to obtain images with sufficient quality to diagnose and evaluate breast lesions [20] [Table 18.2].

18.3.3 Evaluation of Residual Tumor

Many studies have demonstrated that residual tumor size measured on MRI after NAC correlates well with residual tumor size at pathology. A meta-analysis of 19 studies revealed that residual tumor size on MRI and US agrees with that at pathology, with a mean difference of 0.1 cm (slight overestimation) for both modalities, while clinical examination tended to underestimate with a mean difference of −0.3 cm. It should be noted, however, that even MRI is liable to under- or overestimation [9]. When differences of within 30 % were defined as equal, the size of residual tumor on MRI agreed with that of pathology in 71 %, better than clinical examination, mammography, and US. They discussed that causes of overestimation by MRI may be increased vascularity by taxane, chemotherapy-induced fibrosis, or reactive inflammation by tumor response and healing. On the other hand, possible reasons for underestimation included very small (<0.1 cm) foci of cancer and cancers with lobular features [7]. MRI seems unable to detect small residual tumor foci that may persist after neoadjuvant chemotherapy. It should be noted as the patient may wish to have breast-conserving surgery after a near complete response.

As pathological complete response (pCR) is a surrogate marker of long-term survival, identification of cases achieving pCR is important. In a meta-analysis, overall area under the curve (AUC) of MRI was 0.88. Specificity was higher with negative MRI defined as contrast enhancement less than or equal to normal tissue (0.83). Radiological complete response is not the pathological complete response (pCR) even with the use of MRI.

Morphological characteristics of the initial and/or treated tumor may have an impact on accuracy in treatment response. Under treatment, two types of tumor shrinkage have been described on MR images: a concentric one that selects good candidates for breast-conserving surgery and a dendritic type that indicates a high risk of positive margins after a lumpectomy [21] (Fig. 18.1). Our analysis including

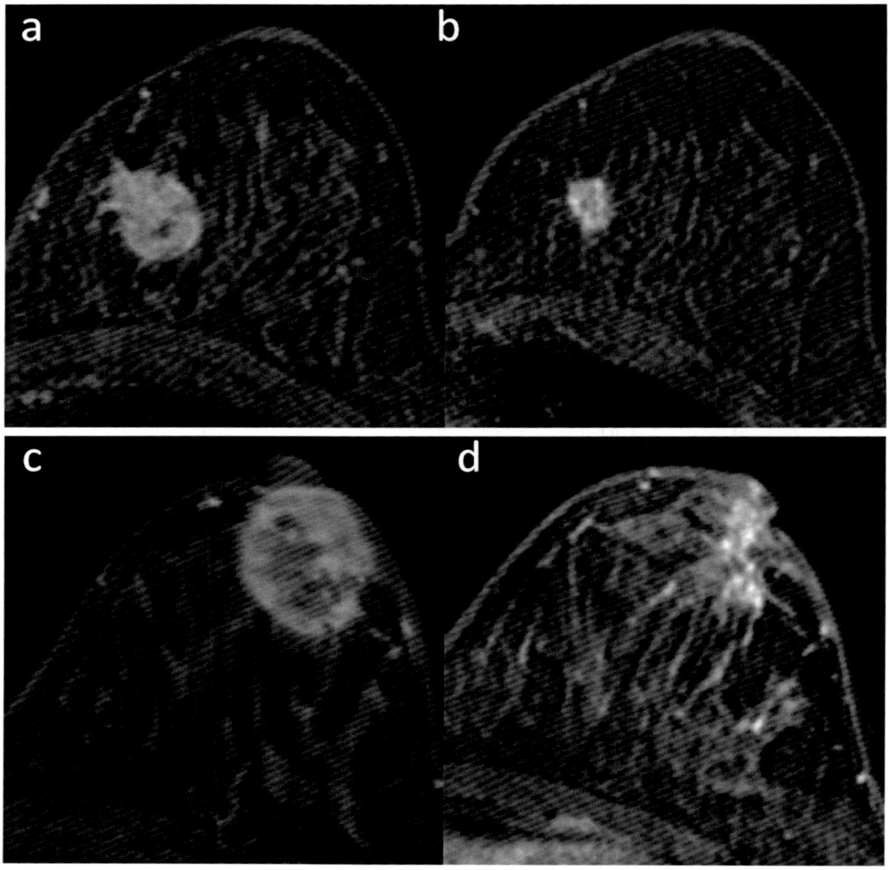

Fig. 18.1 Representative image of concentric shrinkage (CS) and dendritic shrinkage (DS). *Upper row* images are DCE-MRI of breast cancer before (**a**) and after (**b**) PST showing a concentric shrinkage. *Oval-shaped* mass kept its shape but diminished in size. Patients with this pattern of shrinkage are good candidates for breast-conserving surgery. *Lower row* images are DCE-MRI of breast cancer before (**c**) and after (**d**) PST showing a dendritic shrinkage. The *round* mass shrank to small and spiculated mass, almost non-mass enhancement. This type of shrinkage indicates a high risk of positive margins after a lumpectomy

both NAC and NAE patients showed that dendritic shrinkage was associated with underestimation when compared to surgical specimen [22]. Underestimation occurs frequently and has been reported in patients with residual in situ components and residues of invasive carcinomas (multifocal or diffuse initial disease presentation, dendritic shrinkage pattern, absent or low enhancement, patchy mild enhancement); overestimation also has been described and was related to induced fibrosis and resorptive inflammation. Residual disease tended to be underestimated in case of lesions presenting as non-mass enhancement. Another data came from the American College of Radiology Imaging Network (ACRIN) 6657 trial – a prospective study to test MRI for its ability to predict response to treatment and to stratify the risk of recurrence in patients with stage II or III breast cancer receiving NAC. Data of 174 women demonstrated that concordance between MRI-based tumor size and tumor size on surgical pathology was higher in well-defined tumors, especially with those with a triple-negative subtype [14].

Volumetry can help in reducing the influence of tumor morphology in evaluating tumor response. Since the DCE-MRI data are obtained as three-dimensional (3D) data, 3D volumetry is considered to be more accurate in estimating tumor burden and thus treatment response. With the use of sophisticated software, 3D volume data can be measured relatively easily. Early change of MR tumor volume was significantly correlated with the final MRI volume change and more predictive of recurrence-free survival than tumor diameter. Volumetric changes measured using MRI may provide a more sensitive assessment of treatment efficacy [23] (Fig. 18.2). Because MRI can easily handle 3D digital data, volumetry combined with enhancement kinetic information is also possible. Computer-aided detection-generated tumor volume can provide total enhancing volumes and washout volumes, i.e., enhanced areas with more than 100 % signal increase on early DCE and signal reduction by 10 % or more on delayed DCE phase. This CAD-generated volume had significantly higher interobserver concordance than conventional RECIST-based longest diameter measurement. Washout volume measurement after the completion chemotherapy is significantly better in differentiating pCR and non-pCR patients [24].

Finally, treatment regimen can have an impact on evaluation of residual tumor. Some studies suggested that the type of chemotherapy agent should be taken into account when using MRI for evaluating the tumor response. Residual disease was frequently underestimated in patients treated with taxane-containing regimens and in HER-2-negative patients treated with bevacizumab. A recent study investigating the influence of taxanes on response assessment of DCE-MRI demonstrated that an almost complete suppression of contrast enhancement occurred in cancers, benign enhancing lesions, and normal fibroglandular tissue after taxane-containing chemotherapy, while lower reduction of enhancement was observed after non-taxane-containing chemotherapy [12]. Conventional RECIST criteria may not be appropriate for immunotherapeutic agents as response is observed after initial apparent PD, leading to the development of immune-related response criteria [25, 26].

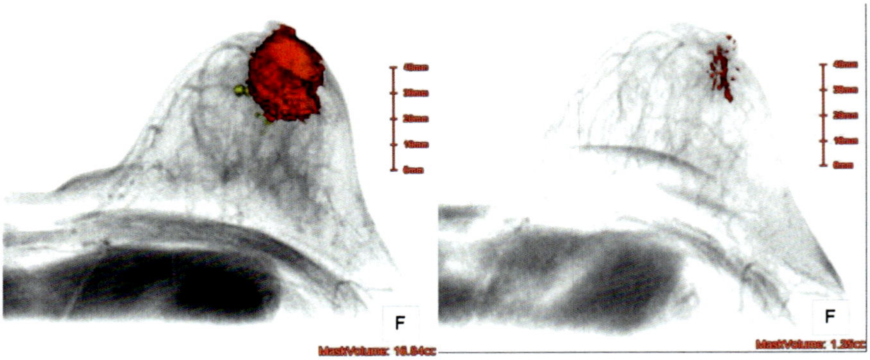

	Pre treatment	After treatment	
Diameter	42mm	34mm (-21%)	SD (<30%)
Volume	16.84cc	1.28cc (-94%)	PR (>65%)

Fig. 18.2 3D volumetry and volume rendering image in evaluating tumor response. 3D volume image is created from DCR-MRI of the case in Fig. 18.1c, d. The longest diameter changes from 42 to 34 mm. According to the RECIST criteria, the therapeutic effect is SD. Volume changes from 16 to 1 cc. According to the modified RECIST criteria, the therapeutic effect is PR (more than 65% decrease in volume)

18.3.4 Prediction of Treatment Response

Another aim of MR imaging is to find parameters that could predict the pathological response at surgery. At this time, the most relevant ones are morphological changes under treatment. Multivariate analysis revealed that a >65 % reduction in the tumor volume after two cycles of chemotherapy was associated with a major histopathological response (small cluster of dispersed residual cancer cells or no residual viable cancer cell) at surgery [27]. Cheung et al. evaluated MRI in 33 patients with locally advanced breast cancers (one study before treatment, one after one course of chemotherapy, and one before surgery). Twelve of the 23 responders (complete and partial response) had reached the criteria for partial response (greater than or equal to 30 % size reduction; RECIST criteria) after the first course of chemotherapy; all complete responses had a marked early size reduction of more than 45 % [28]. The most solid evidence comes from the recent data of 216 women from the ACRIN 6657 trial. In their analysis, MRI size measurements were superior to clinical examination at all time points. Tumor volume change showed the greatest benefit at MRI after one cycle of anthracycline-based treatment; AUC is better than other measurements including the longest diameter, signal enhancement ratio, and clinical examination [3]. Prediction of tumor response using pharmacokinetic parameters including K^{trans} and Kep has been investigated with mixed results [29, 30].

18.3.5 *Diffusion-Weighted Imaging and Other MR-Related Topics*

In addition to DCE-MRI, diffusion-weighted imaging (DW-MRI) is an emerging new method of evaluating breast cancer. Diffusion-weighted MR imaging uses motion-sensitizing gradients to measure the mobility of water in tissue and therefore can assess the cellular density of the tissue. This sequence is the most sensitive non-contrast MR imaging, and many institutions use DW-MRI as a routine clinical practice. Some researchers reported usefulness of DW-MRI in NAC setting. At least DW-MRI can delineate tumors without using a contrast agent [31]. Changes of apparent diffusion coefficient (ADC) may be observed earlier than tumor size or vascularity during treatment due to tumor cell death and necrosis and may be valuable early indicators of treatment efficacy. Proton MR spectroscopy had reported some favorable results which are yet to be established.

18.3.6 *Evaluation of NAE by MRI*

Endocrine (NAE) treatment is recently used as a treatment of hormone receptor-positive large or aggressive tumor. Tumor extent evaluated by MRI in the neoadjuvant endocrine (NAE) treatment setting is in good correlation with pathology. Although some researchers reported that the underestimation of lesion size in luminal-type breast cancer is worse than that of non-luminal-type cancer, we reported that the underestimation was affected more by the pattern of shrinkage (i.e., concentric versus dendritic) than the choice of treatment [22]. Another important feature of NAE is that the pCR rate is lower than that in NAC. Evaluation of accurate partial response and residual tumor extent is important because of low pCR rate. At the moment, evidence on imaging evaluation for NAE is limited.

18.4 Evaluation and Prediction of Tumor Response by FDG-PET

Nuclear medicine is different from other imaging modalities discussed above in reflecting the metabolic/functional aspect of the disease. Breast scintigraphy using 99mTc-sestamibi has been investigated and may be preferred to evaluate breast cancer treatment response due to lower cost [32]. However, positron emission tomography (PET) using ^{18}F-fluorodeoxyglucose (FDG) is becoming more commonly used. Wider use of FDG-PET/CT enabled more accurate detection of the tumor.

^{18}F-FDG consists of ^{18}F as a positron-emitting radionuclide and FDG that is taken into the cells by glucose transporters. Cancer cells generally overexpress glucose transporters and therefore uptake ^{18}F-FDG. In contrast to morphological imaging using diameter or 3D volume, ^{18}F-FDG-PET quantifies tracer uptake in tumor. Standard uptake value (SUV), calculated value to show FDG uptake within a volume of interest, is used as an index to measure tumor metabolic function [11]. Therefore, it should be emphasized that FDG-PET evaluates the functional aspect of tumor different from the morphological aspect used by other imaging modalities, and therefore it is possible that "responses" in these two aspects may disagree.

One of the main purposes of FDG-PET post-PST in breast cancer is to identify cases achieving pCR. Many studies examine the value of FDG-PET after the completion of chemotherapy and demonstrated that residual FDG uptake predicts residual disease. On the contrary, absence of FDG uptake does not mean pCR [33–36]. These results can be influenced by several factors. Difference in threshold SUV can affect the final judgment of positive/negative FDG uptake [37]. Certain types of breast cancer, including luminal A subtype or ductal carcinoma in situ (DCIS), are known to have low SUV. Smaller uptake cannot be identified due to limited spatial resolution. The recently developed breast PET scanner dedicated to breast scan may overcome these limitations [38, 39].

Prediction of tumor response earlier in the course of treatment is another interest. Studies evaluating FDG-PET mid-therapy or early (i.e., after a single cycle) in the therapy suggested that changes in FDG uptake from the baseline scan are a good predictor to identify responder and nonresponders. Decrease of SUV in 50 % or more at mid-therapy suggested good response and lesser reduction indicated poor response [10, 33]. Research on tumor response prediction early in the treatment has shown promising results. Initially Wahl et al. reported rapid decrease of uptake in responders as early as day 8 and no reduction in nonresponders, while tumor diameter showed no significant change [40]. Similar results were reported from other groups [41, 42].

Some researchers are interested in predicting mid- or long-term survival of the patients using FDG uptake. Small study of 40 patients (all but one patient had FDG-avid tumor) by Emmering et al. demonstrated that FDG uptake in the primary tumor was inversely associated with disease-free survival [43]. With these results, new response assessment criteria using PET (PERCIST) have been advocated [44]. Yet, evidence was still limited to understand the significance of FDG uptake in tumor response and, more importantly, patient survival.

Acknowledgments We appreciate Dr. Yuji Nakamoto, Kyoto University, for his constructive comments and advice regarding FDG-PET.

References

1. Fisher B, Costantino JP, Wickerham DL, Redmond CK, Kavanah M, Cronin WM, Vogel V, Robidoux A, Dimitrov N, Atkins J, Daly M, Wieand S, Tan-Chiu E, Ford L, Wolmark N (1998) Tamoxifen for prevention of breast cancer: report of the National Surgical Adjuvant Breast and Bowel Project P-1 Study. J Natl Cancer Inst 90(18):1371–1388
2. Wolmark N, Wang J, Mamounas E, Bryant J, Fisher B (2001) Preoperative chemotherapy in patients with operable breast cancer: nine-year results from National Surgical Adjuvant Breast and Bowel Project B-18. J Natl Cancer Inst Monogr 30:96–102
3. Hylton NM, Blume JD, Bernreuter WK, Pisano ED, Rosen MA, Morris EA, Weatherall PT, Lehman CD, Newstead GM, Polin S, Marques HS, Esserman LJ, Schnall MD, Team AT, Investigators IST (2012) Locally advanced breast cancer: MR imaging for prediction of response to neoadjuvant chemotherapy – results from ACRIN 6657/I-SPY TRIAL. Radiology 263(3):663–672. doi:10.1148/radiol.12110748
4. Rastogi P, Anderson SJ, Bear HD, Geyer CE, Kahlenberg MS, Robidoux A, Margolese RG, Hoehn JL, Vogel VG, Dakhil SR, Tamkus D, King KM, Pajon ER, Wright MJ, Robert J, Paik S, Mamounas EP, Wolmark N (2008) Preoperative chemotherapy: updates of National Surgical Adjuvant Breast and Bowel Project Protocols B-18 and B-27. J Clin Oncol 26 (5):778–785. doi:10.1200/JCO.2007.15.0235
5. Eisenhauer EA, Therasse P, Bogaerts J, Schwartz LH, Sargent D, Ford R, Dancey J, Arbuck S, Gwyther S, Mooney M, Rubinstein L, Shankar L, Dodd L, Kaplan R, Lacombe D, Verweij J (2009) New response evaluation criteria in solid tumours: revised RECIST guideline (version 1.1). Eur J Cancer 45(2):228–247. doi:10.1016/j.ejca.2008.10.026
6. von Minckwitz G, Blohmer JU, Costa SD, Denkert C, Eidtmann H, Eiermann W, Gerber B, Hanusch C, Hilfrich J, Huober J, Jackisch C, Kaufmann M, Kummel S, Paepke S, Schneeweiss A, Untch M, Zahm DM, Mehta K, Loibl S (2013) Response-guided neoadjuvant chemotherapy for breast cancer. J Clin Oncol 31(29):3623–3630. doi:10.1200/JCO.2012.45.0940
7. Yeh E, Slanetz P, Kopans DB, Rafferty E, Georgian-Smith D, Moy L, Halpern E, Moore R, Kuter I, Taghian A (2005) Prospective comparison of mammography, sonography, and MRI in patients undergoing neoadjuvant chemotherapy for palpable breast cancer. AJR Am J Roentgenol 184(3):868–877. doi:10.2214/ajr.184.3.01840868
8. Marinovich ML, Houssami N, Macaskill P, Sardanelli F, Irwig L, Mamounas EP, von Minckwitz G, Brennan ME, Ciatto S (2013) Meta-analysis of magnetic resonance imaging in detecting residual breast cancer after neoadjuvant therapy. J Natl Cancer Inst 105 (5):321–333. doi:10.1093/jnci/djs528
9. Marinovich ML, Macaskill P, Irwig L, Sardanelli F, von Minckwitz G, Mamounas E, Brennan M, Ciatto S, Houssami N (2013) Meta-analysis of agreement between MRI and pathologic breast tumour size after neoadjuvant chemotherapy. Br J Cancer 109 (6):1528–1536. doi:10.1038/bjc.2013.473
10. Rosen EL, Eubank WB, Mankoff DA (2007) FDG PET, PET/CT, and breast cancer imaging. Radiographics 27(Suppl 1):S215–S229. doi:10.1148/rg.27si075517
11. Groheux D, Espie M, Giacchetti S, Hindie E (2013) Performance of FDG PET/CT in the clinical management of breast cancer. Radiology 266(2):388–405. doi:10.1148/radiol.12110853
12. Schrading S, Kuhl CK (2015) Breast cancer: influence of taxanes on response assessment with dynamic contrast-enhanced MR imaging. Radiology 150006. doi:10.1148/radiol.2015150006
13. Cureton EL, Yau C, Alvarado MD, Krontiras H, Ollila DW, Ewing CA, Monnier S, Esserman LJ (2014) Local recurrence rates are low in high-risk neoadjuvant breast cancer in the I-SPY 1 Trial (CALGB 150007/150012; ACRIN 6657). Ann Surg Oncol 21(9):2889–2896. doi:10.1245/s10434-014-3721-7
14. Mukhtar RA, Yau C, Rosen M, Tandon VJ, I-Spy T, Investigators A, Hylton N, Esserman LJ (2013) Clinically meaningful tumor reduction rates vary by prechemotherapy MRI phenotype

and tumor subtype in the I-SPY 1 TRIAL (CALGB 150007/150012; ACRIN 6657). Ann Surg Oncol 20(12):3823–3830. doi:10.1245/s10434-013-3038-y
15. Li JJ, Chen C, Gu Y, Di G, Wu J, Liu G, Shao Z (2014) The role of mammographic calcification in the neoadjuvant therapy of breast cancer imaging evaluation. PLoS One 9(2): e88853. doi:10.1371/journal.pone.0088853
16. Huber S, Wagner M, Zuna I, Medl M, Czembirek H, Delorme S (2000) Locally advanced breast carcinoma: evaluation of mammography in the prediction of residual disease after induction chemotherapy. Anticancer Res 20(1B):553–558
17. Keune JD, Jeffe DB, Schootman M, Hoffman A, Gillanders WE, Aft RL (2010) Accuracy of ultrasonography and mammography in predicting pathologic response after neoadjuvant chemotherapy for breast cancer. Am J Surg 199(4):477–484. doi:10.1016/j.amjsurg.2009.03.012
18. Atkins JJ, Appleton CM, Fisher CS, Gao F, Margenthaler JA (2013) Which imaging modality is superior for prediction of response to neoadjuvant chemotherapy in patients with triple negative breast cancer? J Oncol 2013:964863. doi:10.1155/2013/964863
19. Marinovich ML, Houssami N, Macaskill P, von Minckwitz G, Blohmer JU, Irwig L (2015) Accuracy of ultrasound for predicting pathologic response during neoadjuvant therapy for breast cancer. Int J Cancer 136(11):2730–2737. doi:10.1002/ijc.29323
20. Mann RM, Kuhl CK, Kinkel K, Boetes C (2008) Breast MRI: guidelines from the European Society of Breast Imaging. Eur Radiol 18(7):1307–1318. doi:10.1007/s00330-008-0863-7
21. Tozaki M, Kobayashi T, Uno S, Aiba K, Takeyama H, Shioya H, Tabei I, Toriumi Y, Suzuki M, Fukuda K (2006) Breast-conserving surgery after chemotherapy: value of MDCT for determining tumor distribution and shrinkage pattern. AJR Am J Roentgenol 186 (2):431–439. doi:10.2214/AJR.06.0317
22. Takeda K, Kanao S, Okada T, Ueno T, Toi M, Ishiguro H, Mikami Y, Tanaka S, Togashi K (2012) MRI evaluation of residual tumor size after neoadjuvant endocrine therapy vs. neoadjuvant chemotherapy. Eur J Radiol 81(9):2148–2153. doi:10.1016/j.ejrad.2011.05.013
23. Partridge SC, Gibbs JE, Lu Y, Esserman LJ, Tripathy D, Wolverton DS, Rugo HS, Hwang ES, Ewing CA, Hylton NM (2005) MRI measurements of breast tumor volume predict response to neoadjuvant chemotherapy and recurrence-free survival. AJR Am J Roentgenol 184 (6):1774–1781. doi:10.2214/ajr.184.6.01841774
24. Takeda K, Kanao S, Okada T, Kataoka M, Ueno T, Toi M, Ishiguro H, Mikami Y, Togashi K (2012) Assessment of CAD-generated tumor volumes measured using MRI in breast cancers before and after neoadjuvant chemotherapy. Eur J Radiol 81(10):2627–2631. doi:10.1016/j.ejrad.2011.12.013
25. Wolchok JD, Hoos A, O'Day S, Weber JS, Hamid O, Lebbe C, Maio M, Binder M, Bohnsack O, Nichol G, Humphrey R, Hodi FS (2009) Guidelines for the evaluation of immune therapy activity in solid tumors: immune-related response criteria. Clin Cancer Res 15 (23):7412–7420. doi:10.1158/1078-0432.CCR-09-1624
26. Nishino M, Giobbie-Hurder A, Gargano M, Suda M, Ramaiya NH, Hodi FS (2013) Developing a common language for tumor response to immunotherapy: immune-related response criteria using unidimensional measurements. Clin Cancer Res 19(14):3936–3943. doi:10.1158/1078-0432.CCR-13-0895
27. Martincich L, Montemurro F, De Rosa G, Marra V, Ponzone R, Cirillo S, Gatti M, Biglia N, Sarotto I, Sismondi P, Regge D, Aglietta M (2004) Monitoring response to primary chemotherapy in breast cancer using dynamic contrast-enhanced magnetic resonance imaging. Breast Cancer Res Treat 83(1):67–76. doi:10.1023/B:BREA.0000010700.11092.f4
28. Cheung YC, Chen SC, Su MY, See LC, Hsueh S, Chang HK, Lin YC, Tsai CS (2003) Monitoring the size and response of locally advanced breast cancers to neoadjuvant chemotherapy (weekly paclitaxel and epirubicin) with serial enhanced MRI. Breast Cancer Res Treat 78(1):51–58

29. Drisis S, Metens T, Ignatiadis M, Stathopoulos K, Chao SL, Lemort M (2015) Quantitative DCE-MRI for prediction of pathological complete response following neoadjuvant treatment for locally advanced breast cancer: the impact of breast cancer subtypes on the diagnostic accuracy. Eur Radiol. doi:10.1007/s00330-015-3948-0
30. Yu HJ, Chen JH, Mehta RS, Nalcioglu O, Su MY (2007) MRI measurements of tumor size and pharmacokinetic parameters as early predictors of response in breast cancer patients undergoing neoadjuvant anthracycline chemotherapy. J Magn Reson Imaging 26(3):615–623. doi:10.1002/jmri.21060
31. Woodhams R, Kakita S, Hata H, Iwabuchi K, Kuranami M, Gautam S, Hatabu H, Kan S, Mountford C (2010) Identification of residual breast carcinoma following neoadjuvant chemotherapy: diffusion-weighted imaging – comparison with contrast-enhanced MR imaging and pathologic findings. Radiology 254(2):357–366. doi:10.1148/radiol.2542090405
32. Tiling R, Linke R, Untch M, Richter A, Fieber S, Brinkbaumer K, Tatsch K, Hahn K (2001) 18F-FDG PET and 99mTc-sestamibi scintimammography for monitoring breast cancer response to neoadjuvant chemotherapy: a comparative study. Eur J Nucl Med 28(6):711–720
33. Lee JH, Rosen EL, Mankoff DA (2009) The role of radiotracer imaging in the diagnosis and management of patients with breast cancer: part 2 – response to therapy, other indications, and future directions. J Nucl Med 50(5):738–748. doi:10.2967/jnumed.108.061416
34. Bassa P, Kim EE, Inoue T, Wong FC, Korkmaz M, Yang DJ, Wong WH, Hicks KW, Buzdar AU, Podoloff DA (1996) Evaluation of preoperative chemotherapy using PET with fluorine-18-fluorodeoxyglucose in breast cancer. J Nucl Med 37(6):931–938
35. Burcombe RJ, Makris A, Pittam M, Lowe J, Emmott J, Wong WL (2002) Evaluation of good clinical response to neoadjuvant chemotherapy in primary breast cancer using [18F]-fluorodeoxyglucose positron emission tomography. Eur J Cancer 38(3):375–379
36. Kim SJ, Kim SK, Lee ES, Ro J, Kang S (2004) Predictive value of [18F]FDG PET for pathological response of breast cancer to neo-adjuvant chemotherapy. Ann Oncol 15 (9):1352–1357. doi:10.1093/annonc/mdh345
37. Dose-Schwarz J, Tiling R, Avril-Sassen S, Mahner S, Lebeau A, Weber C, Schwaiger M, Janicke F, Untch M, Avril N (2010) Assessment of residual tumour by FDG-PET: conventional imaging and clinical examination following primary chemotherapy of large and locally advanced breast cancer. Br J Cancer 102(1):35–41. doi:10.1038/sj.bjc.6605427
38. Miyake KK, Nakamoto Y, Kanao S, Tanaka S, Sugie T, Mikami Y, Toi M, Togashi K (2014) Journal Club: diagnostic value of (18)F-FDG PET/CT and MRI in predicting the clinicopathologic subtypes of invasive breast cancer. AJR Am J Roentgenol 203(2):272–279. doi:10.2214/AJR.13.11971
39. Iima M, Nakamoto Y, Kanao S, Sugie T, Ueno T, Kawada M, Mikami Y, Toi M, Togashi K (2012) Clinical performance of 2 dedicated PET scanners for breast imaging: initial evaluation. J Nucl Med 53(10):1534–1542. doi:10.2967/jnumed.111.100958
40. Wahl RL, Zasadny K, Helvie M, Hutchins GD, Weber B, Cody R (1993) Metabolic monitoring of breast cancer chemohormonotherapy using positron emission tomography: initial evaluation. J Clin Oncol 11(11):2101–2111
41. Schelling M, Avril N, Nahrig J, Kuhn W, Romer W, Sattler D, Werner M, Dose J, Janicke F, Graeff H, Schwaiger M (2000) Positron emission tomography using [(18)F]Fluorodeoxyglucose for monitoring primary chemotherapy in breast cancer. J Clin Oncol 18 (8):1689–1695
42. Rousseau C, Devillers A, Sagan C, Ferrer L, Bridji B, Campion L, Ricaud M, Bourbouloux E, Doutriaux I, Clouet M, Berton-Rigaud D, Bouriel C, Delecroix V, Garin E, Rouquette S, Resche I, Kerbrat P, Chatal JF, Campone M (2006) Monitoring of early response to neoadjuvant chemotherapy in stage II and III breast cancer by [18F]fluorodeoxyglucose positron emission tomography. J Clin Oncol 24(34):5366–5372. doi:10.1200/JCO.2006.05.7406

43. Emmering J, Krak NC, Van der Hoeven JJ, Spreeuwenberg MD, Twisk JW, Meijer S, Pinedo HM, Hoekstra OS (2008) Preoperative [18F] FDG-PET after chemotherapy in locally advanced breast cancer: prognostic value as compared with histopathology. Ann Oncol 19 (9):1573–1577. doi:10.1093/annonc/mdn185
44. Wahl RL, Jacene H, Kasamon Y, Lodge MA (2009) From RECIST to PERCIST: evolving considerations for PET response criteria in solid tumors. J Nucl Med 50(Suppl 1):122S–150S. doi:10.2967/jnumed.108.057307

Part VI
Preoperative Anti-HER2 Therapy

Chapter 19
Human Epidermal Growth Factor Receptor (HER) Family Molecular Structure

Mark D. Pegram and Ralf Landgraf

Abstract ERBB receptors and their cognate ligands provide a rich and complex multilayered network of signaling control. Multiple layers of control act to safeguard against unwanted ERBB receptor activation, including the "closed" conformations of ligand-unbound EGFR, ERBB3, and ERBB4, auto-inhibited interactions among "open" conformation extracellular domains (ECDs), a vast repertoire of receptor-specific ligands (with, in some cases, a myriad of isoforms), the potential to form high-order complexes with associated proxy phosphorylation, and receptor-mediated endocytosis with associated recycling and degradation pathways. Despite these extensive safeguards, the deregulation of ERBB receptors is observed in multiple tumor types. In the case of ERBB2, the use of therapeutic antibodies aimed at distinct epitopes within the extracellular domain has resulted in marked improvements in clinical efficacy, and greater understanding of biology of ERBB2 receptor trafficking following receptor-mediated endocytosis has led to important insights in the development of an antibody-drug conjugate targeting this receptor. The multilayered nature of ERBB signaling offers a broad spectrum of future points for consideration of therapeutic interventions.

Keywords Neoadjuvant • Pathological complete response • Chemotherapy • Survival

19.1 Evolution of ERBB Receptors

In evolutionary terms, dating back approximately 100 million years to the nematode *Caenorhabditis elegans*, the human epidermal growth factor receptor (HER; a.k.a. ERBB receptor) system is an ancient receptor kinase pathway. *C. elegans* and *Drosophila* each contain just a single ERBB receptor homologue (Let-23 and DER,

M.D. Pegram (✉)
Stanford Cancer Institute, Stanford University School of Medicine, G2021B Lorey I. Lokey Building, 265 Campus Drive West, Stanford, CA 94305-5456, USA
e-mail: mpegram@stanford.edu

R. Landgraf
Department of Biochemistry and Molecular Biology, Sylvester Comprehensive Cancer Center, University of Miami Miller School of Medicine, Miami, FL, USA

M. Toi et al. (eds.), *Personalized Treatment of Breast Cancer*,
DOI 10.1007/978-4-431-55552-0_19

respectively), with Lin-3 being the only EGF-like ligand of *C. elegans*, whereas there are four ligands in *Drosophila* [74]. All ERBB receptor species feature an extracellular domain (ECD), a single transmembrane span, an intracellular tyrosine kinase domain, and a C-terminal tail [10, 21]. The ECD has four sub-domains consisting of two L regions (sub-domains I and III) and two cysteine-rich regions (sub-domains II and IV) [10, 21]. In *C. elegans*, development of the vulva is dependent upon Lin-3/Let-23 signaling, which binds to a juxtaposed receptor, triggering cell division and progression to a differentiated phenotype. Loss-of-function mutations in the receptor result in a vulvaless phenotype, sterility, abnormal male tail development, and lethality (reviewed in [74]). The *Drosophila* EGF receptor (DER) is used repeatedly in several stages of development, including oogenesis, embryogenesis, and wing and eye development [74]. In higher organisms, the ERBB receptor system has evolved into a complex network consisting of four receptor species – EGFR/ERBB1/HER1, ERBB2/HER2, ERBB3/HER3, and ERBB4/HER4 [8, 34] – and more than a dozen ligands, including the epidermal growth factor (EGF), transforming growth factor-α (TGFα), and neuregulins [74]. The mechanisms of activation are more complex than initially believed, but molecular details for some of the stages involved have emerged. Receptor activation involves a single ligand molecule binding simultaneously to ECD sub-domains I and III, thus stabilizing and activating homo- and heterodimers that interact primarily through a dimerization hairpin loop structure contained within sub-domain II [10, 11, 15, 43, 49], as shown in Fig. 19.1. In the absence of ligand, the receptor can assume an alternative stable configuration that is incompatible with ligand binding. In this so-called "tethered" or "closed" auto-inhibited conformation, the ß-hairpin loop sub-domain II, involved in ligand-dependent dimerization, is not exposed, being buried away via an intramolecular interaction with sub-domain IV [10, 11, 20, 43]. While loss of tethering alone does not lead to autoactivation [47], artificially stabilized tethered states, for example, binding of chimeric anti-EGFR monoclonal antibody cetuximab to EGFR [45], do result in signal inhibition. The relative contribution of tethered and extended states or dimers at various stages of activation remains an open question.

Although a similar domain organization is shared among the four vertebrate ERBB receptors, functional and structural studies have demonstrated that the ERBB2 does not bind any of the known ERBB family ligands and is constitutively in the "untethered" (open) conformation – suitable for dimerization [27]. Interestingly, a similar conformation has been observed in DER, which, though capable of ligand binding, exists in an auto-inhibited state incapable of dimerization in the absence of ligand binding [2]. In contrast, ERBB3 has a catalytically *impaired* kinase domain, although the ECD is capable of ligand binding and heterodimerization, and when activated, multiple C-terminal phosphotyrosine residues are generated capable of docking the p85 regulatory subunit of phosphoinositide 3-kinase (PI3K) – promoting downstream signaling events [8, 39, 58]. It is notable that while ERBB2 and ERBB3 may be functionally incomplete on their own, their heterodimers are potent activators of cellular signaling events [32, 53, 69].

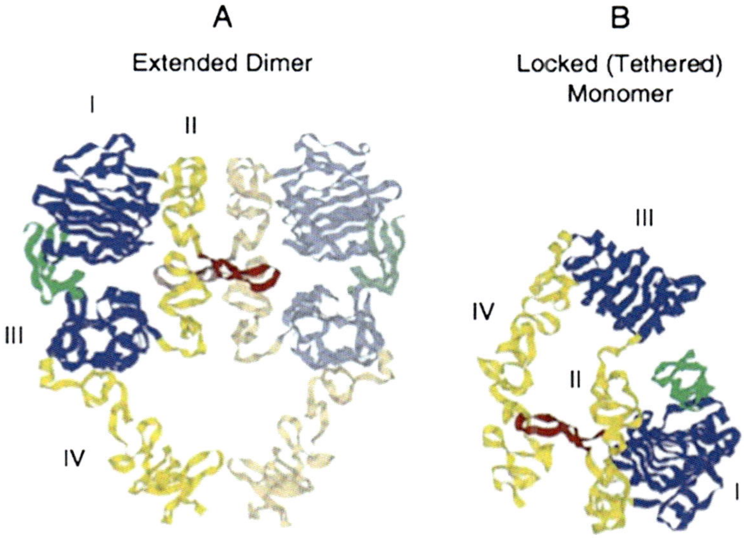

Fig. 19.1 (**a**) Structure of the homodimer of the ECD of EGFR with bound ligand (TGFα), including a model for sub-domain IV, which was modeled after the ERBB2 crystal structure. The putative dimerization loop is colored in *red* and TGFα is colored in *green*. (**b**) In the "closed" or "locked" monomer structure of EGFR ECD, the putative dimerization loop interacts with domain IV and the dimerization interface is not accessible (Modified from [26, 71 (with permission])

While the ERBB receptors have been shown to be critical regulators of normal growth and development in a myriad of cell types, their *deregulation* has been implicated in tumorigenesis and cancer progression [8, 35, 60]. Indeed, RNA tumor viruses, such as the avian erythroblastosis virus, co-opt a divergent strategy to harness ERBB signaling by encoding a truncated form of ERBB1 lacking most of the ectodomain (and harboring additional intracellular mutations). Accordingly, the oncoprotein v-ErbB is capable of forming ligand-independent covalent dimers at the cell surface [23]. In human tumors, gene amplification leading to receptor overexpression, as well as activating somatic mutations, is well known to occur in ERBB2 and EGFR in various tumor types [35, 60, 70, 73]. These seminal observations have led to the development of multiple small-molecule and antibody-based therapeutics that target EGFR and ERBB2 [3, 8]. Recently, ERBB3 has emerged as a potential cancer therapeutic target, given that it plays an important role in ERBB2 signaling and acquired resistance to some existing therapeutics [4, 8]. ERBB3 amplification and/or overexpression in isolation does not likely play a significant role as an oncogene, but it does occur in some cancers in the context of ERBB2 overexpression and acts as a potent amplifier, while only sporadic occurrence of oncogenic ERBB3 somatic mutations has been reported [17, 30, 36, 41, 63, 65]. Finally, transforming somatic mutations in ERBB4 have been reported in melanoma [54]. Thus remarkably, all four ERBB receptors are implicated in malignant transformation of various human tumors [37].

19.2 ERBB Family Ligands

All ERBB ligands share an EGF-like domain of approximately 60 amino acids that are necessary and sufficient for activation [6]. Ligands that bind to EGFR include EGF, the heparin-binding EGF-like growth factor (HB-EGF), epiregulin, amphiregulin, TGFα, and betacellulin. Ligands for ERBB3 and ERBB4, commonly named neuregulins (NRG) [68], comprise a large family arising from alternative splice variants of the four neuregulin genes [61]. Arguably the most well studied, NRG1 gives rise to more than 15 splicing isoforms [18]. NRG1 type I ligands (α, β1, β2, β3) are often referred to as heregulins. Despite the multiplicity of ligands capable of binding the ERBB receptor family, efficient activation can be achieved without the ECD. ERBB2 without its ECD is constitutively active [7, 16], as is truncated EGFR [33]. Indeed, discovery of the constitutively active v-ErbB oncogene, lacking much of the ERBB ECD [29, 56], preceded the discovery of EGFR (ERBB1). This indicates that regions other than the ECD must contribute significantly to interactions that are sufficient for activation [71]. It also suggests that the primary role of the ECD may not be to facilitate ERBB receptor interactions but rather to impose ligand control on the receptors.

19.3 Endocytosis and Receptor Trafficking

Once activation has occurred, ERBB receptor kinase signal attenuation can principally be achieved by two means, (1) by dephosphorylation of key residues by phosphatases and (2) removal of the receptor from signaling processes altogether by receptor trafficking. Phosphatases form a very large and highly specialized family of enzymes [67], and in the case of the EGFR, for example, disturbing the balance between phosphorylation and dephosphorylation can result in receptor activation that is comparable in scale and timing to that induced by ligand [55]. ERBB kinase signal attenuation through receptor endocytosis and degradation is a very complex process which has been extensively studied for EGFR. For clathrin-mediated endocytosis, key steps involve the interaction of EGFR with clathrin via AP2 adapters, mediated by EPS15 and epsin, endocytosis, and sorting to early endosomes and multivesicular bodies toward late endosomes for degradation or to recycling endosomes (reviewed in [71]). The ubiquitin ligase CBL directs poly-ubiquitination of EGFR [31], which acts as a routing signal for lysosomal degradation [46]. Upon activation with high concentrations of EGF, caveolae provide an alternate route of EGFR which can alter signaling outcomes through the exposure to distinct subsets of signaling scaffolds [59]. Interestingly, mechanisms of signal attenuation are nonuniform among ERBB receptors and for a given receptor differ depending on the ligand [72]. For example, while activated EGFR and ERBB3 are primarily directed toward degradation, ERBB2 is to a much larger extent dephosphorylated and recycled, contributing to its exceptionally long half-life. The differential routing of ERBB receptors in turn can influence signaling potency and present a level of targeted intervention exemplified by the impact of geldanamycin on EGFR [64] and ERBB2 [5]. Such findings have implications with respect to the development of ERBB receptor-directed antibody-drug conjugates (ADCs) and may influence selection of particular linker chemistry to optimize delivery of cytotoxic payloads [44].

19.4 Exploiting Ligand-Induced ERBB2 Heterodimer Formation

Ligand-activated dimers provide the normal downstream signaling mechanism for the ERBBs [10], but does ligand-associated signaling participate in disease pathogenesis of human tumors, and could blocking heterodimer formation uniquely affect disease outcome? ERBB2 overexpression in breast cancer correlates well with increased tumor growth rates, higher metastatic potential, and poorer long-term overall survival rates for patients whose tumors harbor ERBB2 gene amplification/overexpression [32, 50, 57, 62]. A number of therapeutic approaches have been developed to block the effects of ERBB2 overexpression, including small-molecule ERBB2 kinase inhibitors, antibody-drug conjugates, and the humanized monoclonal antibodies trastuzumab and pertuzumab. Trastuzumab and pertuzumab bind to distinct epitopes in the ERBB2 ECD, as has been seen both functionally [19] and structurally [12, 22]. Pertuzumab mediates the same antibody-dependent cytotoxic effects as does trastuzumab [14], although it does not block ERBB2 shedding like trastuzumab [48]. As shown in Fig. 19.2, pertuzumab binding directly inhibits ERBB2 ECD-directed heterodimerization with its partner receptors, thus blocking ligand-dependent signaling at its source [1], while it fails to suppress the ligand-independent activation of ERBB2 or constitutive activation of ERBB3/AKT under conditions of overexpression [38] and Fig. 19.2.

To more fully understand the mechanism of action of pertuzumab, Franklin and colleagues have determined the co-crystal structure of the pertuzumab Fab fragment bound to the extracellular domain of ERBB2. The overlap between the pertuzumab binding site on sub-domain II of the ERBB2 ECD and the heterodimer interface suggests that the binding of pertuzumab uniquely sterically interferes with ERBB2 heterodimerization and is consistent with the potent inhibition of ligand-dependent signaling by pertuzumab [22].

By contrast, other groups have focused efforts on the formation of ERBB3-ERBB2 heterodimers by directing antibodies against ERBB3 [24]. For instance, LJM716 is a novel ERBB3 monoclonal antibody that neutralizes multiple modes of

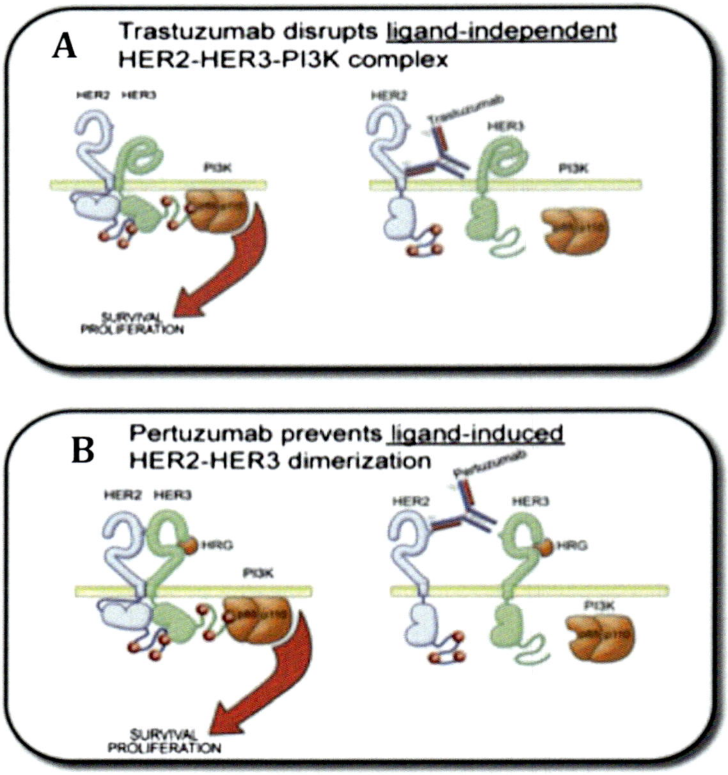

Fig. 19.2 Schematic representation of the mechanism of action for trastuzumab and pertuzumab. (**a**) Amplification of ERBB2 leads to ligand-*independent* ERBB2/ERBB3 interaction and resulting ERBB3 phosphorylation. Phosphorylated ERBB3 activates the PI3K pathway promoting cell survival and proliferation. Trastuzumab disrupts ligand-independent ERBB2/ERBB3 interaction, leading to rapid ERBB3 dephosphorylation and inhibition of the PI3K/AKT pathway, thereby inhibiting cell proliferation. (**b**) Pertuzumab is efficient in preventing *ligand-induced* ERBB2/ERBB3 heterodimerization, distinguishing its mechanism of action from that of trastuzumab (Modified from [38], with permission)

ERBB3 activation. LJM716 is a potent inhibitor of ERBB3/AKT phosphorylation and proliferation in ERBB2-amplified and NRG1-expressing cancer cells, and it displays single-agent efficacy in tumor xenograft models [25]. Moreover, combining LJM716 with agents that target ERBB2 or EGFR produced synergistic antitumor activity in vitro and in vivo [25]. Indeed, combining LJM716 with trastuzumab produced a more potent inhibition of signaling and cell proliferation than trastuzumab/pertuzumab combination, with similar activity in vivo [25]. Remarkably, the solved structure of LJM716 bound to ERBB3 indicates that LJM716 binds an epitope including sub-domains II and IV that trap ERBB3 in an inactive or "closed" conformation [25], a mode of action comparable to that proposed for cetuximab binding to EGFR [45]. Taken together, the above findings suggest that ERBB receptor-directed antibodies with unique epitopes may possess novel mechanism(s) of action that, alone or in combination with other ERBB2- or EGFR-targeted agents, may further leverage clinical efficacy in ERBB-driven cancers [28].

19.5 The Problem of ERBB2 Homodimers

In their elegant work, solving the ERBB2 ECD structure, Cho and colleagues noted that "The exposed domain II loop that mediates inter-receptor dimers of sHER1 [soluble EGFR] is also exposed in sHER2 [soluble ERBB2] but does not mediate a similar HER2 dimer,.…indicating a dimerization constant greater than about 10 mM" [12]. The failure of ERBB2 ECD and unliganded DER ECD to form stable, conventional dimers, despite both having an exposed dimerization arm, argues for an "inactive" dimerization-*incompetent* sub-domain II conformation – one that is stringently auto-inhibited [2]. Such a model argues against the prevailing notion that ERBB2 is "poised" to dimerize via its "open" conformation [12]. Nonetheless, cross-linking and co-immunoprecipitation studies show that intact ERBB2 can form complexes in mammalian cells [9, 13, 52]. One hypothesis is that ERBB2 relies uniquely on interactions outside its extracellular region to drive complex formation, perhaps within the transmembrane domain or in the cytoplasmic domain (or both). A second remaining (yet elusive) possibility is that as yet unknown cellular ligand(s) promote ERBB2 activation when it is overexpressed in mammalian cells [40]. A third model was proposed by Junttila et al. based on the comparison of trastuzumab and pertuzumab activity, suggesting the existence of a second, presumably highly transient interface in ERBB2 homodimerization [38].

19.6 High-Order ERBB Complexes

Higher-order complexes of ERBB receptors have been observed biophysically and offer a theoretical framework to help explain ERBB2 phosphorylation, but it remains unclear as to whether higher-order ERBB complexes provide functionality beyond the scope of constituent dimers [51]. Landgraf et al. have previously shown that a selected inhibitory RNA aptamer that targets the ERBB3 ECD acts by sterically disrupting higher-order interactions [51]. Ligand binding, ERBB2 heterodimerization, phosphorylation of ERBB3, and AKT signaling are only minimally affected in the presence of the inhibitory RNA aptamer, whereas ERBB2 phosphorylation and MAPK signaling are selectively strongly inhibited [75]. Mapping of the binding site and the creation of aptamer-resistant point mutants suggest an entirely new model of side-to-side oriented dimers of heterodimers (i.e.,

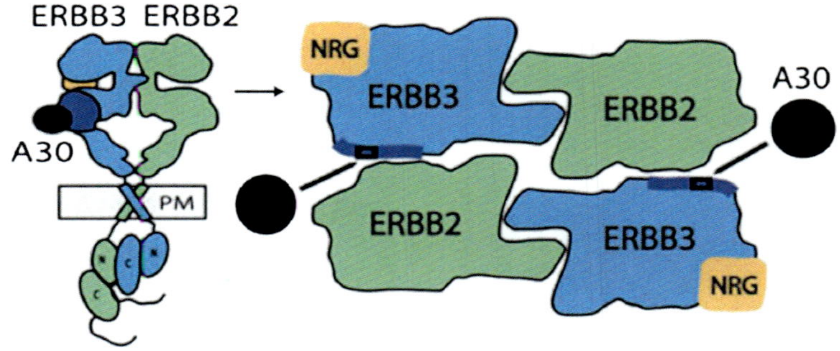

Fig. 19.3 A new model of side-to-side antiparallel dimer of dimers (heterotetramer) proposed to explain ERBB3-directed RNA aptamer A30 Action. At *left*, cartoon of the heterodimer in the plasma membrane (PM) with indicated RNA aptamer (called A30) binding site and charge complimentary interface on ERBB3 in *dark blue*. Allosteric cytoplasmic interactions are not drawn to scale. On the *right*, the structure-derived cartoon outline for the *top* view highlights the interlocking canonical dimer interface (as a side-to-side heterotetramer), the charge complimentary interface on ERBB3 (*blue*), and the binding sites for A30 and NRG (Modified from [75], with permission)

heterotetramers) to facilitate proxy receptor tyrosine phosphorylation (see Fig. 19.3).

Additional modes of signaling with relevance to pathological ERBB expression states, in theory, emerge at high receptor levels potentially resulting in heterotetramers or even higher-order ERBB-containing complexes. Such a model of ERBB receptor activation has implications for allosteric control mechanisms, specificity of interactions, and possible mechanisms of cross talk and suggests the possibility of future therapeutic intervention and clinical outcomes that do not reconcile with the current purely canonical, dimer-based models.

19.7 Conclusion

ERBB receptors and their cognate ligands provide a rich and complex multilayered network of signaling control. Multiple layers of control act to safeguard against unwanted ERBB receptor activation, including the "closed" conformations of ligand-unbound EGFR, ERBB3, and ERBB4 [42], auto-inhibited interactions among ERBB2 (and DER), "open" conformation ECDs, a vast repertoire of receptor-specific ligands (with, in some cases, a myriad of isoforms), the potential to form high-order complexes with associated proxy phosphorylation, and receptor-mediated endocytosis with associated recycling and degradation pathways [71]. Despite these extensive safeguards, the deregulation of ERBB receptors is observed in multiple tumor types. However, the causes and mechanisms of uncontrolled signaling by different ERBB receptors appear to be distinct, consistent with the observation that nuances in epitope selection could have profound clinical consequences [66]. The multilayered nature of ERBB signaling offers a broader spectrum for future points of therapeutic intervention than previously imagined.

References

1. Agus DB, Akita RW, Fox WD, Lewis GD, Higgins B, Pisacane PI, Lofgren JA, Tindell C, Evans DP, Maiese K, Scher HI, Sliwkowski MX (2002) Targeting ligand-activated ErbB2 signaling inhibits breast and prostate tumor growth. Cancer Cell 2(2):127–137
2. Alvarado D, Klein DE, Lemmon MA (2009) ErbB2/HER2/Neu resembles an autoinhibited invertebrate EGF receptor. Nature 461(7261):287–291. doi:10.1038/nature08297
3. Alvarez RH, Valero V, Hortobagyi GN (2010) Emerging targeted therapies for breast cancer. J Clin Oncol 28:3366–3379
4. Amin DN, Campbell MR, Moasser MM (2010) The role of HER3, the unpretentious member of the HER family, in cancer biology and cancer therapeutics. Semin Cell Dev Biol 21:944–950
5. Austin CD, De Maziere AM, Pisacane PI, van Dijk SM, Eigenbrot C, Sliwkowski MX et al (2004) Endocytosis and sorting of ErbB2 and the site of action of cancer therapeutics trastuzumab and geldanamycin. Mol Biol Cell 15(12):5268–5282. PubMed
6. Barbacci EG, Guarino BC, Stroh JG, Singleton DH, Rosnack KJ, Moyer JD, Andrews GC (1995) The structural basis for the specificity of epidermal growth factor and heregulin binding. J Biol Chem 270:9585
7. Bargmann CI, Weinberg RA (1988) Increased tyrosine kinase activity associated with the protein encoded by the activated neu oncogene. Proc Natl Acad Sci U S A 85:5394
8. Baselga J, Swain SM (2009) Novel anticancer targets: revisiting ERBB2 and discovering ERBB3. Nat Rev Cancer 9:463–475
9. Brennan PJ, Kumagai T, Berezov A, Murali R, Greene MI (2000) HER2/neu: mechanisms of dimerization/oligomerization. Oncogene 19:6093–6101
10. Burgess AW, Cho HS, Eigenbrot C, Ferguson KM, Garrett TP, Leahy DJ, Lemmon MA, Sliwkowski MX, Ward CW, Yokoyama S (2003) An open-and-shut case? Recent insights into the activation of EGF/ErbB receptors. Mol Cell 12:541–552
11. Cho HS, Leahy DJ (2002) Structure of the extracellular region of HER3 reveals an interdomain tether. Science 297:1330–1333
12. Cho HS, Mason K, Ramyar KX, Stanley AM, Gabelli SB, Denney DW Jr et al (2003) Structure of the extracellular region of HER2 alone and in complex with the Herceptin Fab. Nature 421:756–760
13. Citri A, Skaria KB, Yarden Y (2003) The deaf and the dumb: the biology of ErbB-2 and ErbB-3. Exp Cell Res 284:54–65
14. Clynes RA, Towers TL, Presta LG, Ravetch JV (2000) Inhibitory Fc receptors modulate in vivo cytotoxicity against tumor targets. Nat Med 6(4):443–446
15. Dawson JP, Berger MB, Lin CC, Schlessinger J, Lemmon MA, Ferguson KM (2005) Epidermal growth factor receptor dimerization and activation require ligand-induced conformational changes in the dimer interface. Mol Cell Biol 25:7734–7742
16. Di Fiore PP, Pierce JH, Kraus MH, Segatto O, King CR, Aaronson SA (1987) erbB-2 is a potent oncogene when overexpressed in NIH/3T3 cells. Science 237:178
17. Ding L, Getz G, Wheeler DA, Mardis ER, McLellan MD, Cibulskis K, Sougnez C, Greulich H, Muzny DM, Morgan MB et al (2008) Somatic mutations affect key pathways in lung adenocarcinoma. Nature 455:1069–1075
18. Falls DL (2003) Neuregulins: functions, forms, and signaling strategies. Exp Cell Res 284:14

19. Fendly BM, Winget M, Hudziak RM, Lipari MT, Napier MA, Ullrich A (1990) Characterization of murine monoclonal antibodies reactive to either the human epidermal growth factor receptor or HER2/neu gene product. Cancer Res 50(5):1550–1558
20. Ferguson KM, Berger MB, Mendrola JM, Cho H-S, Leahy DJ, Lemmon MA (2003) EGF activates its receptor by removing interactions that autoinhibit ectodomain dimerization. Mol Cell 11:507–517
21. Ferguson KM (2008) Structure-based view of epidermal growth factor receptor regulation. Annu Rev Biophys 37:353–373
22. Franklin MC, Carey KD, Vajdos FF, Leahy DJ, de Vos AM, Sliwkowski MX (2004) Insights into ErbB signaling from the structure of the ErbB2-pertuzumab complex. Cancer Cell 5(4):317–328
23. Frykberg L, Palmieri S, Beug H, Graf T, Hayman MJ, Vennstrom B (1983) Transforming capacities of avian erythroblastosis virus mutants deleted in the erbA or erbB oncogenes. Cell 32:227–238
24. Gala K, Chandarlapaty S (2014) Molecular pathways: HER3 targeted therapy. Clin Cancer Res 20(6):1410–1416
25. Garner AP, Bialucha CU, Sprague ER, Garrett JT, Sheng Q, Li S, Sineshchekova O, Saxena P, Sutton CR, Chen D, Chen Y, Wang H, Liang J, Das R, Mosher R, Gu J, Huang A, Haubst N, Zehetmeier C, Haberl M, Elis W, Kunz C, Heidt AB, Herlihy K, Murtie J, Schuller A, Arteaga CL, Sellers WR, Ettenberg SA (2013) An antibody that locks HER3 in the inactive conformation inhibits tumor growth driven by HER2 or neuregulin. Cancer Res 73(19):6024–6035. doi:10.1158/0008-5472.CAN-13-1198. Epub 2013 Aug 8
26. Garrett TP, McKern NM, Lou M, Elleman TC, Adams TE, Lovrecz GO, Zhu HJ, Walker F, Frenkel MJ, Hoyne PA, Jorissen RN, Nice EC, Burgess AW, Ward CW (2002) Crystal structure of a truncated epidermal growth factor receptor extracellular domain bound to transforming growth factor alpha. Cell 110:763
27. Garrett TP, McKern NM, Lou M, Elleman TC, Adams TE, Lovrecz GO, Kofler M, Jorissen RN, Nice EC, Burgess AW, Ward CW (2003) The crystal structure of a truncated ErbB2 ectodomain reveals an active conformation, poised to interact with other ErbB receptors. Mol Cell 11:495
28. Garrett JT, Sutton CR, Kurupi R, Bialucha CU, Ettenberg SA, Collins SD, Sheng Q, Wallweber J, Defazio-Eli L, Arteaga CL (2013) Combination of antibody that inhibits ligand-independent HER3 dimerization and a p110α inhibitor potently blocks PI3K signaling and growth of HER2+ breast cancers. Cancer Res 73(19):6013–6023
29. Gilmore T, DeClue JE, Martin GS (1985) Protein phosphorylation at tyrosine is induced by the v-erbB gene product in vivo and in vitro. Cell 40:609
30. Greenman C, Stephens P, Smith R, Dalgliesh GL, Hunter C, Bignell G, Davies H, Teague J, Butler A, Stevens C et al (2007) Patterns of somatic mutation in human cancer genomes. Nature 446:153–158
31. Haglund K, Sigismund S, Polo S, Szymkiewicz I, Di Fiore PP, Dikic I (2003) Multiple monoubiquitination of RTKs is sufficient for their endocytosis and degradation. Nat Cell Biol 5:461
32. Holbro T, Beerli RR, Maurer F, Koziczak M, Barbas CF III, Hynes NE (2003) The ErbB2/ErbB3 heterodimer functions as an oncogenic unit: ErbB2 requires ErbB3 to drive breast tumor cell proliferation. Proc Natl Acad Sci U S A 100:8933–8938
33. Honegger AM, Schmidt A, Ullrich A, Schlessinger J (1990) Evidence for epidermal growth factor (EGF)-induced intermolecular autophosphorylation of the EGF receptors in living cells. Mol Cell Biol 10:4035
34. Hynes NE, Lane HA (2005) ERBB receptors and cancer: the complexity of targeted inhibitors. Nat Rev Cancer 5:341–354
35. Hynes NE, MacDonald G (2009) ErbB receptors and signaling pathways in cancer. Curr Opin Cell Biol 21:177–184
36. Jeong EG, Soung YH, Lee JW, Lee SH, Nam SW, Lee JY, Yoo NJ, Lee SH (2006) ERBB3 kinase domain mutations are rare in lung, breast and colon carcinomas. Int J Cancer 119:2986–2987

37. Jaiswal BS et al (2013) Oncogenic ERBB3 mutations in human cancers. Cancer Cell 23:603–617
38. Junttila TT, Akita RW, Parsons K, Fields C, Lewis Phillips GD, Friedman LS, Sampath D, Sliwkowski MX (2009) Ligand-independent HER2/HER3/PI3K complex is disrupted by trastuzumab and is effectively inhibited by the PI3K inhibitor GDC-0941. Cancer Cell 15:429–440
39. Jura N, Shan Y, Cao X, Shaw DE, Kuriyan J (2009) Structural analysis of the catalytically inactive kinase domain of the human EGF receptor 3. Proc Natl Acad Sci U S A 106:21608–21613
40. Komatsu M, Jepson S, Arango ME, Carothers Carraway CA, Carraway KL (2001) Muc4/sialomucin complex, an intramembrane modulator of ErbB2/HER2/Neu, potentiates primary tumor growth and suppresses apoptosis in a xenotransplanted tumor. Oncogene 20(4):461–470
41. Kan Z, Jaiswal BS, Stinson J, Janakiraman V, Bhatt D, Stern HM, Yue P, Haverty PM, Bourgon R, Zheng J et al (2010) Diverse somatic mutation patterns and pathway alterations in human cancers. Nature 466:869–873
42. Landgraf R (2007) HER2 (ERBB2): functional diversity from structurally conserved building blocks. Breast Cancer Res 9:202
43. Lemmon MA, Schlessinger J (2010) Cell signaling by receptor tyrosine kinases. Cell 141:1117–1134
44. Lewis Phillips GD, Li G, Dugger DL, Crocker LM, Parsons KL, Mai E et al (2008) Targeting HER2-positive breast cancer with trastuzumab-DM1, an antibody-cytotoxic drug conjugate. Cancer Res 68:9280–9290
45. Li S, Schmitz KR, Jeffrey PD, Wiltzius JJ, Kussie P, Ferguson KM (2005) Structural basis for inhibition of the epidermal growth factor receptor by cetuximab. Cancer Cell 7(4):301–311. PubMed
46. Marmor MD, Yarden Y (2004) Role of protein ubiquitylation in regulating endocytosis of receptor tyrosine kinases. Oncogene 23:2057
47. Mattoon D, Klein P, Lemmon MA, Lax I, Schlessinger J (2004) The tethered configuration of the EGF receptor extracellular domain exerts only a limited control of receptor function. Proc Natl Acad Sci U S A 101(4):923–928. PubMed
48. Molina MA, Codony-Servat J, Albanell J, Rojo F, Arribas J, Baselga J (2001) Trastuzumab (herceptin), a humanized anti-Her2 receptor monoclonal antibody, inhibits basal and activated Her2 ectodomain cleavage in breast cancer cells. Cancer Res 61(12):4744–4749
49. Ogiso H, Ishitani R, Nureki O, Fukai S, Yamanaka M, Kim JH, Saito K, Sakamoto A, Inoue M, Shirouzu M, Yokoyama S (2002) Crystal structure of the complex of human epidermal growth factor and receptor extracellular domains. Cell 110:775–787
50. Paik S, Liu ET (2000) HER2 as a predictor of therapeutic response in breast cancer. Breast Dis 11:91–102
51. Park E, Baron R, Landgraf R (2008) Higher-order association states of cellular ERBB3 probed with photo-cross-linkable aptamers. Biochemistry 47(46):11992–12005
52. Penuel E, Akita RW, Sliwkowski MX (2002) Identification of a region within the ErbB2/HER2 intracellular domain that is necessary for ligand-independent association. J Biol Chem 277:28468–28473
53. Pinkas-Kramarski R, Soussan L, Waterman H, Levkowitz G, Alroy I, Klapper L, Lavi S, Seger R, Ratzkin BJ, Sela M, Yarden Y (1996) Diversification of Neu differentiation factor and epidermal growth factor signaling by combinatorial receptor interactions. EMBO J 15:2452
54. Prickett TD, Agrawal NS, Wei X, Yates KE, Lin JC, Wunderlich JR, Cronin JC, Cruz P, Rosenberg SA, Samuels Y (2009) Analysis of the tyrosine kinome in melanoma reveals recurrent mutations in ERBB4. Nat Genet 41:1127–1132
55. Reynolds AR, Tischer C, Verveer PJ, Rocks O, Bastiaens PI (2003) EGFR activation coupled to inhibition of tyrosine phosphatases causes lateral signal propagation. Nat Cell Biol 5:447
56. Riedel H, Schlessinger J, Ullrich A (1987) A chimeric, ligand-binding v-erbB/EGF receptor retains transforming potential. Science 236:197
57. Ross JS, Fletcher JA (1998) The HER-2/neu oncogene in breast cancer: prognostic factor, predictive factor, and target for therapy. Stem Cells 16(6):413–428

58. Shi F, Telesco SE, Liu Y, Radhakrishnan R, Lemmon MA (2010) ErbB3/HER3 intracellular domain is competent to bind ATP and catalyze auto-phosphorylation. Proc Natl Acad Sci U S A 107:7692–7697
59. Sigismund S, Woelk T, Puri C, Maspero E, Tacchetti C, Transidico P, Di Fiore PP, Polo S (2005) Clathrin-independent endocytosis of ubiquitinated cargos. Proc Natl Acad Sci USA 102 (8):2760–2765
60. Sithanandam G, Anderson LM (2008) The ERBB3 receptor in cancer and cancer gene therapy. Cancer Gene Ther 15:413–448
61. Stove C, Bracke M (2004) Roles for neuregulins in human cancer. Clin Exp Metastasis 21:665
62. Slamon DJ, Godolphin W, Jones LA, Holt JA, Wong SG, Keith DE, Levin WJ, Stuart SG, Udove J, Ullrich A et al (1989) Studies of the HER-2/neu proto-oncogene in human breast and ovarian cancer. Science 244(4905):707–712
63. Stransky N, Egloff AM, Tward AD, Kostic AD, Cibulskis K, Sivachenko A, Kryukov GV, Lawrence MS, Sougnez C, McKenna A et al (2011) The mutational landscape of head and neck squamous cell carcinoma. Science 333:1157–1160
64. Supino-Rosin L, Yoshimura A, Yarden Y, Elazar Z, Neumann D (2000) Intracellular retention and degradation of the epidermal growth factor receptor, two distinct processes mediated by benzoquinone ansamycins. J Biol Chem 275(29):21850–21855. PubMed
65. TCGA Cancer Genome Atlas Network (2012) Comprehensive molecular portraits of human breast tumours. Nature 490:61–70
66. Swain SM, Baselga J, Kim SB, Ro J, Semiglazov V, Campone M, Ciruelos E, Ferrero JM, Schneeweiss A, Heeson S, Clark E, Ross G, Benyunes MC, Cortés J, CLEOPATRA Study Group (2015) Pertuzumab, trastuzumab, and docetaxel in HER2-positive metastatic breast cancer. N Engl J Med 372(8):724–734
67. Tonks NK, Neel BG (2001) Combinatorial control of the specificity of protein tyrosine phosphatases. Curr Opin Cell Biol 13:182
68. Tzahar E, Levkowitz G, Karunagaran D, Yi L, Peles E, Lavi S, Chang D, Liu N, Yayon A, Wen D, Yarden Y (1994) ErbB-3 and ErbB-4 function as the respective low and high affinity receptors of all NDF/heregulin isoforms. J Biol Chem 269:25226–25233
69. Tzahar E, Waterman H, Chen X, Levkowitz G, Karunagaran D, Lavi S, Ratzkin BJ, Yarden Y (1996) A hierarchical network of interreceptor interactions determines signal transduction by neu diferentiation factor/neuregulin and epidermal growth factor. Mol Cell Biol 16(10): 5276–5287
70. Wang SE, Narasanna A, Perez-Torres M, Xiang B, Wu FY, Yang S, Carpenter G, Gazdar AF, Muthuswamy SK, Arteaga CL (2006) HER2 kinase domain mutation results in constitutive phosphorylation and activation of HER2 and EGFR and resistance to EGFR tyrosine kinase inhibitors. Cancer Cell 10:25–38
71. Warren CM, Landgraf R (2006) Signaling through ERBB receptors: multiple layers of diversity and control. Cell Signal 18:923–933
72. Waterman H, Sabanai I, Geiger B, Yarden Y (1998) Alternative intracellular routing of ErbB receptors may determine signaling potency. J Biol Chem 273:13819
73. Yamauchi M, Gotoh N (2009) Theme: oncology–molecular mechanisms determining the efficacy of EGF receptor-specific tyrosine kinase inhibitors help to identify biomarker candidates. Biomark Med 3:139–151
74. Yarden Y, Sliwkowski MX (2001) Untangling the ErbB signalling network. Nat Rev Mol Cell Biol 2:127–137
75. Zhang Q, Park E, Kani K, Landgraf R (2012) Functional isolation of activated and unilaterally phosphorylated heterodimers of ERBB2 and ERBB3 as scaffolds in ligand-dependent signaling. Proc Natl Acad Sci U S A 109(33):13237–13242

Chapter 20
Locoregional Therapy Following Neoadjuvant Therapy for HER-2+ Breast Cancer: Opportunities and Challenges

Stephen R. Grobmyer, Stephanie A. Valente, Sheen Cherian, Holly J. Pederson, and Jame Abraham

Abstract Advances in the management of patients with HER-2+ breast cancer with combinatorial targeted therapies are leading to unprecedented rates of pathologic complete response. The high rates of complete pathologic response in the breast and the axillary lymph nodes following neoadjuvant therapy are raising new questions about the role of local therapies (surgery and radiation therapy) in treating these patients. The safe elimination of surgery and radiation therapy for selected breast cancer patients would ultimately reduce the short- and long-term morbidity associated with traditional breast cancer treatments and would represent a major step forward. However, numerous technical and clinical challenges remain which will be discussed in this chapter. Collaborative efforts to address these challenges are essential to improving current therapeutic approaches for patients with HER-2+ breast cancer.

Keywords Breast cancer • Surgery • Neoadjuvant chemotherapy • HER-2+ • Radiation therapy • Breast imaging

20.1 Introduction

HER-2+ breast cancer is caused by a gene mutation that results in an overexpression of the HER-2 receptor on the cell membrane of breast cancer cells. This overexpression is seen in approximately 15–30 % of all breast cancers [1]. Advances in HER-2-directed therapy have resulted in unprecedented favorable response rates for patients with HER-2+ breast cancer who undergo therapy in the neoadjuvant setting [2]. Traditionally, neoadjuvant chemotherapy is followed by

S.R. Grobmyer (✉)
Cleveland Clinic Comprehensive Breast Cancer Program, Cleveland, OH, USA

Cleveland Clinic, 9500 Euclid Ave. Desk A81, Cleveland, OH 44195, USA
e-mail: GROBMYS@ccf.org

S.A. Valente • S. Cherian • H.J. Pederson • J. Abraham
Cleveland Clinic Comprehensive Breast Cancer Program, Cleveland, OH, USA

M. Toi et al. (eds.), *Personalized Treatment of Breast Cancer*,
DOI 10.1007/978-4-431-55552-0_20

locoregional therapy (surgical excision of the tumor and lymph node evaluation with or without adjuvant radiotherapy). However, high observed complete response rates to neoadjuvant chemotherapy in patients with HER-2+ breast cancer raise new issues regarding the optimal role of locoregional therapy in this setting. The critical question is: "do selected patients following neoadjuvant chemotherapy for HER-2+ breast cancer lack additional benefit from surgery or radiation therapy, and can these modalities be safely omitted or limited in selected patients?"

Defining optimal approaches to locoregional therapy relies heavily on breast imaging interpretation to assess response to therapy in the breast and regional nodes. Defining these optimal approaches to locoregional therapy also relies on an understanding of the relationships between response rates, locoregional recurrence-free survival, and overall survival. Continued refinement in our understanding of these concepts provides hope for the future safe elimination of all or some components of locoregional therapies for HER-2+ breast cancer patients. Ultimately this paradigm shift would reduce the impact of current locoregional therapies on patient quality of life and cosmesis without compromising oncologic outcomes.

20.2 Increasing Pathologic Complete Response Rates Are Being Achieved with Dual-Targeted HER-2-Directed Agents

The development of HER-2-targeted therapy for the adjuvant therapy of patients with HER-2+ breast cancer in the late 1990s and early 2000s represented a breakthrough in the management of patients with HER-2+ breast cancer [3]. HER-2-targeted adjuvant therapies have dramatically improved the overall survival of patients with HER-2+ breast cancer [4].

Recent studies have focused on the development of dual HER-2-targeted therapies in the neoadjuvant setting. The goal of these studies has been to evaluate the impact of dual-targeted therapies on pathologic complete response rates in HER-2+ breast cancer. Pathologic complete response has been associated with improved outcomes in some intrinsic subtypes of breast cancer, particularly HER-2+ nonluminal and triple-negative breast cancers [5]. A summary of several recently published studies is outlined in Table 20.1. Observed complete response rates with dual-targeted therapy are significantly higher than have been observed with single-agent targeted therapy for HER-2+ breast cancer and higher than complete response rates observed in other types of breast cancer [6–10]. The high complete response rates with dual-targeted therapies are what lead to US Food and Drug Administration approval of the combination of pertuzumab and trastuzumab for use in the neoadjuvant setting for patients with HER-2+ breast cancer [11].

Several studies have also analyzed the association of dual-targeted HER-2-directed therapy with post-chemotherapy pathologic nodal status (Table 20.2).

Table 20.1 Pathologic complete response rate in trials of dual HER-2-targeted therapy

Trial (year)	#	Pathologic complete response Single-agent HER-2-targeted agent (%)	Dual-agent HER-2-targeted agent (%)
NeoSphere (2012) [6]	417	26	46
NeoALTTO (2012) [7]	455	30	51
CHER-LOB (2012) [8]	121	25	47
NSABP B-41 (2013) [9]	519	49	60
TRYPHAENA (2013) [10]	225	–	57–66

Table 20.2 Rate of post-neoadjuvant therapy pathologic N0 nodal status in patients treated with single- or dual-targeted HER-2-directed therapy

	Single agent (%)	Dual agent (%)
NeoALTTO (2012) [7]	59	73
CHER-LOB (2102) [8]	71	84
NeoSphere (2011) [6]	54	71

Patients treated with dual-targeted therapies are observed to have high rates of post-chemotherapy N0 status (71–84 %). These high rates of pathologically clear nodal status suggest the opportunity to reduce the extent and morbidity of axillary surgery and radiotherapy through improvements in predicting pathologic nodal complete response, improvements in understanding the relationship of post-NAC nodal status and outcomes, and improvements in lymph node imaging.

20.3 Assessment of Response Rates to Neoadjuvant Chemotherapy in Breast and Axillary Nodes

While complete response rates to dual HER-2-targeted therapies are high, preoperative determination of which patients have had a complete pathologic response remains a significant challenge. Ideally, if imaging study results were highly correlated with pathologic complete response, then selected patients *might* be suitable for consideration of omitting surgical and/or radiotherapeutic management for breast cancer. However, there are currently no absolutely reliable imaging studies to assess complete pathologic response to neoadjuvant HER-2-directed chemotherapy [12]. Some patients following complete imaging response to NAC are still found to have residual microscopic disease at the time of surgery [13]. This fear of leaving unknown residual disease without surgical resection is the main reason adjuvant surgery continues to be recommended. Breast magnetic resonance imaging (MRI) has been demonstrated to be accurate in estimating tumor size following NAC [12]. However, reported specificity rates of breast MRI in the post-NAC setting have varied widely [13]. Recent studies have suggested that changes seen on PET-CT are associated with complete response rates to NAC, but again PET-CT cannot reliably predict which patients have had a pathologic complete response [14]. Similarly mammography following NAC has not been demonstrated to be highly predictive of pathologic complete response [13]. Continued efforts to improve imaging for prediction of complete pathologic response following HER-2-targeted NAC are clearly warranted. Such improvements could serve as an important platform for advancing the treatment of patients with HER-2+ breast cancer. Additionally, there are currently no bioassays to assess the response to NAC, but development of accurate bioassays to assess response would represent a major breakthrough.

Assessment of the axilla with imaging presents similar challenges. MRI has been demonstrated to have limited value in the evaluation of axillary nodal disease [15]. Loss of fatty hilum in axillary nodes has been most associated with the presence of axillary nodal disease, but detection of low-volume axillary disease remains a challenge with MRI [15]. Axillary ultrasound (AUS) has been extensively studied for the evaluation of axillary nodes in breast cancer patients [16]. AUS is effective at detecting more advanced nodal disease but lacks sensitivity for the detection of small-volume axillary nodal disease [16]. Studies have shown that with physical exam, mammogram, ultrasound, and MRI all being negative, there still exists approximately a 14 % chance of lymph node metastasis at the time of surgery, necessitating continued surgical lymph node evaluation [17]. New emerging technologies aimed at preoperative nodal imaging and assessment such as optoacoustic tomography [18], particularly aimed at detecting small-volume nodal disease, might enable transformation of current approaches to axillary management in patients with HER-2+ breast cancer.

20.4 Surgical Management Following HER-2-Directed Neoadjuvant Chemotherapy

A traditional indication for NAC in patients with breast cancer is downstaging of larger primary tumors to facilitate breast-conserving surgery [19]. Downstaging of tumors with NAC followed by conservative surgery and whole breast radiation therapy has been demonstrated to be a safe therapeutic approach [19].

In spite of observed high complete response rates and the demonstrated safety of breast-conserving therapy following NAC, observed rates of breast conservation in patients treated with HER-2-targeted NAC have varied widely (Table 20.3). There is clearly a lack of uniformity in approaches to surgical management to patients

Table 20.3 Breast-conserving therapy rates following NAC for breast cancer

Trial	Pathologic complete response rate (%)	Breast-conserving therapy rate (%)
GeparQuattro (2010) [20]	32	63
TECHNO (2011) [21]	39	64
NOAH (2011) [22]	38	23
KCSG BR 07-01 (2012) [23]	59	79
ACOSOG Z1041 (2013) [24]	60	38
NeoALTTO (2013) [7]	43	44

following an observed excellent response to NAC that are related to a combination of patient- and provider-related factors.

A study recently analyzed objective factors associated with the choice of breast-conserving therapy in patients treated in the NeoALTTO study [25]. Factors associated (hazard ratio) with breast-conserving therapy and relative risk for breast-conserving therapy were planned BCT at diagnosis (0.46), < cT3 size (1.97), developed country (1.62), no complete clinical response to NAC (0.41), estrogen receptor negative (0.50), and tumor multicentricity (0.21). Factors not significantly associated with breast-conserving therapy were age, tumor grade, clinical nodal stage, and radiological response. This study suggests the need to develop more standardized approaches to surgery following highly effective dual HER-2-targeted NAC.

20.5 Locoregional Control in Patients Being Treated with Neoadjuvant HER-2-Directed Therapy

Several studies have evaluated rates of locoregional control in patients treated with neoadjuvant HER-2-directed therapy, and locoregional control is excellent in these patients. In the NOAH study which compared neoadjuvant chemotherapy to chemotherapy plus trastuzumab, excellent local control was demonstrated in patients receiving chemotherapy plus trastuzumab [22]. A small percentage in the trial was treated with BCT: patients receiving chemotherapy only, 13 % BCT rate, and patients receiving chemotherapy plus trastuzumab, 23 % BCT rate. At a median follow-up of 39 months, the rates of locoregional recurrence in chemotherapy plus trastuzumab-treated patients were BCT, 0 %, and mastectomy, 3 %. These recurrence rates compared favorably to patients with chemotherapy only: BCT, 21 %, and mastectomy, 3 %.

The Korean neoadjuvant study (Korean 07-01) which was a neoadjuvant phase 2 study of paclitaxel, gemcitabine, and trastuzumab in HER-2+ patients similarly demonstrated excellent locoregional control [23]. Most patients in this trial were

Table 20.4 Relationship of post-NAC stage and locoregional recurrence [28]

Stage	LRR (%)
ypT0	4.7
ypTis	11.8
ypT1	9.1
ypT2	8.2
ypT3	13.8
ypT4a-c	20
ypT4d	31.2

treated with BCT (79 %) and median follow-up was 40 months. Among patients having BCT, the locoregional recurrence rate was excellent at 5 %.

Arsenault et al. have evaluated predictors of locoregional control in a series of 157 HER-2 patients being treated with neoadjuvant chemotherapy followed by mastectomy (90 %) [26]. With a median follow-up of 43 months, the authors reported a locoregional recurrence rate of 8 %. The factors most associated with locoregional recurrence were no adjuvant radiation therapy and lymph node positive status.

Pathologic complete response in HER-2+ patients has been associated with significant improvements in overall survival [27]. von Minckwitz et al. have also importantly evaluated the relationship of pathologic response with locoregional recurrence in patients receiving neoadjuvant chemotherapy by analyzing the results of seven prospective trials [28]. In these trials, adjuvant radiation therapy was given to all patients having BCT as well as those having mastectomy with stage cN1 or cT3-4 tumors. At a median follow-up of 46 months, the investigators reported the lowest rate of locoregional recurrence among those with a pathologic complete response (Table 20.4). Further, the authors demonstrated that the rates of locoregional control in patients having a pathologic complete response varied by the intrinsic subtype of breast cancer. The reported locoregional recurrence rate associated with pathologic complete response was lower in HER-2+ nonluminal cancers (1.9 %) compared to HER-2+ luminal B cancers (8.2 %).

20.6 Can Operation Be Omitted Following NAC for Breast Cancer?

An ultimate goal of advances in NAC for HER-2+ breast cancer would be totally eliminating the need for surgery. Nonoperative therapy following NAC has been studied and reported in a series by Ring et al. [29]. The investigators performed a retrospective analysis of patients who had operative therapy ($n = 67$) versus those who did not have operative therapy ($n = 69$). All patients in the series received adjuvant radiation therapy. The investigators reported no significant difference in overall survival comparing the groups ($p = 0.9$). A trend was noted, however, toward an improvement in local recurrence-free survival in those having surgery

($p = 0.09$). Further, in nonsurgical patients with complete response noted on ultrasound, local recurrence-free survival was >90 % at 8 years of follow-up. This study, although retrospective, suggests the future possibility of nonoperative therapy for selected patients receiving modern HER-2-directed therapy.

20.7 Can Radiotherapy Be Safely Omitted Following NAC for HER-2+ Breast Cancer?

Axillary node involvement has traditionally been an indication for adjuvant radiation therapy in patients following mastectomy for breast cancer [30]. As noted above, modern combinatorial approaches to neoadjuvant therapy for HER-2+ breast cancer patients are leading to higher observed responses in the axillary nodal basin. The high complete nodal response rates have raised questions regarding the role of adjuvant radiation therapy in the setting of complete pathologic nodal response [31]. The role of adjuvant radiation therapy is currently being evaluated in a phase 3 randomized trial (NSABP B-51) in which patients having a complete pathologic axillary nodal response are randomized to adjuvant radiation versus no axillary radiation [31]. Results from this trial should contribute significantly to optimizing approaches to adjuvant therapy in HER-2+ breast cancer patients following NAC.

20.8 Opportunities and Challenges for the Future

The exciting advances being made in neoadjuvant therapy for HER-2+ breast cancer suggest the opportunity to improve outcome for patients and possibly reduce the need for aggressive local therapies including surgery and radiation. Challenges still remain in advancing the care of patients including the need for improved imaging to detect the presence of residual disease in the breast and axilla following NAC, the need to better understand the relationships between pathologic complete response and locoregional control, the need to better assess the axilla to exclude the presence of metastatic disease following NAC, and the need to understand the role of radiation therapy in selected patients who have had excellent response to NAC. It is expected that ongoing and future studies aimed at understanding these concepts will continue to transform the care of patients with HER-2+ breast cancer.

References

1. Mitri Z, Constantine T, O'Regan R (2012) The HER2 receptor in breast cancer: pathophysiology, clinical use, and new advances in therapy. Chemother Res Pract 2012:743193

2. Johnston SR (2013) Dual HER2 targeting for early breast cancer. Lancet Oncol 14:1145–1146
3. Slamon DJ, Leyland-Jones B, Shak S et al (2001) Use of chemotherapy plus a monoclonal antibody against HER2 for metastatic breast cancer that overexpresses HER2. N Engl J Med 344:783–792
4. Romond EH, Perez EA, Bryant J et al (2005) Trastuzumab plus adjuvant chemotherapy for operable HER2-positive breast cancer. N Engl J Med 353:1673–1684
5. von Minckwitz G, Untch M, Blohmer JU et al (2012) Definition and impact of pathologic complete response on prognosis after neoadjuvant chemotherapy in various intrinsic breast cancer subtypes. J Clin Oncol 30:1796–1804
6. Gianni L, Pienkowski T, Im YH et al (2012) Efficacy and safety of neoadjuvant pertuzumab and trastuzumab in women with locally advanced, inflammatory, or early HER2-positive breast cancer (NeoSphere): a randomised multicentre, open-label, phase 2 trial. Lancet Oncol 13:25–32
7. Baselga J, Bradbury I, Eidtmann H et al (2012) Lapatinib with trastuzumab for HER2-positive early breast cancer (NeoALTTO): a randomised, open-label, multicentre, phase 3 trial. Lancet 379:633–640
8. Guarneri V, Frassoldati A, Bottini A et al (2012) Preoperative chemotherapy plus trastuzumab, lapatinib, or both in human epidermal growth factor receptor 2-positive operable breast cancer: results of the randomized phase II CHER-LOB study. J Clin Oncol 30:1989–1995
9. Robidoux A, Tang G, Rastogi P et al (2013) Lapatinib as a component of neoadjuvant therapy for HER2-positive operable breast cancer (NSABP protocol B-41): an open-label, randomised phase 3 trial. Lancet Oncol 14:1183–1192
10. Schneeweiss A, Chia S, Hickish T et al (2013) Pertuzumab plus trastuzumab in combination with standard neoadjuvant anthracycline-containing and anthracycline-free chemotherapy regimens in patients with HER2-positive early breast cancer: a randomized phase II cardiac safety study (TRYPHAENA). Ann Oncol 24:2278–2284
11. Amiri-Kordestani L, Wedam S, Zhang L et al (2014) First FDA approval of neoadjuvant therapy for breast cancer: pertuzumab for the treatment of patients with HER2-positive breast cancer. Clin Cancer Res 20:5359–5364
12. Marinovich ML, Macaskill P, Irwig L et al (2013) Meta-analysis of agreement between MRI and pathologic breast tumour size after neoadjuvant chemotherapy. Br J Cancer 109:1528–1536
13. Marinovich ML, Houssami N, Macaskill P et al (2013) Meta-analysis of magnetic resonance imaging in detecting residual breast cancer after neoadjuvant therapy. J Natl Cancer Inst 105:321–333
14. Gebhart G, Gamez C, Holmes E et al (2013) 18F-FDG PET/CT for early prediction of response to neoadjuvant lapatinib, trastuzumab, and their combination in HER2-positive breast cancer: results from Neo-ALTTO. J Nucl Med 54:1862–1868
15. Mortellaro VE, Marshall J, Singer L et al (2009) Magnetic resonance imaging for axillary staging in patients with breast cancer. J Magn Reson Imaging 30:309–312
16. Henry-Tillman R, Glover-Collins K, Preston M et al (2015) The SAVE review: sonographic analysis versus excision for axillary staging in breast cancer. J Am Coll Surg 220:560–567
17. Valente SA, Levine GM, Silverstein MJ et al (2012) Accuracy of predicting axillary lymph node positivity by physical examination, mammography, ultrasonography, and magnetic resonance imaging. Ann Surg Oncol 19:1825–1830
18. Akers WJ, Kim C, Berezin M et al (2011) Noninvasive photoacoustic and fluorescence sentinel lymph node identification using dye-loaded perfluorocarbon nanoparticles. ACS Nano 5:173–182
19. Teshome M, Hunt KK (2014) Neoadjuvant therapy in the treatment of breast cancer. Surg Oncol Clin N Am 23:505–523
20. von Minckwitz G, Rezai M, Loibl S et al (2010) Capecitabine in addition to anthracycline- and taxane-based neoadjuvant treatment in patients with primary breast cancer: phase III GeparQuattro study. J Clin Oncol 28:2015–2023

21. Untch M, Fasching PA, Konecny GE et al (2011) Pathologic complete response after neoadjuvant chemotherapy plus trastuzumab predicts favorable survival in human epidermal growth factor receptor 2-overexpressing breast cancer: results from the TECHNO trial of the AGO and GBG study groups. J Clin Oncol 29:3351–3357
22. Semiglazov V, Eiermann W, Zambetti M et al (2011) Surgery following neoadjuvant therapy in patients with HER2-positive locally advanced or inflammatory breast cancer participating in the NeOAdjuvant Herceptin (NOAH) study. Eur J Surg Oncol 37:856–863
23. Im SA, Lee KS, Ro J et al (2012) Phase II trial of preoperative paclitaxel, gemcitabine, and trastuzumab combination therapy in HER2 positive stage II/III breast cancer: the Korean Cancer Study Group BR 07-01. Breast Cancer Res Treat 132:589–600
24. Buzdar AU, Suman VJ, Meric-Bernstam F et al (2013) Fluorouracil, epirubicin, and cyclophosphamide (FEC-75) followed by paclitaxel plus trastuzumab versus paclitaxel plus trastuzumab followed by FEC-75 plus trastuzumab as neoadjuvant treatment for patients with HER2-positive breast cancer (Z1041): a randomised, controlled, phase 3 trial. Lancet Oncol 14:1317–1325
25. Criscitiello C, Azim HA Jr, Agbor-tarh D et al (2013) Factors associated with surgical management following neoadjuvant therapy in patients with primary HER2-positive breast cancer: results from the NeoALTTO phase III trial. Ann Oncol 24:1980–1985
26. Arsenault D, Hurley J, Takita C, et al (2015) Predictors of locoregional outcome in HER2-overexpressing breast cancer treated with neoadjuvant chemotherapy. Am J Clin Oncol 38 (4):348–352
27. Cortazar P, Zhang L, Untch M et al (2012) Meta-analysis results from the Collaborative Trials in Neoadjuvant Breast Cancer (CTNeoBC). Cancer Res 72:P1-14-20
28. von Minckwitz G, Kaufmann M, Kümmel S et al (2011) Local recurrence risk in 6377 patients with early breast cancer receiving neoadjuvant anthracycline-taxane +/− trastuzumab containing chemotherapy. Cancer Res 71:S3-2
29. Ring A, Webb A, Ashley S et al (2003) Is surgery necessary after complete clinical remission following neoadjuvant chemotherapy for early breast cancer? J Clin Oncol 21:4540–4545
30. Bernier J (2015) Post-mastectomy radiotherapy after neodjuvant chemotherapy in breast cancer patients: a review. Crit Rev Oncol Hematol 93:180–189
31. Garg AK, Buchholz TA (2015) Influence of neoadjuvant chemotherapy on radiotherapy for breast cancer. Ann Surg Oncol 22:1434–1440

Part VII
Mathematical Prediction/ Assessment Model

Chapter 21
Nomograms to Predict Positive Resection Margin and to Predict Three or More Positive Lymph Nodes

Eunshin Lee and Wonshik Han

Abstract A nomogram is a graphical calculating device, a two-dimensional diagram designed to allow the approximate graphical computation of a function. Nomograms have been developed for various purposes in clinical use of cancer managements. We will introduce some good examples of useful nomograms for breast cancer surgeons.

The first one is a nomogram that can predict the probability of having tumor-positive resection margins in breast-conserving surgery. Factors included in this nomogram are the presence of microcalcification in mammography, high mammographic density, high tumor size discrepancy between MRI and ultrasonography (>5 mm), the presence of DCIS component in needle biopsy specimen, and the presence of lobular carcinoma on needle biopsy. The AUC of ROC curves was excellent in the training set and the validation set. The efficacy of this nomogram was proved in a prospective cohort and was validated in another institution. This tool is useful for surgeons to reduce frozen section biopsy (FSB) without increasing the reoperation rate. Also, it can provide useful information about the possibility of tumor-positive resection margin for surgeons who are not performing FSB.

The second one is a nomogram that can predict the probability of having three or more positive sentinel lymph nodes. Factors included in this nomogram are imaging findings such as axillary lymph node grading by ultrasonography and chest CT finding of axillary lymph node. The AUC was also excellent in the training set and the validation set. When we applied this nomogram to patients who met the criteria of ACOSOG Z0011 trial, 88.3 % of the patients could be spared FSB of sentinel node, and reoperation rate was only 1.6 %. This nomogram is useful for surgeons especially who follow the Z0011 trial result and who want to do selective intraoperative analysis of SLN.

Keywords Breast cancer • Nomogram • Resection margin • Sentinel lymph node

---

E. Lee • W. Han (✉)
Department of Surgery, Seoul National University College of Medicine, 101 Daehak-ro, Jongno-gu, Seoul 110-744, South Korea
e-mail: hanw@snu.ac.kr

M. Toi et al. (eds.), *Personalized Treatment of Breast Cancer*,
DOI 10.1007/978-4-431-55552-0_21

21.1 Nomogram for Predicting Positive Resection Margins After Breast-Conserving Surgery (BCS)

21.1.1 Introduction of Nomogram for Predicting Positive Resection Margins After BCS

Positive resection margin(s) after breast-conserving surgery (BCS) is the most important risk factor for ipsilateral breast tumor recurrence [1, 2]. Reoperation is inevitable in most cases if tumor cells are found on inked resection margin(s) in pathologic examination after BCS. However, wider excision after initial surgery or multiple re-excisions could result in a poorer cosmetic outcome. Multiple re-excisions also increase the patients' anxiety and medical costs. One option to reduce reoperation is intraoperative assessment of resection margins using frozen section biopsy (FSB). However, false negative rate is high, and even false positive result is possible with the FSB. In addition, FSB usually makes the surgery time longer and the cost higher. So, it is not widely used in breast cancer surgery. In these perspectives, a tool to predict the risk of positive resection margins after BCS is very useful to perform selective FSB in patients with predicted high probability for positive resection margins. It might be advantageous for both surgeons and patients.

Several factors have been reported to be associated with positive resection margins in previous studies, including lobular histology, size of tumor on pathology, tumor grade, multifocality, the presence of extensive intraductal component (EIC), and lymphovascular invasion (LVI) [3]. However, many of these factors' information are available after the evaluation of paraffin-embedded surgical specimens (Fig. 21.1).

21.1.2 Development of Nomogram for Predicting Positive Resection Margins After BCS

Data from 1,034 consecutive breast cancer patients with invasive or in situ breast cancer who initially underwent BCS in single institution (Seoul National University Hospital, Seoul, Korea) between January 2008 and December 2009 were used to develop a nomogram for predicting positive resection margins. The nomogram was then validated independently using a cohort of 563 patients who underwent breast surgery in 2010. Multivariate logistic regression analysis showed that microcalcifications in mammography (OR 1.57, $P = 0.034$), grade 4 mammographic density (OR 4.51, $P = 0.005$), >0.5 cm difference in tumor size between magnetic resonance imaging (MRI) and ultrasonography (OR 10.00, $P < 0.0001$), the presence of ductal carcinoma in situ (DCIS) on needle biopsy (OR 1.57, $P = 0.044$), and lobular component on needle biopsy (OR 3.98, $P = 0.015$) were independent predictors of positive resection margins (Table 21.1). These significant variables were used to

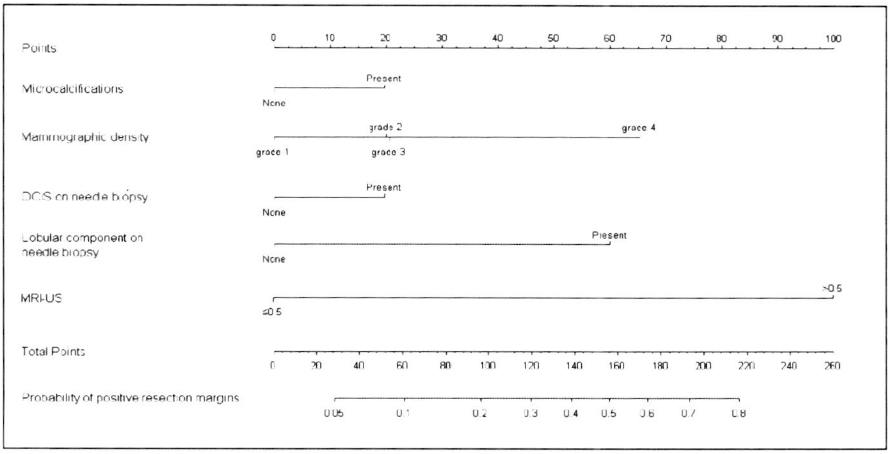

Fig. 21.1 Nomogram for predicting positive resection margins after breast-conserving surgery. This nomogram includes five imaging or pathologic factors: the presence of microcalcification in mammography; high mammographic density; tumor size discrepancy between MRI and ultrasonography (>5 mm); the presence of DCIS component in needle biopsy specimen; and the presence of lobular carcinoma on needle biopsy

Table 21.1 Multivariate logistic regression model for positive resection margins in the validation cohort

Variables	N	Odds ratio	*p*-value
Microcalcifications			
None	678		
Present	356	1.574	0.034
Mammographic density			
1	69		
2	220	1.590	0.411
3	482	1.611	0.376
4	263	4.515	0.005
MRI-US (cm)			
≤0.5	867		
>0.5	167	10.001	<0.001
DCIS on needle biopsy			
None	773		
Present	261	1.575	0.044
Lobular component on needle biopsy			
None	1014		
Present	20	3.985	0.015

develop a nomogram for predicting positive resection margins. The AUC of receiver operating characteristic (ROC) curve of the study and the validation cohort were 0.823 [95 % confidence interval (CI), 0.785–0.862] and 0.846 (95 % CI, 0.800–0.892), respectively (Fig. 21.2).

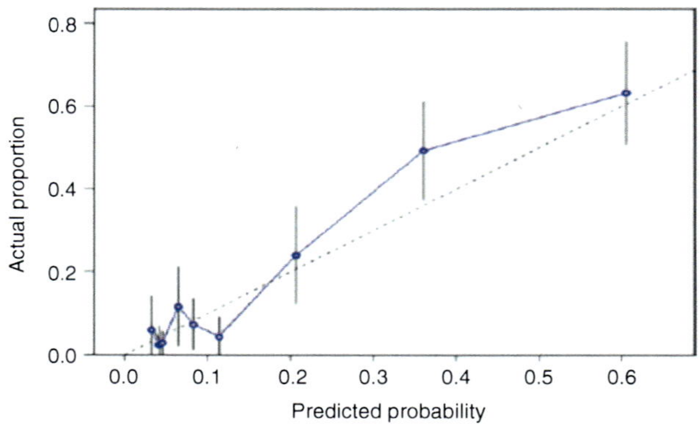

Fig. 21.2 Calibration plot of the nomogram using the validation cohort

21.1.3 Prospective Study of the Nomogram in SNUH and Validation Study in Kyoto University

We conducted a prospective study to investigate the clinical usefulness of the nomogram. The aim of this investigation was to compare the reoperation rate and surgery time between surgeries using this nomogram and the past control group without this nomogram. In the past, we conducted routine intraoperative frozen section biopsy (FSB) in almost all patients. After application of the nomogram, we omitted the intraoperative FSB in patients who presented low nomogram score. About 62 % of all BCS patients during the study period presented low nomogram score and avoided FSB. Surgical decision using the nomogram did not significantly increase reoperation rate due to positive RM compared with control FSB group (4.6 % vs. 3.8 %, $p = 0.47$). The surgery time was significantly reduced by 18.1 % (mean 14.7 min) in nomogram group ($p < 0.001$).

In the Kyoto University Hospital, the reoperation rate was significantly lower in patients with low score than in patients with high score (2.7 % vs. 11.4 %, $p < 0.001$) (Tables 21.2 and 21.3).

21.1.4 Use of Nomogram for Predicting Positive Resection Margins After BCS

Below is an example of application of this nomogram to a clinical case (Fig. 21.5).

A woman had infiltrating ductal carcinoma in her breast. Mammography showed microcalcification in the tumor and grade 3 density. Tumor size was 23 and 25 mm

Table 21.2 Mean operation time and reoperation rate due to tumor cell-positive resection margin in the control group and the nomogram group

	Control group N = 266	Nomogram group N = 260	p-value
Frozen section biopsy			
Yes	258 (97 %)	99 (38.1 %)	
No	8 (3 %)	161 (61.9 %)	
Mean operation time (min)	81.2	66.5	$p < 0.001$
High-score group (frozen bx. yes)		82.8	
Low-score group (frozen bx. no)		56.4	
Reoperation (%)	10 (3.76 %)	12 (4.61 %)	$p = 0.465$
High-score group (N = 99)		6 (6.1 %)	
Low-score group (N = 161)		6 (3.7 %)	

Table 21.3 Reoperation rate of low- vs. high-score group in the validation set of Kyoto University Hospital

	Low-score group[a] N = 111	High-score group N = 70	p-value
Reoperation (%)	3 (2.7 %)	8 (11.4 %)	<0.001

[a]Score in our nomogram <80, low-score group, ≥80 high-score group

in ultrasonography and MRI, respectively. The pathology in needle biopsy did not show DCIS or lobular component. The nomogram total score was 40, and as a result the probability of positive resection margin was below 10 %. This patient did not need intraoperative FSB based on this nomogram.

Let us see another case (Fig. 21.6).

The patient had 15 mm invasive carcinoma in breast US and core needle biopsy. On mammography, density grade was 4 and there was no microcalcification. There was lobular carcinoma component in the needle biopsy specimen. Total extent of the tumor was 38 mm in MRI. The nomogram score was calculated to be 220, and the probability of positive resection margin was above 80 %. For this patient, intraoperative FSB would be helpful to reduce reoperation.

21.1.5 Considerations Using the Nomogram for Prediction of Positive Resection Margins

A disadvantage to use this nomogram in routine clinical practice is that both of preoperative breast ultrasonography and MRI are compulsory. The clinical benefit of routine use of breast ultrasonography or MRI is controversial [4, 5] besides this nomogram.

Another issue is the core biopsy method. The use of a larger gauge vacuum-assisted biopsy would have more chances to find DCIS component in the biopsy specimen than that of a 14-gauge gun [6, 7]. The higher incidence of finding DCIS would result in a higher nomogram score. The cutoff of the nomogram score should be adjusted for each individual site for use.

21.2 Nomogram for Predicting Three or More Axillary Lymph Node Involvement Before Breast Cancer Surgery

21.2.1 Introduction of Nomogram for Predicting Three or More Axillary Lymph Node Involvement Before Breast Cancer Surgery

There have been major changes in the standard management of axilla in invasive breast cancer, progressing from axillary lymph node dissection (ALND) to sentinel lymph node biopsy (SLNB). Recently, a result from American College of Surgeons Oncology Group (ACOSOG) Z0011 study indicates that women with one or two involved axillary nodes and clinical T1–T2 tumors undergoing lumpectomy with radiation therapy followed by systemic therapy do not benefit from completion of ALND in terms of recurrence and survival [8]. As a result, it now appears that a significant proportion of patients may not require ALND at all.

Knowledge of the status of axillary lymph node involvement before surgical intervention might be able to allow informed discussion of management options with the patients and make individualized multidisciplinary treatment feasible [9]. We hypothesized that it would be possible to select patients predicted to have high tumor burden in axillary lymph node, as to select patients who needs intraoperative analysis of SLN by using preoperative imaging and preoperatively gathered clinicopathological information.

We developed a nomogram to predict the probability of having three or more axillary nodes involvement for usage in clinical practice (Fig. 21.3). Our data suggested that patients with a high probability of having three or more axillary lymph nodes can be identified using the preoperative images and patient's characteristics. The nomogram that we developed will be useful for surgeons especially who follow the ACOSOG Z0011 trial result and who want to do selective intraoperative analysis of SLN.

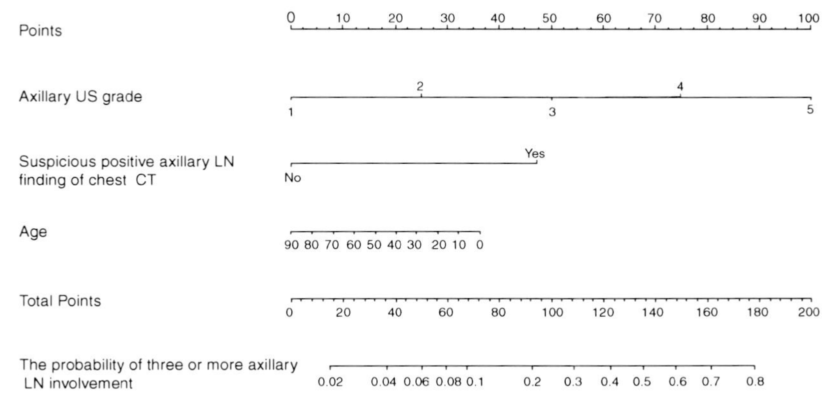

Total Points	15	37	50	60	67	92	109	123	135	148	161	178
Likelihood	0.02	0.04	0.06	0.08	0.1	0.2	0.3	0.4	0.5	0.6	0.7	0.8

Fig. 21.3 Nomogram for predicting the probability of having three or more involved axillary lymph nodes

21.2.2 Development of Nomogram for Predicting Three or More Axillary Lymph Node Involvement Before Breast Cancer Surgery

We reviewed the records of 1,917 patients with clinical T1–T2 and clinical node-negative invasive breast cancer. Patients who received neoadjuvant chemotherapy were excluded. Factors associated with having three or more involved axillary nodes were evaluated by univariate and multivariate logistic regression analysis. A nomogram was developed and validated in 378 independent patients. Two hundred four of 1917 patients (10.6 %) had three or more positive nodes. On a multivariate analysis, three or more nodes involvement was associated with the axillary lymph node category assessed by ultrasonography and the presence of suspicious axillary lymph node on chest CT. Area under ROC curve for the multivariate logistic regression model involving ultrasonography and CT finding was 0.852 (95 % CI: 0.820–0.883) and 0.896 (95 % CI: 0.836–0.957) in the training set and a validation set of 378 patients, respectively (Fig. 21.4). A nomogram to predict the probability of having three or more axillary nodes involvement was developed (Table 21.4).

21.2.3 Prospective Application of the Established Nomogram

We applied our nomogram prospectively to 512 invasive breast cancer patients who were operated between January, 2012 and June, 2014 and who met the criteria of

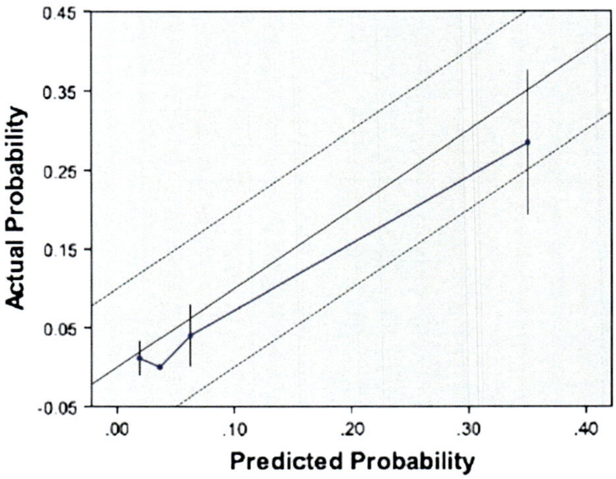

Fig. 21.4 Calibration plot of the nomogram using validation cohort

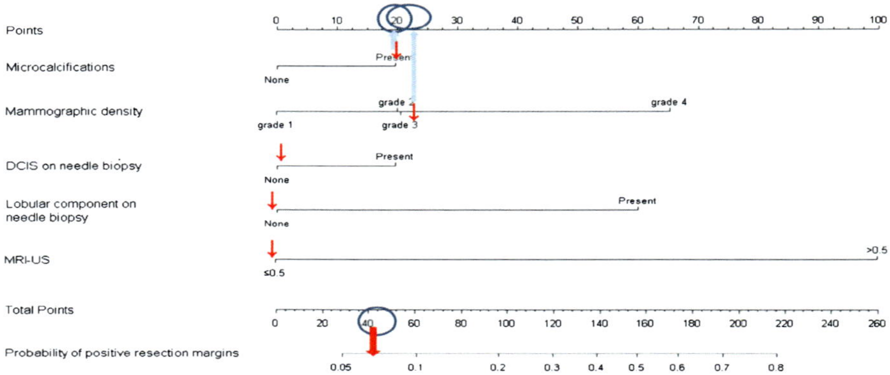

Fig. 21.5 Example of application of nomogram for predicting positive resection margins after BCS

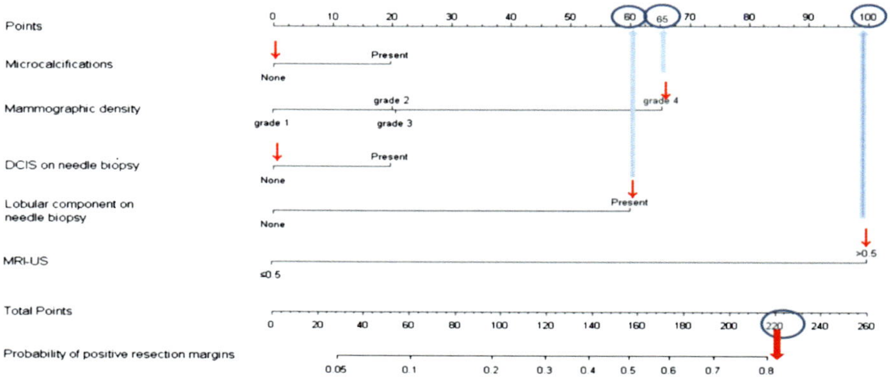

Fig. 21.6 Example of application of nomogram for predicting positive resection margins after BCS

Table 21.4 Multivariate logistic regression analysis of factors associated with involvement of three or more axillary lymph nodes

Variable	Odds ratio	95 % CI	P
Age	0.99	0.97–1.00	0.097
Tumor size by preop. US(cm)	1.08	0.91–1.28	0.392
Axillary US grade	2.13	1.80–2.52	<0.001
Chest CT-ALN positive	4.78	3.07–7.45	<0.001

Z0011 trial. Four hundred fifty two patients (88.3 %) had nomogram score below the cutoff and could be spared intraoperative frozen analysis of SLN. As a result, we could save the cost of frozen biopsy and operation time (data not shown). In these patients with low score and without frozen biopsy, only eight patients (1.6 % of all 512 patients) needed reoperation for completion ALND with three or more positive SLNs. If we had applied no-frozen biopsy strategy for all of these patients without using the nomogram, 22 patients (4.3 %) would have been received reoperation.

21.2.4 *Use of Nomogram for Predicting Three or More Axillary Lymph Node Involvement Before Breast Cancer Surgery*

Preoperative ultrasonography (US) and chest CT are required for this nomogram. Axillary US examination was performed 1 day before surgery. The lymph node was classified according to the maximum thickness of the cortex and the appearance of the fatty hilum as follows: grade 1, cortical thickness of $\leq$1.5 mm; grade 2, 1.5 mm< cortical thickness $\leq$2.5 mm; grade 3, 2.5 mm< cortical thickness $\leq$3.5 mm; grade 4, cortical thickness >3.5 mm with an intact fatty hilum; and grade 5, cortical thickness >3.5 mm with a loss of the fatty hilum. The maximum cortical thickness was measured perpendicular to the long axis of the lymph node on a cross-sectional plane [10]. In chest CT, axillary lymph node was considered as positive with one or more of the following CT findings of axillary lymph nodes: shortest diameter more than 1 cm, loss of fatty hilum, or the presence of central necrosis.

Below is an example of application of this nomogram to a clinical case (Fig. 21.7).

A 40-year-old woman had infiltrating ductal carcinoma. In US, the axillary LN was classified as Gr 3 (2.5 mm< cortical thickness $\leq$3.5 mm) by the criteria of Cho et al. The chest CT showed no suspicious axillary LN. The nomogram score was about 70 and the probability of having three or more axillary lymph node involvement was about 10 %. Intraoperative FSB of SLN was skipped in this patient.

Let us see another case (Fig. 21.8).

The patient was 70 years old with invasive breast cancer. Axillary LN was not palpable in physical examination. She had Gr 4 (cortical thickness >3.5 mm with

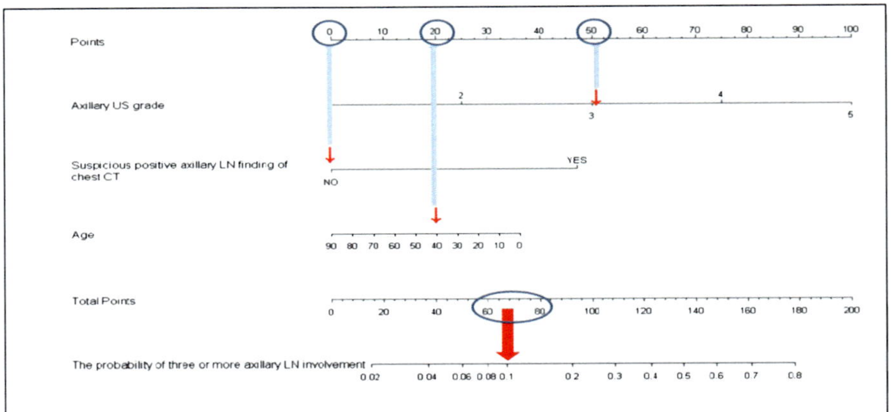

Total Points	15	37	50	60	67	92	109	123	135	148	161	178
Likelihood	0.02	0.04	0.06	0.08	0.1	0.2	0.3	0.4	0.5	0.6	0.7	0.8

Fig. 21.7 Example of application of nomogram for predicting three or more axillary lymph node involvement

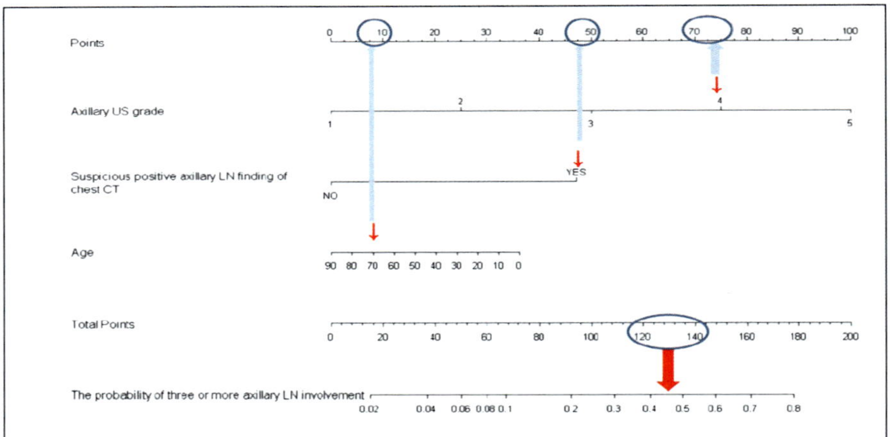

Total Points	15	37	50	60	67	92	109	123	135	148	161	178
Likelihood	0.02	0.04	0.06	0.08	0.1	0.2	0.3	0.4	0.5	0.6	0.7	0.8

Fig. 21.8 Example of application of nomogram for predicting three or more axillary lymph node involvement

an intact fatty hilum) LN in axillary US. In chest CT, there were enhanced and enlarged LNs (more than 1 cm) in the axilla. The score in nomogram was 130–140, the probability of predicting three or more axillary lymph node involvement before breast cancer surgery was about 50 %. For this patient, intraoperative FSB would be helpful to reduce reoperation.

21.2.5 Considerations of Using the Nomogram for Predicting Three or More Axillary Lymph Node Involvement

There are several issues with this nomogram. US classification of axillary LN could be subjective. Chest CT is not a routine imaging modality for breast cancer metastasis work-up in most institutions.

Also, our nomogram could not be so useful for surgeons who do not follow the Z0011 trial result in clinical practice. As evolution of image modality is rapid, further investigations are warranted to improve our nomogram by adding other image modalities.

References

1. Shin HC, Han W, Moon HG, Cho N, Moon WK, Park IA, Park SJ, Noh DY (2012) Nomogram for predicting positive resection margins after breast-conserving surgery. Breast Cancer Res Treat 134(3):1115–1123
2. Kreike B, Hart AA et al (2008) Continuing risk of ipsilateral breast relapse after breast-conserving therapy at long-term follow-up. Int J Radiat Oncol Biol Phys 71:1014–1021
3. Mechera R, Viehl CT et al (2009) Factors predicting inbreast tumor recurrence after breast-conserving surgery. Breast Cancer Res Treat 116:171–177
4. Lovrics PJ, Cornacchi SD et al (2009) The relationship between surgical factors and margin status after breast-conservation surgery for early stage breast cancer. Am J Surg 197:740–746
5. Saslow D, Boetes C et al (2007) American Cancer Society guidelines for breast screening with MRI as an adjunct to mammography. CA Cancer J Clin 57(2):75–89
6. Bilimoria KY, Cambic A et al (2007) Evaluating the impact of preoperative breast magnetic resonance imaging on the surgical management of newly diagnosed breast cancers. Arch Surg (Chicago, Ill: 1960) 142(5):441–445; discussion 445-447
7. Rakha EA, Ellis IO (2007) An overview of assessment of prognostic and predictive factors in breast cancer needle core biopsy specimens. J Clin Pathol 60(12):1300–1306
8. Giuliano AE, Hunt KK, Ballman KV et al (2011) Axillary dissection vs no axillary dissection in women with invasive breast cancer and sentinel node metastasis: a randomized clinical trial. JAMA 305:569–575
9. Valente SA, Levine GM, Silverstein MJ et al (2012) Accuracy of predicting axillary lymph node positivity by physical examination, mammography, ultrasonography, and magnetic resonance imaging. Ann Surg Oncol 19:1825–1830
10. Cho N, Moon WK, Han W et al (2009) Preoperative sonographic classification of axillary lymph nodes in patients with breast cancer: node-to-node correlation with surgical histology and sentinel node biopsy results. AJR Am J Roentgenol 193:1731–1737

Chapter 22
Practical Use of Nomograms

José Luiz B. Bevilacqua, Paulo R. de Alcantara Filho, Lillian Fraianella, and Carla Curi

Abstract To predict an event or create predictive models, parameters that are associated with the final outcome ("end-points") are usually used. Although medical literature presents a myriad of studies on disease predictors, it is very difficult to accurately and numerically answer many questions that are often raised by physicians and patients themselves. Statistical modeling, especially regressions, can help answer these questions in a more objective fashion. Nonetheless, clinical judgment should not be underestimated but may be improved, if necessary, with the aid of statistical models. Decision to diagnose or treat in any clinical scenario must undergo medical judgment and physician-patient relationship; thus, statistical models should be used only to support decision-making.

Keywords Breast cancer • Nomogram • Predicting tools

22.1 Introduction

To predict an event or create predictive models, parameters that are associated to the final outcome ("end-point") are usually used. Nevertheless, our predictive ability is generally limited when compared to statistical models. This stems from the multifactorial nature of natural and biological events in which there are numerous associations and correlations between these events; the nonlinearity of outcomes and the rarity of perfection between causality and effect make it difficult to predict with perfection. The fashion in which study results are generally expressed – the odds ratio or relative risk in respect to a sub-variable – is of difficult clinical application. The results should be easily applicable, presented in a practical and measurable way, preferably in the form of percentage figures. Nevertheless, the decision to diagnose or treat in any clinical scenario must undergo medical judgment and physician-patient relationship; thus, statistical models should be used only to support decision-making.

J.L.B. Bevilacqua (✉) • P.R. de Alcantara Filho • L. Fraianella • C. Curi
Department of Breast Surgery, A. C. Camargo Cancer Center, São Paulo, Brazil
e-mail: jose.bevilacqua@accamargo.org.br

M. Toi et al. (eds.), *Personalized Treatment of Breast Cancer*,
DOI 10.1007/978-4-431-55552-0_22

In recent years, predictive risk models of cancer, including breast cancer, have grown substantially in number as they gained great attention of researchers, physicians, and the public in general, including cancer government agencies of the United States, such as the National Cancer Institute (NCI), which funds numerous researches on the subject. Recently, three other statistical models have been developed in the form of a nomogram which has been quite useful in predicting axillary metastases in breast cancer: a nomogram for prediction of metastasis in sentinel lymph nodes (SLN), a nomogram for prediction of metastasis in non-SLN, and nomograms for prediction of lymphedema in patients undergoing axillary dissection for breast cancer.

Statistical modeling, which integrates clinical information and gene expression, has great potential to significantly improve the prognostic ability of predictive models in oncology. No statistical model is perfect, and thus, the models need to be continuously developed, improved, and validated. Validation of a statistical model, in a separate, distinct sample from the one in which it was developed, is of utmost importance to show the power of the model. Unfortunately, most published models do not have prospective validation in different samples.

This chapter will address nomograms for predicting lymph node metastases and lymphedema. It is divided in two parts: the first addresses the predictive factors of axillary lymph node metastases and lymphedema and the other addresses nomograms. An extensive review of the literature on predictors of metastases and lymphedema is presented.

22.2 Predictive Factors of Axillary Node Metastases and Lymphedema

22.2.1 Predictive Factors of Axillary Lymph Node and Axillary SLN Metastasis

Information on the presence of lymph node metastasis is a major prognostic factor in patients with invasive breast carcinoma [1–7]. Axillary lymphadenectomy (ALND) has been used in the treatment of this disease for centuries [8–13]. Until the 1980s, the importance of systematic ALND as part of the surgical treatment was unquestionable. The NSABP-B04 study is the first to question the therapeutic value of axillary dissection placed exclusively as a prognostic factor of postoperative progression of the disease [14–16]. With the widespread use of mammography for early diagnosis of breast cancer, there has been a significant increase in the number of cases diagnosed at an early stage of the disease, i.e., non-palpable small tumors. Consequently, diagnoses can now be made in situations in which the frequency of axillary metastases is much smaller. Therefore, many authors have questioned the necessity of the realization of ALND in these small tumors, since this procedure is not without morbidity [17]. In an attempt to better select patients for ALND, several

Table 22.1 Predictive factors of SLN metastasis – Pre-SLN era

Variables	Number of studies	References
Size	20	[17–36]
Age	10	[20, 23–26, 34, 35, 37, 38]
LVI (lymphatic vascular invasion)	7	[18, 19, 23–25, 33, 36]
Histological type	7	[23, 26, 30–33, 38]
Tumor location	4	[25, 26, 32, 38]
Palpability	3	[18, 25, 33]
Nuclear grade	4	[18, 25, 36, 39]
Histological grade	3	[22, 32, 35]
Tumor grade	2	[26, 40]
Multifocality	2	[23, 24]
Estrogen receptor	2	[26, 34]
Clinical lymph node status	2	[24, 33]
Menopause status	1	[24]
Progesterone receptor	1	[26]
Her-2/neu	1	[28]
Margin status	1	[37]
Spiculated margins	1	[23]
S-phase	1	[34]
Ploidy	1	[26]
Race	1	[26]
Microcalcifications	1	[40]
Number of lymph nodes analyzed	1	[38]
Nipple invasion	1	[38]
Parity	1	[24]

retrospective studies have attempted to identify predictive factors of lymph node metastasis [17–36] (Table 22.1). The most frequent variables independently associated with axillary metastases are tumor size, age, lymphatic vascular invasion (LVI), and histological subtype of the tumor. Table 22.1 summarizes the independent factors associated with lymph node metastases in breast cancer described in the literature.

The advent of the SLN concept [36, 41], as well as its application in the staging of the axilla in breast cancer [29–31], enabled patient selection for ALND, proposed only in cases of metastasis in SLN. The SLN biopsy has gained importance in that it proved to be technically simple, a very effective procedure in the staging of the axilla and associated with minimal morbidity [21, 22, 38, 42–44]. This biopsy has been adopted as a standard procedure in axillary staging. It replaces systematic ALND, when the excised SLN is negative for metastases. SLN biopsy has high accuracy in axillary staging and is at least equal to ALND.

The study of Bevilacqua et al. [35] demonstrates that age, palpability, tumor location within the breast, lymph vascular invasion (LVI), multifocality, positive progesterone receptor, tumor size, histological subtype, histological grade, and nuclear grade are predictors of SLN metastases in the univariate analysis. However, multivariate analysis revealed that the independent predictors of SLN metastases in breast cancer were histological type, LVI, tumor size, tumor location, age, nuclear grade (+ lobular), and multifocality. Therefore, the inclusion of lobular histology in nuclear grade was needed so as not to automatically exclude it from the logistic regression. As might be expected, other studies in the pre-SLN era [24–26, 32, 33, 37, 45] also demonstrated that the factors are predictors of axillary metastases (Table 22.1).

The variables associated with lymph node metastases have not changed dramatically with the advent of the SLN, strengthening confidence in the SLN biopsy procedure in breast cancer.

Only a minority of published studies identified nuclear grade and histological grade as predictors of lymph node metastasis (Table 22.1). These variables may be absent in the results of other studies, since many pathologists and institutions, including MSKCC, do not classify invasive lobular carcinoma neither in nuclear nor in histological grade. In Bevilacqua et al.'s [35] study, multifocality is an independent predictor of metastases in SLN. Only a few studies show multifocality as a predictor of lymph node metastasis [23, 24]. Another explanation for this finding is that multifocal carcinomas generally have a greater tumor volume than similar staged unifocal tumors, and tumor size is a predictor of lymph node metastasis. Perhaps, multifocality contributes to determine the best volume in multifocal tumors. Another study conducted at MSKCC revealed that multifocality is also an independent factor of worse disease-free survival [46]. Moreover, tumor location also proved to be an independent SLN metastasis factor in the multivariate analysis [35]. Furthermore, four of these studies cite the location of the tumor as an independent predictor of lymph node metastasis and report a higher frequency of lymph node metastasis associated with lateral tumors [25, 26, 32, 47, 48]. Gann et al. [26] analyzed 18,000 patients from the American College database. The lesser frequency of metastases in axillary lymph nodes, including SLN, observed in medial tumors in our study and identified in the literature, supports the hypothesis of alternative routes of lymphatic flow at that location. Lohrish et al. [49], Asaga et al. [50], and Zucali et al. [51] demonstrate a worse prognosis in terms of disease-free and overall survival, associated with medial quarter tumors compared to lateral quadrant tumors. Israel et al. [52] reported differences in patterns of distant metastases in medial tumors. These studies [49, 52–54] all explain that the differences may be due to the greater likelihood of metastases to the lymph nodes of the internal mammary artery associated with medial tumors. This is also confirmed by Bevilacqua et al. [53] in an extensive review of the literature related to the approach of metastases in the internal mammary chain in breast cancer. Another curious fact noted by Bevilacqua is the apparent differences in the rates of metastases in SLN between ductal and lobular carcinomas, respectively 31.5 % and 40.3 % ($P < 0.0001$) [53]. A possible explanation would be the differences associated with other variables, such as multifocality, known to be more frequent in lobular tumor histology. This author has identified differences in the following variables: age, represented by the median and the age distribution; tumor size, represented by

T stage and the median; positivity of estrogen receptors and HER-2/neu; distribution of the location of the tumor; LVI; and multifocality. Nevertheless, in multivariate analysis, the difference between ductal and lobular carcinoma ceased to exist; i.e., there is no statistical difference in relation to metastasis between SLN in ductal and lobular carcinoma ($P = 0.142$). The difference observed in the univariate analysis is not independent and can be explained by differences in other variables. Thus, the developed logistic regression tumor models of ductal and lobular histology were grouped into a single group and compared with the tumors.

22.2.2 *Predictive Factors of Metastasis in Non-SLN (Additional Axillary Lymph Nodes)*

The number of affected axillary lymph nodes is an important prognostic factor and is even adopted in the current version of TNM. Therefore, SLN information only as positive or negative is somewhat limited. The information on the number of lymph nodes may in some circumstances assist in therapeutic decision of radiotherapy or adjuvant chemotherapy. In MKSCC's series, in 38 % of cases in which the SLN was positive, other axillary lymph nodes (non-SLN) were also affected, as opposed to rates as high as 50 % in the literature [29–31, 55–60]. This can be explained by the number of patients in these studies, lower than in the MSKCC study [61].

According to the above findings, 62 % of patients with a positive SLN should not have any additional positive axillary lymph node, which makes mandatory ALND in all cases questionable. Several clinical pathologic factors are associated with the presence of additional non-SLN disease (Table 22.2). We can observe that the series of some studies are limited, since many neither perform multivariate analysis of the observations nor validate the results from different samples. Tumor size and the size of SLN metastasis are the most commonly analyzed factors. However, none of these studies included in Table 22.2 is able to safely identify a group exempt at risk for metastasis in non-SLN [55, 57–59, 62–67]. Table 22.3 summarizes the literature that demonstrates the influence of tumor size on the incidence of metastasis in non-SLN. As expected, the larger the tumor, the greater the probability of metastasis in non-SLN, as seen in Table 22.4, which shows the impact of LVI positivity existing in non-SLN information. The influence of the size of SLN metastasis as a predictor of non-SLN metastasis is evident in the literature data summarized in Table 22.5. The larger the metastasis, or the greater the number of metastatic foci identified in the SLN, the greater the risk of impairment of non-SLN. Although the sample is small, even in cases where metastasis is uniquely identified by immunohistochemistry (IHC), the incidence of non-SLN metastasis is relevant, ranging from 8 % to 16 % (Table 22.6). Bevilacqua et al. [35] demonstrate that multifocality is predictive of metastasis in SLN. The finding that this factor is also an independent non-SLN metastasis factor does not surprise us for the same reasons previously described [68]. The independent inverse association of metastasis in

Table 22.2 Predictors of axillary metastases in univariate or multivariate analyses of non-SLN and SN (the numbers of the table are the P values reported in the original literature)

Study			Subjects		Primary tumor characteristics								SLN characteristics				
Author	Year	Multivariate analysis	N	Age	Size (cm)	Nuclear grade	Histologic grade	Histologic type	LVI	Multifocality	ER	PR	Detection method	Metastasis size in SLN	Extranodal extension	N° of Positive SLN	Total N° of negative SLN
Chu [62]	1999	Yes	157	NS	0.01	NS	–	NS	NS	–	NS	NS	NS	<0.0001	–	NS	–
Reynolds [58]	1999	Yes	60	NS	0.0004	NS	–	NS	NS	–	0.03	NS	–	0.002	–	–	–
Teng [59]	2000	Yes	26	–	0.001	–	–	–	–	–	–	–	0.02	–	–	–	–
Turner [71]	2000	Yes	194	NS	0.03	NS	NS	–	0.03	–	NS	NS	–	0.01	0.0001	NS	–
Abdessalam [55]	2001	No	100	NS	NS	NS	–	NS	0.004	–	NS	NS	–	0.01	<0.001	NS	–
Canavese [72]	2001	No	72	–	NR	–	–	–	–	–	–	–	–	NR	–	–	–
Cserni [73]	2001	Yes	69	–	<0.01	–	NS	–	–	–	–	–	–	<0.005	<0.05	–	–
Kamath [66]	2001	No	101	–	0.005	–	–	–	–	–	–	–	0.02	<0.001	–	–	–
Liang [74]	2001	No	78	–	–	–	–	–	–	–	–	–	–	NR	–	–	–
Rahusen [57]	2001	No	93	NS	NS	–	NS	–	NS	–	NS	–	–	0.05	–	0.002	–
Viale [75]	2001	Yes	109	NS	NS	–	NS	NS	NS	–	NS	NS	–	0.02	–	–	–
Weiser [76]	2001	Yes	206	NS	0.007	NS	NS	NS	NS	–	–	–	–	0.0002	–	–	–
Wong [70]	2001	Yes	389	NS	<0.001	–	–	NS	–	–	–	–	–	–	–	<0.001	–
den Bakker [77]	2002	No	32	–	0.03	NR	–	NR	–	–	–	–	–	–	–	–	–
Jakub [69]	2002	No	62	–	NS	–	–	–	–	–	–	–	–	–	–	0.06	–
Mignotte [78]	2002	No	120	–	NR	–	–	–	–	–	–	–	NR	NR	–	–	–
Sachdev [67]	2002	Yes	55	NS	0.0001	–	–	NS	0.001	–	–	–	–	0.02	–	–	–
Hwang [65]	2003	Yes	131	NS	0.009	NS	–	NS	0.03		NS	NS	–	0.024	NS	NS	0.04
Fleming [64]	2004	Yes	54	NS	NS	–	NS	NS	–	–	–	–	–	0.02	0.02	–	–
Van Zee [61, 79]		Yes	702+373	–	0.001	NS	–	NS	0.003	0.02	0.08	–	<0.001	–	–	<0.001	<0.001

SLN sentinel lymph node, *Non-SLN* non-sentinel axillary lymph node, *LVI* lymphatic vascular invasion, *ER* estrogen receptor, *PR* progesterone receptor, *N* number of subjects with positive SLN who underwent axillary dissection, – not analyzed, *NS* not significant, *NR* statistics not reported

Table 22.3 Literature of incidence of metastasis in Non-SLN with positive SLN, per primary tumor size

Study	T1a (≤5 cm)	T1b (0.6–1.0 cm)	T1c (1.1–2.0 cm)	T2 (2.1–5.0 cm)	T3 (>5.0 cm)
Chu [62]	0 %	13 %	29 %	38 %	71 %
Reynolds [58]	[——25 % for T1——]			[—— 79 % for T2/3 ——]	
Turner [71]	17 %	20 %	46 %	48 %	73 %
Kamath [66]	25 %	30 %	40 %	46 %	80 %
Rahusen [57]	50 %	50 %	49 %	50 %	–
Weiser [76]	8 %	21 %	37 %	48 %	–
Wong [70]	14 %	22 %	30 %	45 %	57 %
Viale [75]	100 %	14 %	25 %	24 %	–
Sachdev [67]	[—— 13 % for T1——]			[——33 % for ≥T2——]	
Mignotte [78]	[—— 14 % ——]		54 %	52 %	–

Non-SLN non-sentinel axillary lymph node, *SLN* sentinel lymph node

Table 22.4 Studies that report metastasis incidence in Non-SLN in positive axillary SLN with LVI in primary tumor

Study	Absence of LVI (%)	Presence of LVI (%)
Reynolds [58]	43	62
Turner [71]	37	65
Abdessalam [55]	31	62
Rahusen [57]	42	30
Weiser [76]	26	41
Viale [75]	21	26
Sachdev [67]	12	32

Non-SLN non-sentinel axillary lymph node, *SLN* sentinel lymph node, *LVI* lymphatic vascular invasion

Table 22.5 Studies that report metastasis incidence in Non-SLN with positive SLN, by size of SLN metastasis

Study	<1 mm	≥1 mm	<2 mm	>2 mm	>2 cm or "Extensive disease"
Chu [62]	–	–	7 %	55 %	–
Reynolds [58]	–	–	22 %	67 %	–
Turner [71]	–	–	26 %	63 %	–
Abdessalam [55]	–	–	20 %	47 %	75 %
Kamath [66]	–	–	15 %	58 %	65 %
Rahusen [57]	27 %	50 %	–	–	–
Viale [75]	16 %	–	22 %	45 %	–
Weiser [76]	–	–	18 %	45 %	–
Mignotte [78]	–	–	22 %	79 %	–
Sachdev [67]	17 %	49 %	–	–	–

Non-SLN non-sentinel axillary lymph node, *SLN* sentinel lymph node

Table 22.6 Studies that report metastasis incidence in non-SLN in subjects with metastasis in SLN detected exclusively by IHC

Study	Proportion	%
Teng [59]	3/26	12
Kamath [66]	2/26	8
Wong [70]	3/28	11
Mignotte [78]	7/44	16
Jakub [69]	9/62	15

Non-SLN non-sentinel axillary lymph node, *SLN* sentinel lymph node, *IHC* immunohistochemistry

non-SLN and the number of negative SLNs are somewhat intuitive. The finding of a single metastasis in SLN over other resected SLNs induces us to think that the "volume" or "amount" of metastases is not sufficient to affect all SLNs, and therefore, it is much less likely that other axillary lymph nodes may be committed [61]. The direct and independent association of metastasis in non-SLN and the number of positive SLN are also somewhat logical and obvious. By identifying a situation in which multiple SLNs are committed, it seems very likely that other axillary lymph nodes may also be compromised. Other authors also describe this finding [57, 69, 70].

22.2.3 *Predictive Factors of Lymphedema*

Lymphedema of the upper limb particularly after lymphadenectomy is a chronic and incurable disabling condition, which continues to be one of the main sequelae after breast cancer treatment. In addition to the physical problems, lymphedema frequently causes social and psychological problems [80, 81].

In the last decades, extraordinary advances in the treatment of breast cancer have occurred, both in surgery and in adjuvant treatment. Nevertheless, currently in Brazil, 30–50 % of patients still require classical ALND as part of their surgical treatment. Based on breast cancer estimates in Brazil [82], one can calculate that approximately 3000–5000 breast cancer patients per year will develop lymphedema. In 2007, there were approximately 2.6 million women alive who had a history of breast cancer in the United States, which amounted up to an estimated prevalence of 0.58 % [83]. Worldwide [84], this corresponds to an age-standardized prevalence of 0.40 % or about 27.5 million survivors of breast cancer who are at risk for lymphedema (LE) of the upper extremity, which can occur after axillary lymph node dissection (ALND). If lymphedema is an incurable chronic disease and if cancer of the breast generally has a good prognosis (prolonged survival), we can, without a doubt, classify lymphedema as a serious public health problem, which is commonly ignored by society and by physicians as well.

The pathophysiology of lymphedema is characterized by an inadequate and decreased lymphatic transport, necessary for deficit absorption of microvascularization (arterial and venous capillaries) of blood filtrate that normally accumulates in the interstitium and necessary for transportation of macromolecules and excess liquids from capillary filtration. This filtrate is composed mainly of water, proteins, and some cells. In an initial stage, the edema is an exclusive result of the accumulation of fluids (water) in the extracellular space, filtrated plasmatic proteins, extravasation of cells from the blood, and parenchymal cell products. At a second stage, there is proliferation of parenchymal and stromal elements, with excessive deposit of extracellular matrice substances [80].

Nevertheless, not all women who undergo breast cancer treatment develop lymphedema, as a compensatory mechanism between the lymphatic and blood systems [85]. Factors that can trigger the imbalance between these systems [86] may vary from characteristics that are specific to the woman, postoperative complications, routine daily activities, and exposure to traumas and high temperatures.

After ALND for treatment of breast cancer, the prevalence of lymphedema has varied between 6 and 49 % (Table 22.7) and the incidence between 0 and 22 % (Table 22.8). In these tables, we can observe the great variability of prevalence and incidence of lymphedema in post-lymphadenectomy. These differences can be justified by the different methodologies of these studies, such as criteria adopted

Table 22.7 Prevalence of lymphedema post-lymphadenectomy – systematic review (2000–2006)

Study	Year	N	Median follow-up period	Lymphedema prevalence (%)
Edwards et al. [88]	2000	201	37 months	11–23
Kuehn et al. [89]	2000	396	34 months	22
Hojris et al. [90]	2000	84	9 years	14
Johansen et al. [91]	2000	266	7,6 years	11
Petrek et al. [16]	2001	263	20 years	49
Freitas et al. [92]	2001	109	Not available	14
Ververs et al. [93]	2001	400	3 months–5 years	17
Meric et al. [94]	2002	294	1–120 months	14
Almeida et al. [95]	2002	99	3–170 months	38
Beaulac et al. [96]	2002	151	4,8 years	28
Rampaul et al. [97]	2003	677	Not available	6
Deustch et al. [98]	2003	265	61 months	7
Schijven et al. [99]	2003	393	2 years	7
Yap et al. [100]	2003	370	3,3 years	15
Goffman et al. [101]	2004	240	1,5 years	8
Deo et al. [102]	2004	299	2,5 years	34
Ozaslan et al. [103]	2004	240	18–43 months	37
Armer et al. [104]	2004	100	28 months	43
van der V et al. [105]	2004	245	Not available	24
Bergmann et al. [106]	2004	394	59 months	12–31

Table 22.8 Incidence of lymphedema post-lymphadenectomy – systematic review (2000–2006)

Study	Year	N	Median follow-up period	Lymphedema incidence (%)
Isaksson et al. [107]	2000	48	1–2 years	9
Sener et al. [108]	2001	420	24 months	17
Duff et al. [109]	2001	100	1 year	10
Herd-Smith et al. [110]	2001	1278	56 months	16
Swenson et al. [111]	2002	247	12 months	14
Temple et al. [112]	2002	233	12 months	0
Veronesi et al. [38]	2003	200	2 years	12
Silbernam et al. [113]	2004	94	1–14 years	6–22
Ronka et al. [114]	2005	83	12 months	7
Clark et al. [115]	2005	188	3 years	21
Bergmann [116]	2005	1002	24 months	17

for definition and measurement of lymphedema, treatments used (radiotherapy, surgery and chemotherapy), time elapsed between surgery and evaluation, and population characteristics [87].

Table 22.9 Occurrence of lymphedema when compared to SLN biopsy versus axillary lymphadenectomy (ALND)

Study	Lymphedema %(N)		
	Sentinel lymph node	Lymphadenectomy	P
Schrenk 2000 [117]	0 (0/35)	14 % (5/35)	0.0536
Sener 2001 [108]	3 % (9/303)	17 % (20/117)	<0.001
Veronesi 2003 [38]	0 (0/100)	12 % (12/100)	<0.001
Blanchard 2003 [118]	6 % (44/730)	34 % (56/164)	<0.001
Golshan 2003 [119]	3 % (2/77)	27 % (13/48)	<0.001
Armer 2004 [104]	2/9	41 % (33/79)	NS
Langer [120]	0 (0/61)	17 % (10/59)	<0.001
(ALMANAC) Mansel 2006 [121]	5 % (20/412)	13 % (53/403)	<0.001
(Z0011) Lucci 2007 [122]	2 % (6/268)	13 % (37/288)	<0.001
Median	4 % (83/1995)	18 % (239/1293)	<0.001

The SLN biopsy has presented significantly lower estimates of occurrence of lymphedema, about 5 % for biopsy of SLN and 20 % for axillary lymphadenectomy, i.e., four times less (Table 22.9).

The knowledge of the risk factors for the development of lymphedema is essential for establishment of preventive measures, whether preoperative, intraoperative, or postoperative. Various risk factors for lymphedema have already been described and are summarized in Table 22.10.

22.3 Nomograms

Based on a review of previous literature, we observed that there are several predictive factors of lymph node metastasis and lymphedema. Applying this data to calculate the individual probability is somewhat complex. Founded on subjectivism, there is a natural tendency of the physician to estimate the probability by "guessing," which can often fail due to the large number and the interrelationships of these predictors. With the widespread use of the Internet to access information, patients are daily more informed about their health problems, and thus, their questions also require increasingly more accurate answers. Mathematical models, including the nomograms, are developed to facilitate and improve the calculation of these probabilities.

22.3.1 *Nomograms for Predicting Metastasis in SLN*

In 2007, Bevilacqua et al. [35] described the first validated nomogram predictive of metastasis in SLN (Figs. 22.1 and 22.2). The aim of this study was to create a

Table 22.10 Risk factors for development of lymphedema identified in the literature. Study references can be seen in the columns

Risk factors for development of lymphedema	Risk increase	Risk decrease	Risk unaltered
Body mass index (BMI)	[16, 80, 84, 86, 88, 90, 93, 97, 107, 108]		
Radiotherapy of the lymphatic drainage	[94, 95, 97, 108]		
Breast radiotherapy/boost			[94, 96, 97]
Early-onset edema	[108]		
Seroma	[108]		[16, 95, 102, 124, 125]
Chemotherapy on ipsilateral arm	[108]		
Axillary dissection	[81, 82, 87, 90, 101]		
Age (older)	[82, 83, 85, 108]	[116]	[16, 80, 81, 84, 86, 88, 90, 92, 93, 95, 101, 105, 117, 120–122]
Limb infection	[80, 84, 86]		[100, 117]
Trauma of the arm	[86, 95]		
Articular restriction	[84, 86]		
Dominant superior limb	[95]		[80, 107]
SLN biopsy		[89, 102, 104, 109–114]	[94]
Systemic treatment (chemotherapy and/or hormone therapy)			[80, 82, 84, 86, 92, 93, 95, 101, 105, 116, 117, 120, 122]
Axillary metastasis			[81, 82, 84, 86, 91–93, 102–105, 115–117, 120, 122]
Tumor size			[80, 82, 84, 86, 91–93, 95, 101, 105, 107, 112–117, 120, 122]
Final staging			[80, 82, 84, 86, 91–93, 95, 101, 105, 107, 112–117, 120, 122]
Tumor location			[80, 82, 84, 86, 91–93, 95, 101, 105, 107, 112–117, 120, 122]
Type of surgery (of the breast) and reconstruction			[80–82, 84, 86, 95, 100, 101, 105, 116, 120]
Race/ethnicity			[86, 116]
Education			[81, 91, 120]
Smoking			[81, 91]
Age at menopause			[86, 95, 101, 116, 120]
Presence of comorbidities			[88, 92, 93, 116]
Arm exercises			[16, 115, 116, 120]
Elapsed time from cancer treatment			[80, 81, 98, 105]

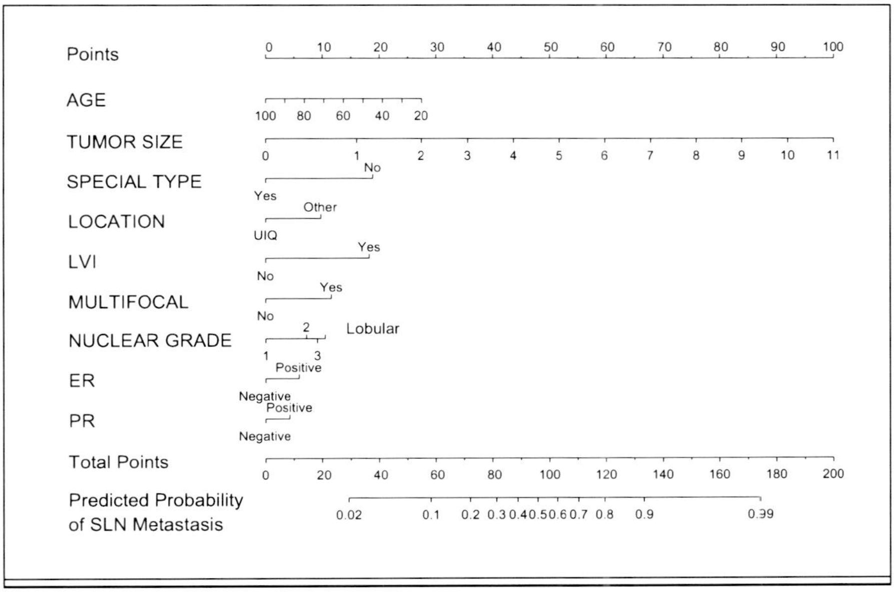

Fig. 22.1 *Definitions*: *AGE*, patient age in years; *TUMOR SIZE*, invasive carcinoma component size in cm; *SPECIAL TYPE*, colloid subtype (or mucinous), medular or tubular "Yes" (if subtype for ductal or lobular, defined as "No"); *LOCATION*, tumor location (UIQ, upper internal quadrant; OTHER, other quadrants); *LVI*, lymphatic vascular invasion; *MULTIFOCAL*, primary tumor multifocality; *NUCLEAR GRADE*, nuclear grade (I, II, II, and lobular); *ER*, estrogen receptor status; *PR*, progesterone receptor status. Reference: Bevilacqua et al. [35]

mathematical model (nomogram) to easily calculate and individualize probability of metastasis in SLN and answer a very common question as: "Doctor, what is my probability of axillary metastasis?"

In this study, the authors developed and validated two nomograms to predict metastasis in SLN based on a large database with over 5,000 SLN biopsies at MSKCC in New York, USA. The demographic and clinical variables of 3786 consecutive SLN biopsies for invasive breast carcinoma, held at that institution between 12/1996 and 7/2002, were collected. The accuracies of the nomograms were quite significant in discriminating patients with and without metastasis in SLN. In both models, the area under the ROC curve (AUC) was 0.754. This accuracy is similar to mammography to detect breast cancer that presents AUC of 0.61 and 0.82, for screen-film and digital mammography, respectively. Free online versions of the nomograms are available at http://nomograms.mskcc.org/breast/index.aspx.

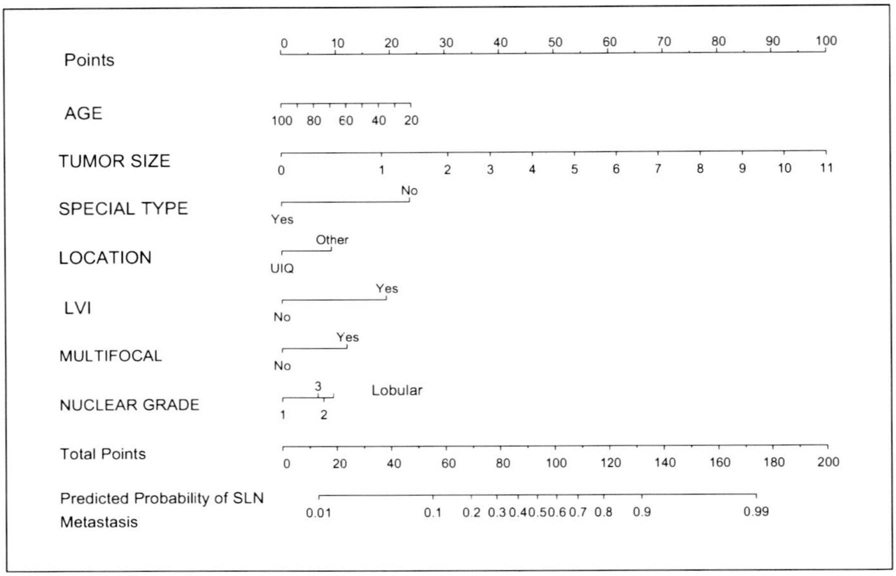

Fig. 22.2 *Definitions*: *AGE*, patient age in years; *TUMOR SIZE*, invasive carcinoma component size in cm; *SPECIAL TYPE*, colloid subtype (or mucinous), medular or tubular "Yes" (if subtype for ductal or lobular, defined as "No"); *LOCATION*, tumor location (UIQ, upper internal quadrant; OTHER, other quadrants); *LVI*, lymphatic vascular invasion; *MULTIFOCAL*, primary tumor multifocality; *NUCLEAR GRADE*, nuclear grade (I, II, II, and lobular); *ER*, estrogen receptor status; *PR*, progesterone receptor status. Reference: Bevilacqua et al. [35]

22.3.2 Nomograms for Predicting Metastasis in Non-SLN (Additional Axillary Lymph Nodes)

In 2003, Van Zee et al. [61, 123] described the first validated nomogram to predict metastasis in non-SLN (Figs. 22.3 and 22.4). The objective of this study was to create a nomogram to easily calculate and individualize probability of metastasis in non-SLN when the SLN was positive, so as to aid in the decision-making process of complete ALND [61, 123]. Clinical and pathological features of the primary tumor and SLN metastases of 702 patients from 12/1996 to 4/2001, who underwent complete ALND, were assessed with multivariable logistic regression to predict the presence of additional disease in the non-SLNs of these patients. All patients underwent ALND with at least ten lymph nodes were resected and examined. Data were analyzed using logistic regression, and two predictive models of metastasis in non-SLN were developed. Both models were applied and validated in other 373 consecutive biopsies performed between 8/2002 and 5/2004, using the same inclusion and exclusion criteria [61, 123].

In these models, the authors added lobular subtype to nuclear grade, so as not to be automatically deleted from logistic regression. They also attempted to eliminate

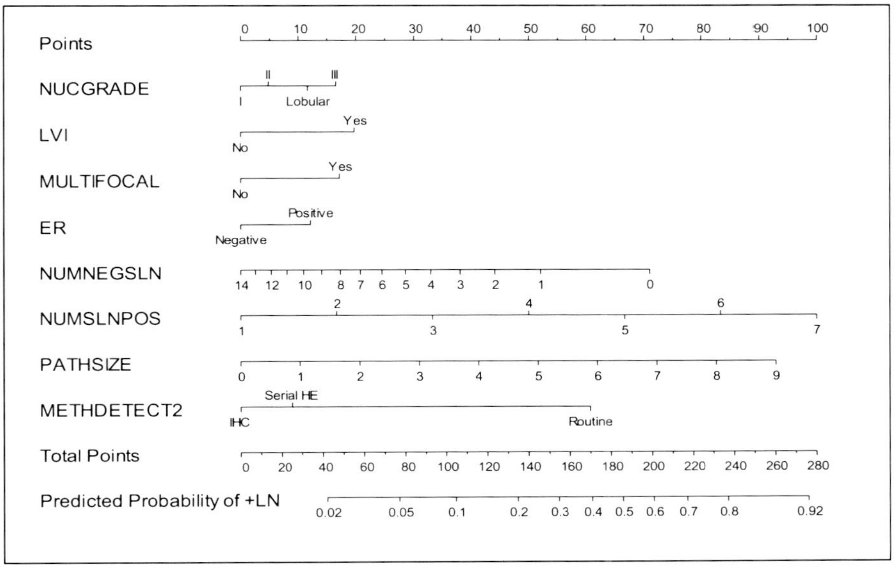

Fig. 22.3 *Definições*: *NUCGRADE*, nuclear grade (I, II, II, and lobular); *LVI*, lymphatic vascular invasion; *MULTIFOCAL*, primary tumor multifocality; *ER*, estrogen receptor status; *NUMNEGSLN*, number of negative sentinel lymph nodes; *NUMSLNPOS* number of positive sentinel lymph nodes; *PATHSIZE*, invasive carcinoma component size in cm; *METHDETECT*, metastasis detection method in SLN – routine, serial sections (Serial H&E) or immunohistochemistry (IHC). Reference: Van Zee et al. [61]

subjectivity of metastases measurement, and hence, the detection method seems to be less subjective, more practical, and reproducible. This way of quantifying metastasis in SLN can be criticized, since the current version of TNM recommends using the size of the lymph node metastasis.

Although the estrogen receptor and the modified nuclear grade (which includes lobular histology) were not identified as independent predictors of metastases in non-SLN in the multivariate analysis, the authors chose to include them in the nomogram since it improved the overall predictive ability of the model [61].

The accuracies of the nomograms were quite significant in discriminating patients with or without metastasis in non-SLN in the validation population. In the model study, which included frozen sections, the area under the ROC curve (AUC) was 0.77; however, in the nonfrozen sections, the AUC was 0.78 [23, 124]. Thus, the predictive ability to detect metastasis in non-LS models is also the same as the predictive value of mammography in breast cancer detection.

Free online versions of the nomograms are available at http://nomograms.mskcc.org/breast/index.aspx.

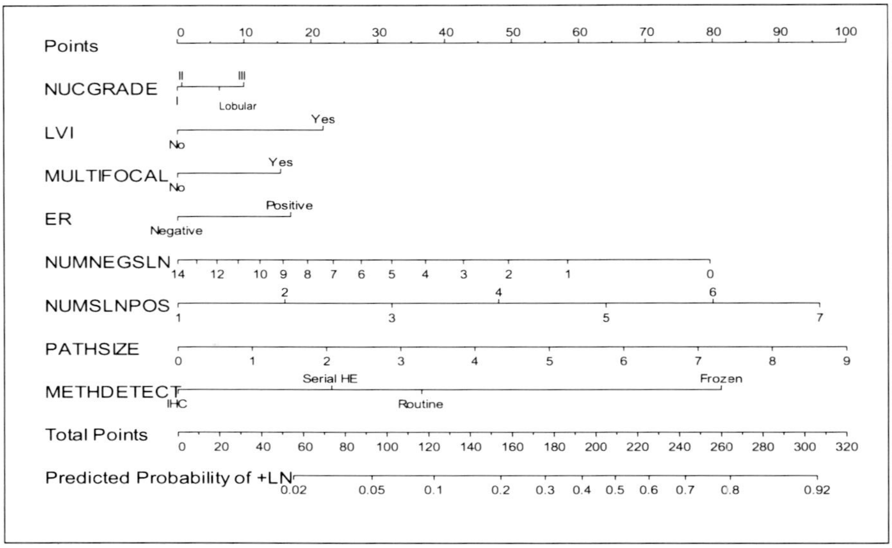

Fig. 22.4 *Definitions*: *NUCGRADE*, nuclear grade (I, II, II, and lobular); *LVI*, lymphatic vascular invasion; *MULTIFOCAL*, primary tumor multifocality; *ER*, estrogen receptor status; *NUMNEGSLN*, number of negative sentinel lymph nodes; *NUMSLNPOS* number of positive sentinel lymph nodes; *PATHSIZE*, invasive carcinoma component size in cm; *METHDETECT*, metastasis detection method in SLN – frozen, routine, serial sections (Serial H&E) or immunohistochemistry (IHC). Reference: Van Zee et al. [61]

22.3.3 Other Predictive Models of Metastasis in Non-SLN

Other predictive models of metastasis in non-SLN were published after the MKSCC nomograms [67, 125–128]. These models differ in the variables used and number of patients included in the sample modeling (Table 22.11). Coutant et al. [129] compared the models described in Tables 22.12 and 22.13, in a study that included 561 patients, all with positive lymph nodes and submitted to ALND. The models were compared to the AUC, to the calibration and the rate of false-negative for metastasis in non-SLN, and to the capacity (number of patients and percentage) of the models. In this cohort, 147 patients (26 %) had metastases in non-SLN. The authors showed that only models of MSKCC [61, 123] and Tenon [130] demonstrated AUC higher than 0.75. Models of MSKCC [61, 123], Mayo [131], and Cambridge [128] were well calibrated. Two models, Tenon and the Stanford, obtained false-negative rates lower than 5 %. The MSKCC model showed a false-negative rate of 6.5 % compared with 4.9 % of the Stanford model and 4.4 % of the Tenon score.

The MSKCC nomogram was the most validated model independently. Nineteen out of 21 validation studies validated this model positively (Table 22.13).

Table 22.11 Variables included in the different predictive models of metastasis in non-SLN and number of subjects included in sampling of the models

	Model (n = model sample size)								
	MSKCC [61, 123]	Tenon [125]	Cambridge [128]	Stanford [133]	Mayo [131]	MD Anderson [65]	Saidi score [134]	RP-ROC [133]	CART [133]
Variables	($n = 702$)	($n = 77$)	($n = 285$)	($n = 362$)	($n = 574$)	($n = 131$)	($n = 34$)	($n = 285$)	($n = 285$)
Metastasis size	X	X	X	X	X	X		X	X
Tumor size	X	X		X	X	X	X	X	X
LVI (lymphatic vascular invasion)	X			X		X	X	X	X
Number of positive SLN	X	X	X		X				
Number of negative SLN	X	X	X		X				
Tumor grade	X		X						
Extra-capsular extension					X		X		
Tumor type	X								
ER status	X								
Multifocality	X								
Age					X				
Number of dissected SLN						X			
Tumor palpability							X		

Table 22.12 Comparison between predictive models of metastasis in Non-SLN. Summary of results obtained by Coutant et al. [129]

	AUC		Calibration	False-negative index	
Model	Value	95 % CI	P	%	95 % CI
Whole cohort $N = 561$					
MSKCC	0.78	0.76–0.81	<0,0001	6.5	3.9–10.3
Mayo	0.74	0.71–0.76	0,08	12.5	3.5–35.6
Cambridge	0.73	0.7–0.75	0,10	10.3	6.2–12.8
Stanford	0.72	0.7–0.74	<0,0001	4.9	2.2–10.7
Tenon	0.81	0.79–0.83	Not evaluable	4.4	2.6–7.1
MD Anderson	0.73	0.7–0.75	Not evaluable	5.7	3–10.5
Saidi	0.65	0.62–0.67	Not evaluable	15.0	10.3–21
RP-ROC	0.68	0.65–0.7	Not evaluable	5.2	2.8–9.2
CART	0.65	0.63–0.67	Not evaluable	6.4	3.8–10.5
Subject subgroup with micrometastasis or tumoral cells isolated in SLN ($N = 246$)					
MSKCC	0.72	0.66–0.79	0.10	3.5	1.6–6.4
Mayo	0.63	0.57–0.7	<0.0001	10.0	1.8–38
Cambridge	0.63	0.57–0.69	<0.0001	4.1	1.4–9.6
Stanford	0.73	0.68–0.79	<0.0001	2.2	0.6–6.4
Tenon	0.81	0.76–0.87	Not evaluable	2.9	1.5–4.8
MD Anderson	0.67	0.62–0.73	Not evaluable	3.8	1.7–7
Saidi	0.62	0.57–0.67	Not evaluable	2.8	0.8–8.2
RP-ROC	0.65	0.59–0.71	Not evaluable	5.2	3.1–7.5
CART	0.60	0.54–0.65	Not evaluable	6.4	4.3–8.3

22.3.4 Nomograms for Predicting the Risk of Arm Lymphedema After Axillary Dissection in Breast Cancer

Lymphedema (LE) after axillary lymph node dissection (ALND) is a multifactorial, chronic, and disabling condition that currently affects an estimated four million people worldwide. Although several risk factors have been described, it is difficult to estimate the risk in individual patients. In 2012, Bevilacqua et al. [132] described the first validated nomogram to predict arm lymphedema after axillary dissection in breast cancer. Descriptive characteristics of the study population are shown in Table 22.14.

In Bevilacqua et al. [132] study, LE was defined as a volume difference of at least 200 mL between arms at 6 months or more after surgery. The volume of each arm was estimated using the formula for the volume of the frustum of a cone (Fig. 22.5). The cumulative incidence of LE was ascertained by the Kaplan–Meier method, and Cox proportional hazard models were used to predict the risk of developing LE on the basis of the available data at each time point: (I) preoperatively, (II) within 6 months from surgery, and (III) 6 months or later after surgery (Table 22.15). The 5-year cumulative incidence of LE was 30.3 %

Table 22.13 Validation of predictive models of metastasis in non-SLN

			AUC								
Study	Year	N	MSKCC [61, 123]	Tenon [125]	Cambridge [128]	Stanford [133]	Mayo [131]	MD Anderson [65]	Saidi score [134]	RP-ROC [133]	CART [133]
Van Zee	2003	373	0.76								
Kocsis	2004	140	Not valid								
Soni	2005	149	0.75								
Degnim	2005	465	0.72								
Mayo clinic dataset apud		462	0.72	0.77							
Michigan dataset apud		89	0.86								
Smidt	2005	222	0.71								
Specht	2005	33	0.72								
Lambert	2005	200	0.71								
Cripe	2006	92	0.82								
Dauphine	2007	39	0.63				0.68	0.70			
Alran	2007	588	0.72								
Alran	2007	213	Not valid								
Ponzone	2007	186	0.71					Not valid			
Zgajnar	2007	276	0.72								
Pal	2007	118	0.68								
Klar	2008	98	0.58								

(continued)

Table 22.13 (continued)

Study	Year	N	AUC								
			MSKCC [61, 123]	Tenon [125]	Cambridge [128]	Stanford [133]	Mayo [131]	MD Anderson [65]	Saidi score [134]	RP-ROC [133]	CART [133]
Kohrt	2008	171	0.77			0.85				0.80	0.80
Coutant	2009	561	0.78	0.74	0.73	0.72	0.81	0.73	0.65	0.68	0.65
Coutant	2009	246	0.72	0.63	0.63	0.73	0.81	0.67	0.62	0.65	0.60
van la Parra	2009	182	0.71								
Coutant	2009	226					0.82				

Subject subgroup with micrometastasis in SLN
N number of subjects submitted to validation, *AUC* area under the curve, *ROC* (receiver operating characteristic), *MSKCC* Memorial Sloan-Kettering Cancer Center, *RP-ROC* recursive partitioning with receiver operating characteristic, *CART* boosted Classification and Regression Trees
Up-dated and adapted from: Coutant et al. [129]

Table 22.14 Descriptive characteristics of the 1054 patients included in the analysis

	N (%)
Age (years)	
≤55 years	582 (55.2)
>55 years	472 (44.8)
Marital status	
Not married	540 (51.2)
Currently married	503 (47.7)
Unavailable data	11 (1.1)
Highest education	
Middle school	705 (66.9)
>Middle school	303 (28.7)
Unavailable data	46 (4.4)
Main occupation	
Home activity	495 (47.0)
Other	310 (29.4)
Unavailable data	249 (23.6)
Body mass index (kg/m^2)	
≥25	716 (67.9)
<25	328 (31.1)
Unavailable data	10 (0.9)
Type of surgery	
Mastectomy	693 (65.7)
Conservative	361 (34.3)
Immediate breast reconstruction	
No	993 (94.2)
Yes	61 (5.8)
Level of axillary lymph node dissection	
Levels I and II	162 (15.4)
Levels I, II, and III	838 (79.5)
Unavailable data	54 (5.1)
Number of lymph nodes dissected	
≤10	132 (12.5)
11–20	606 (57.5)
≥21	316 (30.0)
Number of days with drain	
≤14 days	908 (86.1)
>14 days	90 (8.5)
Unavailable data	56 (5.3)
Axillary lymph node status	
Negative	573 (54.4)
Positive	481 (45.6)

(continued)

Table 22.14 (continued)

	N (%)
Chemotherapy	
None	322 (30.6)
Neoadjuvant	111 (10.5)
Adjuvant	503 (47.7)
Neoadjuvant and adjuvant	118 (11.2)
Neoadjuvant chemotherapy in ipsilateral arm	
No	829 (78.7)
Yes	225 (21.3)
Adjuvant chemotherapy in ipsilateral arm	
No	977 (92.7)
Yes	77 (7.3)
Neoadjuvant or adjuvant chemotherapy in ipsilateral arm	
No	765 (72.6)
Yes	289 (27.4)
Radiotherapy	
No	380 (36.1)
Breast or chest wall	377 (35.8)
Lymph node basins	293 (27.8)
Unavailable data	4 (0.4)
Tumor size (UICC)(68)	
Tis	42 (4.0)
T1	299 (28.4)
T2	464 (44.0)
T3	76 (7.2)
T4	6 (0.6)
Unavailable data	
Staging (UICC)(68)	
0	34 (3.2)
I	200 (19.0)
IIA	335 (31.8)
IIB	246 (23.3)
IIIA	61 (5.8)
IIIB	174 (16.5)
Unavailable data	4 (0.4)
Surgical infection	
No	866 (82.2)
Yes	144 (13.7)
Unavailable data	44 (4.2)
Seroma	
No	373 (35.4)
Yes	634 (60.2)
Unavailable data	47 (4.5)

(continued)

Table 22.14 (continued)

	N (%)
Early edema (volume >200 mL)	
No	1025 (97.2)
Yes	29 (2.8)
Lymphedema	
No	807 (76.6)
Yes	247 (23.4)
Died	
No	827 (78.5)
Yes	171 (16.2)
Probably[a]	56 (5.3)

[a]Patients with untreatable stage IV disease at last follow-up

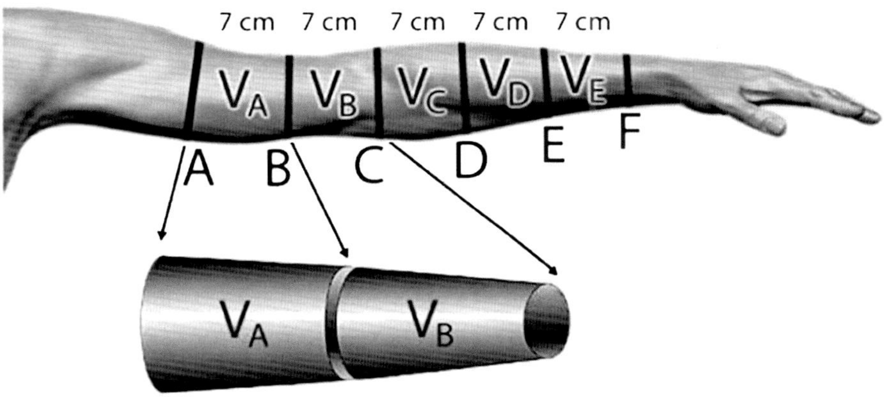

$$V_{Limb} = V_A + V_B + V_C + V_D + V_E$$

Where:

$$V_A = 7\ (A^2 + AB + B^2)/12 \times 3.14$$
$$V_B = 7\ (B^2 + BC + C^2)/12 \times 3.14$$
$$V_C = 7\ (C^2 + CD + D^2)/12 \times 3.14$$
$$V_D = 7\ (D^2 + DE + E^2)/12 \times 3.14$$
$$V_E = 7\ (E^2 + EF + F^2)/12 \times 3.14$$

Fig. 22.5 Arm lymphedema volume estimate: formula for the volume of the frustum of a cone

(Fig. 22.6). These nomograms are shown in Figs. 22.7, 22.8, and 22.9. Independent risk factors for LE were age, body mass index, ipsilateral arm chemotherapy infusions, level of ALND, location of radiotherapy field, development of

Table 22.15 Results of the three multivariable Cox proportional hazards analyses testing the relationship between patient characteristics and the incidence of lymphedema

Predictor variables	P Perioperative nomogram	P Within 6 months from surgery nomogram	P >6-month nomogram
Age	0.0040	0.0002	0.0485
Body mass index	<0.0001	<0.0001	<0.0001
Number of cycles of neoadjuvant or adjuvant chemotherapy	<0.0001	0.0001	0.0338
Level of axillary lymph node dissection	NA	0.0185	0.0836
Radiotherapy field	NA	<0.0001	<0.0001
Seroma	NA	NA	0.0418
Early edema	NA	NA	<0.0001

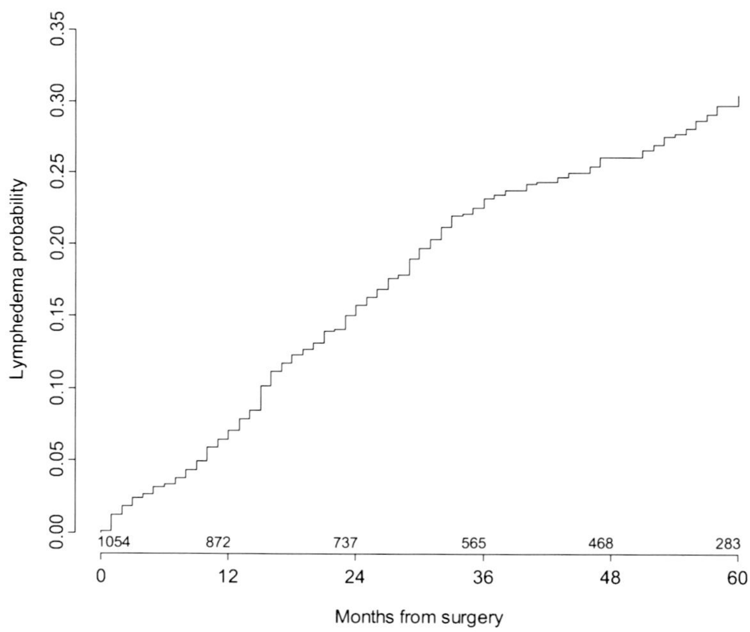

Fig. 22.6 Kaplan–Meier plots of 5-year cumulative incidence of lymphedema in the whole cohort. Numbers above x axis are the numbers of patients at risk at each time point

postoperative seroma, infection, and early edema. When applied to the validation set, the concordance indices were 0.706, 0.729, and 0.736 for models 1, 2, and 3, respectively (Figs. 22.7, 22.8 and 22.9) [132]. Free online versions of the nomograms are available at www.lymphedemarisk.com

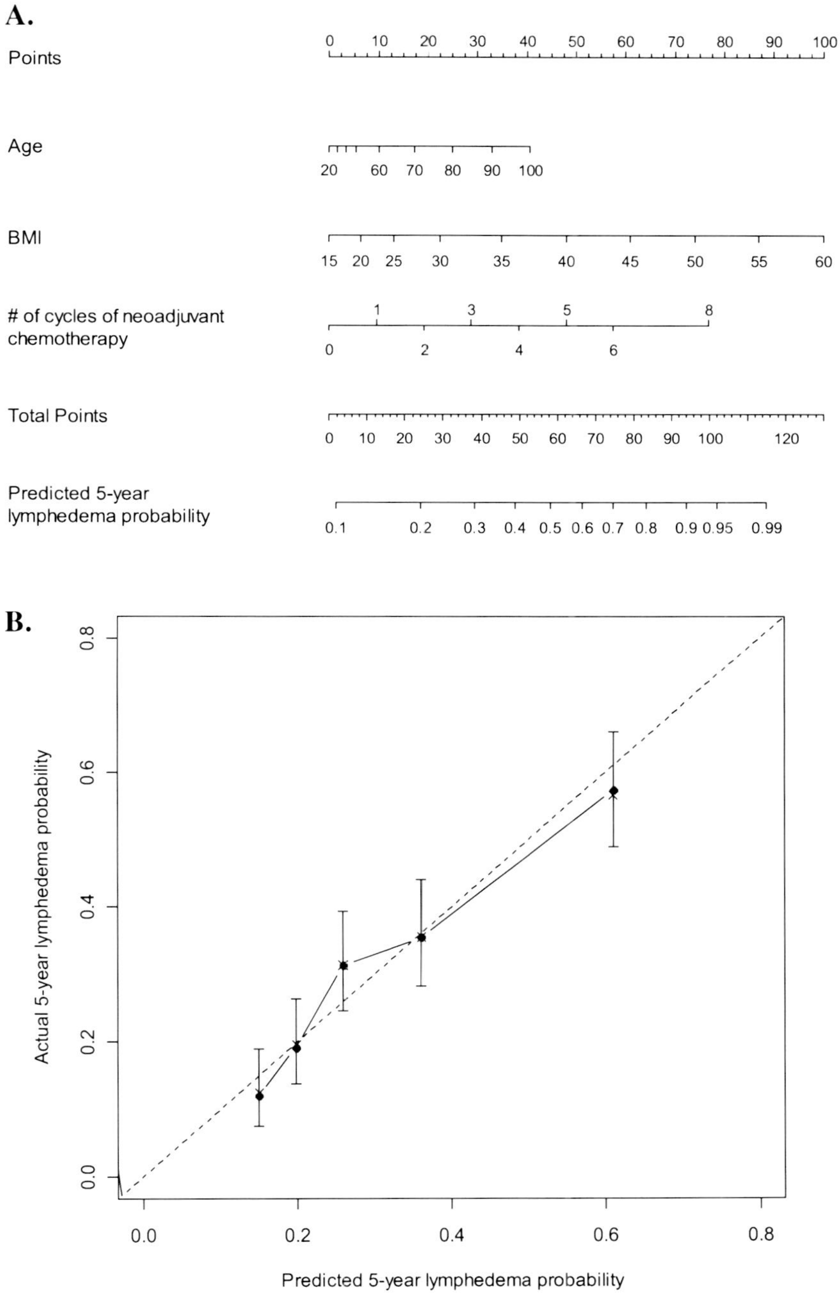

Fig. 22.7 Nomogram to predict probability of arm lymphedema after axillary lymph node dissection, for preoperative use. Below the nomogram (**A**) with its calibration plot (**B**)

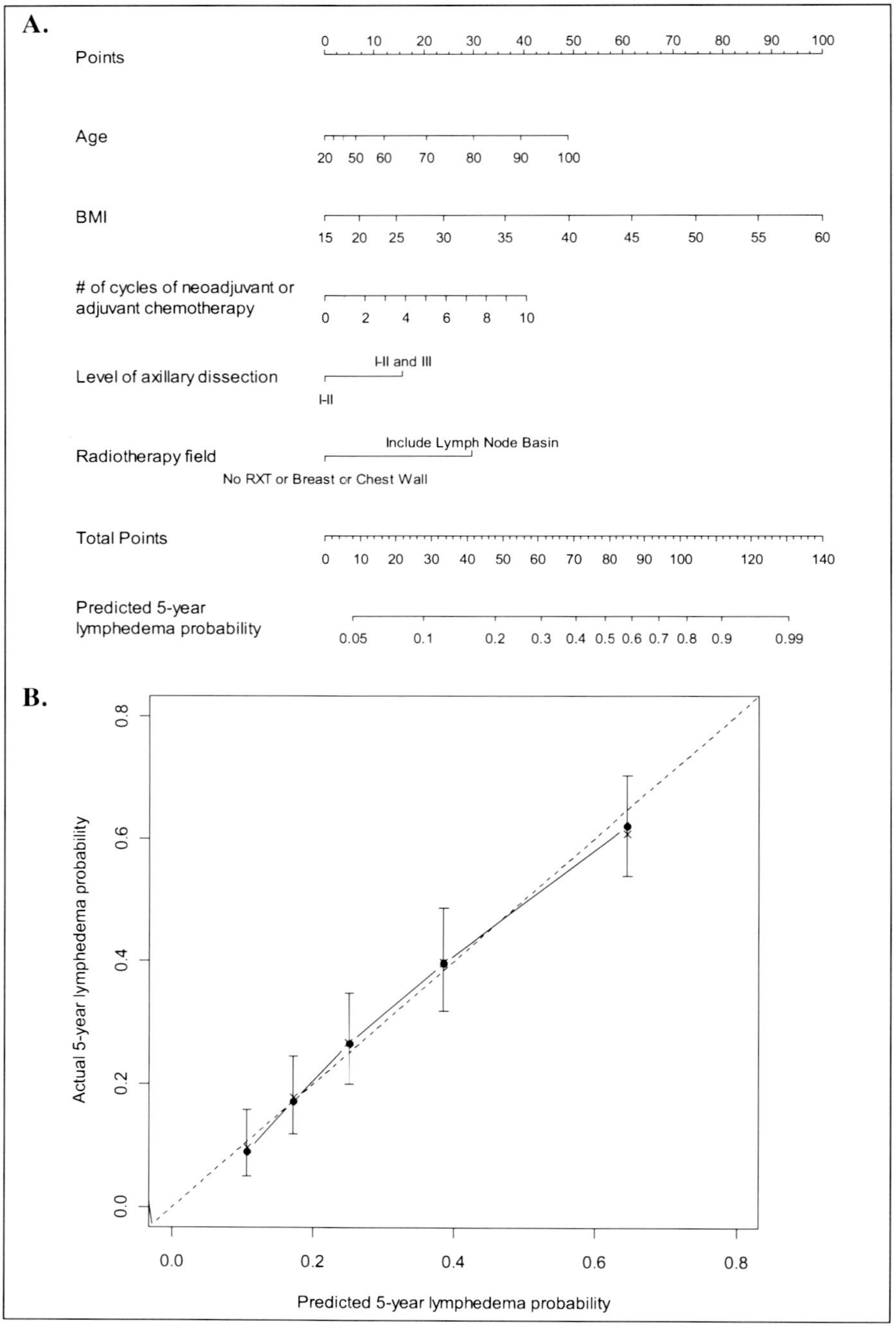

Fig. 22.8 Nomogram to predict probability of arm lymphedema after axillary lymph node dissection, for use within 6 months after surgery. Below the nomogram (**A**) with its calibration plot (**B**)

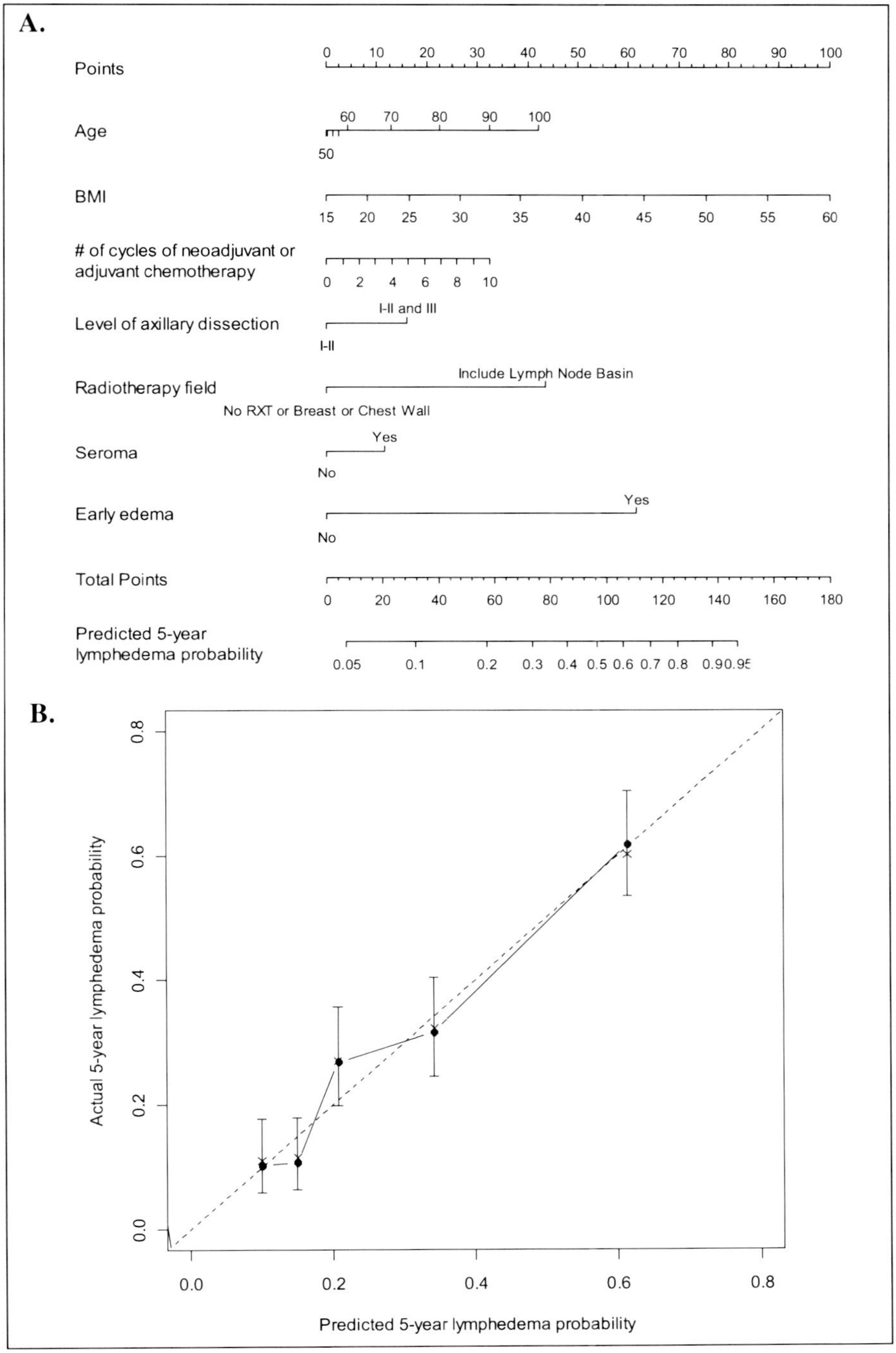

Fig. 22.9 Nomogram to predict probability of arm lymphedema after axillary lymph node dissection, for use 6 months or longer after surgery. Below the nomogram (**A**) with its calibration plot (**B**)

22.3.5 Using the Nomograms

Each version of the nomogram consists of a variable number of rows. The first line (points) is the score given to each variable. Subsequent lines represent the variables included in the models. Based on each patient's individual clinical and/or histopathological characteristics, a value is assigned to each variable in the range of points in the first row. A vertical line drawn between the appropriate value of the variable and the line of points determines the score of each variable scale. For example, in the age variable, patients 40 years of age correspond to 21 points (Fig. 22.1). Then, the points of each variable are added. The value of the sum is identified under "total points." Another vertical line is drawn between the total points and the line of Predicted Probability of SLN Metastasis or Predicted Probability of Non-SLN Metastasis. The corresponding number in the last line is the probability of metastasis in SLN or non-SLN, depending on the nomogram used.

22.4 Conclusions

No model for predicting metastasis in SLN, non-SLN, and lymphedema reaches perfection. In all models, the area under the ROC curve is around 0.70–0.80. To explain what this means, we will use as example the model of metastasis in non-SLN. This means that, if we randomly select two patients, one of whom has at least one positive non-SLN and another has a negative non-SLN, there is a 70–80 % chance that the nomogram will predict a greater likelihood for patients with these outcomes.

Some physicians and patients are reluctant to additional surgery due to the low risk of additional lymph node involvement and the fear of the possible morbidity associated with this procedure. In such cases, nomograms provide an accurate estimate of the risk of additional lymph node disease and future risk of morbidity associated with these procedures, allowing a more conscious, therapeutic decision.

Finally, the models (including nomograms) represent a significant advance to estimate the axillary metastatic disease in breast cancer as well as the risk of lymphedema when compared with our intuition or theory founded on subjectivism.

References

1. Association of Directors of Anatomic and Surgical Pathology; ad hoc committee composed of Connolly JL, Fechner RE, Kempson RL, Livolsi VA, Page DL, Patchefsky AA, Silverberg SG (1996) Recommendations for the reporting of breast carcinoma. Human Pathol 27 (3):220–224
2. Harris J, Lippman ME, Morrow M, Osborne CK (2002) Diseases of the breast. Lippincott Williams & Wilkins, Philadelphia

3. TNM classification of malignant tumors. AJCC 6th edn (2002). Wiley-Blackwell, New York, pp 131–142
4. Mustafa IA et al (1998) Prognostic analysis of survival in small breast cancers. J Am Coll Surg 186(5):562–569
5. Rosen PP et al (1993) Factors influencing prognosis in node-negative breast carcinoma: analysis of 767 T1N0M0/T2N0M0 patients with long-term follow-up. J Clin Oncol 11 (11):2090–2100
6. Rosen PP, Groshen S (1990) Factors influencing survival and prognosis in early breast carcinoma (T1N0M0-T1N1M0). Assessment of 644 patients with median follow-up of 18 years. Surg Clin North Am 70(4):937–962
7. Rosen PR et al (1989) A long-term follow-up study of survival in stage I (T1N0M0) and stage II (T1N1M0) breast carcinoma. J Clin Oncol 7(3):355–366
8. Halsted WS (1894) The results of operation for the cure of cancer the breast performed at Johns Hopkins Hospital from June 1889 to January. Johns Hopkins Hosp Rep 4:297–350
9. Halsted WS (1898) A clinical and histological study of certain adenocarcinomata of the breast: and a brief consideration of the supraclavicular operation and the results of operations for cancer of the breast from 1889 to 1898 at John Hopkins Hospital. Ann Surg 28:557–576
10. Meyer W (1894) An improved method of the radical operation for carcinoma of the breast. Med Rec 46:746–749
11. Patey DH, Dyson WH (1948) Prognosis of carcinoma of the breast in relation to the type of operation performed. Br J Cancer 2:7–13
12. Scarff RW, Handley RS (1938) Prognosis in carcinoma of the breast. Lancet 2:582–583
13. Urban JA, Baker HW (1952) Radical mastectomy in continuity with en bloc resection of the internal mammary lymph node chain – a new procedure for primary operable cancer of the breast. Cancer 5(5):992–1008
14. Fisher B et al (1985) Five-year results of a randomized clinical trial comparing total mastectomy and segmental mastectomy with or without radiation in the treatment of breast cancer. N Engl J Med 312(11):665–673
15. Fisher B et al (2002) Twenty-five-year follow-up of a randomized trial comparing radical mastectomy, total mastectomy, and total mastectomy followed by irradiation. N Engl J Med 347(8):567–575
16. Petrek JA et al (2001) Lymphedema in a cohort of breast carcinoma survivors 20 years after diagnosis. Cancer 92(6):1368–1377
17. Ahlgren J et al (1994) Prediction of axillary lymph node metastases in a screened breast cancer population. South-East Sweden Breast Cancer Group. Acta Oncol 33(6):603–608
18. Barth A, Craig PH, Silverstein MJ (1997) Predictors of axillary lymph node metastases in patients with T1 breast carcinoma [see comments]. Cancer 79(10):1918–1922
19. Chadha M et al (1994) Predictors of axillary lymph node metastases in patients with T1 breast cancer. A multivariate analysis. Cancer 73(2):350–353
20. Choong PL et al (1996) Predicting axillary lymph node metastases in breast carcinoma patients. Breast Cancer Res Treat 37(2):135–149
21. Cody HS III (1999) Sentinel lymph node mapping in breast cancer. Oncology (Huntington) 13(1):25–34
22. Cody HS III (1999) Management of the axilla in early stage breast cancer: will sentinel node biopsy end the debate? [editorial]. J Surg Oncol 71(3):137–139
23. De Laurentiis M et al (1996) A predictive index of axillary nodal involvement in operable breast cancer. Br J Cancer 73(10):1241–1247
24. Fehr MK et al (1995) Multivariate analysis of clinico-pathologic predictors of axillary lymph node metastasis in invasive breast carcinoma. Geburtshilfe Frauenheilkd 55(4):182–188
25. Fein DA et al (1997) Identification of women with T1-T2 breast cancer at low risk of positive axillary nodes. J Surg Oncol 65(1):34–39
26. Gann PH et al (1999) Factors associated with axillary lymph node metastasis from breast carcinoma: descriptive and predictive analyses. Cancer 86(8):1511–1519

27. Giuliano AE et al (1996) Incidence and predictors of axillary metastasis in T1 carcinoma of the breast [see comments]. J Am Coll Surg 183(3):185–189
28. Giuliano AE et al (1997) Sentinel lymphadenectomy in breast cancer. J Clin Oncol 15 (6):2345–2350
29. Giuliano AE et al (1994) Lymphatic mapping and sentinel lymphadenectomy for breast cancer [see comments]. Ann Surg 220(3):391–398
30. Krag D et al (1998) The sentinel node in breast cancer – a multicenter validation study [see comments]. N Engl J Med 339(14):941–946
31. Veronesi U et al (1997) Sentinel-node biopsy to avoid axillary dissection in breast cancer with clinically negative lymph-nodes [see comments]. Lancet 349(9069):1864–1867
32. Maibenco DC et al (1999) Axillary lymph node metastases associated with small invasive breast carcinomas. Cancer 85(7):1530–1536
33. Olivotto IA et al (1998) Prediction of axillary lymph node involvement of women with invasive breast carcinoma: a multivariate analysis [see comments]. Cancer 83(5):948–955
34. Ravdin PM et al (1994) Prediction of axillary lymph node status in breast cancer patients by use of prognostic indicators [see comments]. J Natl Cancer Inst 86(23):1771–1775
35. Bevilacqua JL et al (2007) Doctor, what are my chances of having a positive sentinel node? A validated nomogram for risk estimation. J Clin Oncol 25(24):3670–3679
36. Cabanas RM (1977) An approach for the treatment of penile carcinoma. Cancer 39 (2):456–466
37. Gajdos C et al (2000) Stage 0 to stage III breast cancer in young women. J Am Coll Surg 190 (5):523–529
38. Veronesi U et al (2003) A randomized comparison of sentinel-node biopsy with routine axillary dissection in breast cancer. N Engl J Med 349(6):546–553
39. TNM (2002), Breast, L.H. Sobin, C. Wittekind, and C. International Union Against, Editors. Wiley-Liss: New York. p 131–142
40. Cody HS III, Borgen PI (1999) State-of-the-art approaches to sentinel node biopsy for breast cancer: study design, patient selection, technique, and quality control at Memorial Sloan-Kettering Cancer Center [see comments]. Surg Oncol 8(2):85–91
41. Morton DL et al (1992) Technical details of intraoperative lymphatic mapping for early stage melanoma. Arch Surg 127(4):392–399
42. Giuliano AE et al (1995) Improved axillary staging of breast cancer with sentinel lymphadenectomy [see comments]. Ann Surg 222(3):394–399
43. Naik AM et al (2004) The risk of axillary relapse after sentinel lymph node biopsy for breast cancer is comparable with that of axillary lymph node dissection: a follow-up study of 4008 procedures. Ann Surg 240(3):462–468
44. O'Hea BJ et al (1998) Sentinel lymph node biopsy in breast cancer: initial experience at Memorial Sloan-Kettering Cancer Center [see comments]. J Am Coll Surg 186(4):423–427
45. Mustafa IA et al (1997) The impact of histopathology on nodal metastases in minimal breast cancer. Arch Surg 132(4):384–390
46. Giri D et al (2001) Multifocal versus unifocal node-negative breast carcinomas: are they prognostically different? Mod Pathol 14(1):26A–26A
47. Voogd AC et al (2001) Differences in risk factors for local and distant recurrence after breast-conserving therapy or mastectomy for stage I and II breast cancer: pooled results of two large European randomized trials. J Clin Oncol 19(6):1688–1697
48. International (Ludwig) Breast Cancer Study Group; Writing Committee: Bettelheim R, Price K N, Gelber RD, Davis BW, Castiglione M, Goldhirsch A, Neville AM (1990) Prognostic importance of occult axillary lymph node micrometastases from breast cancers. Lancet 335 (8705):1565–1568
49. Lohrisch C et al (2000) Relationship between tumor location and relapse in 6,781 women with early invasive breast cancer. J Clin Oncol 18(15):2828–2835
50. Asaga T et al (1994) Location of breast cancer as a prognostic factor (meeting abstract). Breast Cancer Res Treat 32:S48

51. Zucali R et al (1998) Early breast cancer: evaluation of the prognostic role of the site of the primary tumor. J Clin Oncol 16(4):1363–1366
52. Israel L et al (1995) Distinct metastatic pattern in breast tumor of inner and central areas (meeting abstract). Proc Annu Meet Am Soc Clin Oncol 14:A110
53. Bevilacqua JL et al (2002) A selection algorithm for internal mammary sentinel lymph node biopsy in breast cancer. Eur J Surg Oncol 28(6):603–614
54. Weaver DL et al (2000) Pathologic analysis of sentinel and nonsentinel lymph nodes in breast carcinoma: a multicenter study [see comments]. Cancer 88(5):1099–1107
55. Abdessalam SF et al (2001) Predictors of positive axillary lymph nodes after sentinel lymph node biopsy in breast cancer. Am J Surg 182(4):316–320
56. Albertini JJ et al (1996) Lymphatic mapping and sentinel node biopsy in the patient with breast cancer. JAMA 276(22):1818–1822
57. Rahusen FD et al (2001) Predictive factors for metastatic involvement of nonsentinel nodes in patients with breast cancer. Arch Surg 136(9):1059–1063
58. Reynolds C et al (1999) Sentinel lymph node biopsy with metastasis: can axillary dissection be avoided in some patients with breast cancer? J Clin Oncol 17(6):1720–1726
59. Teng S et al (2000) Do cytokeratin-positive-only sentinel lymph nodes warrant complete axillary lymph node dissection in patients with invasive breast cancer? Am Surg 66 (6):574–578
60. Veronesi U et al (1999) Sentinel lymph node biopsy and axillary dissection in breast cancer: results in a large series [see comments]. J Natl Cancer Inst 91(4):368–373
61. Van Zee KJ et al (2003) A nomogram for predicting the likelihood of additional nodal metastases in breast cancer patients with a positive sentinel node biopsy. Ann Surg Oncol 10(10):1140–1151
62. Chu KU et al (1999) Do all patients with sentinel node metastasis from breast carcinoma need complete axillary node dissection? [see comments]. Ann Surg 229(4):536–541
63. Cserni G, Szekeres JP (2001) Internal mammary lymph nodes and sentinel node biopsy in breast cancer. Surg Oncol 10(1–2):25–33
64. Fleming FJ et al (2004) Factors affecting metastases to non-sentinel lymph nodes in breast cancer. J Clin Pathol 57(1):73–76
65. Hwang RF et al (2003) Clinicopathologic factors predicting involvement of nonsentinel axillary nodes in women with breast cancer. Ann Surg Oncol 10(3):248–254
66. Kamath VJ et al (2001) Characteristics of the sentinel lymph node in breast cancer predict further involvement of higher-echelon nodes in the axilla: a study to evaluate the need for complete axillary lymph node dissection. Arch Surg 136(6):688–692
67. Sachdev U et al (2002) Predictors of nonsentinel lymph node metastasis in breast cancer patients. Am J Surg 183(3):213–217
68. Silverstein MJ et al (1995) Predicting axillary node positivity in patients with invasive carcinoma of the breast by using a combination of T category and palpability. J Am Coll Surg 180(6):700–704
69. Jakub JW et al (2002) Completion axillary lymph node dissection minimizes the likelihood of false negatives for patients with invasive breast carcinoma and cytokeratin positive only sentinel lymph nodes. Am J Surg 184(4):302–306
70. Wong SL et al (2001) The use of cytokeratin staining in sentinel lymph node biopsy for breast cancer. Am J Surg 182(4):330–334
71. Turner RR et al (2000) Pathologic features associated with nonsentinel lymph node metastases in patients with metastatic breast carcinoma in a sentinel lymph node. Cancer 89 (3):574–581
72. Canavese G et al (2001) Technical issues and pathologic implications of sentinel lymph node biopsy in early-stage breast cancer patients. J Surg Oncol 77(2):81–87; discussion 88
73. Cserni G (2001) Sentinel lymph-node biopsy-based prediction of further breast cancer metastases in the axilla. Eur J Surg Oncol 27(6):532–538

74. Liang WC, Sickle-Santanello BJ, Nims TA (2001) Is a completion axillary dissection indicated for micrometastases in the sentinel lymph node? Am J Surg 182(4):365–368
75. Viale G et al (2001) Histologic detection and clinical implications of micrometastases in axillary sentinel lymph nodes for patients with breast carcinoma. Cancer 92(6):1378–1384
76. Weiser MR et al (2001) Lymphovascular invasion enhances the prediction of non-sentinel node metastases in breast cancer patients with positive sentinel nodes. Ann Surg Oncol 8 (2):145–149
77. den Bakker MA et al (2002) Non-sentinel lymph node involvement in patients with breast cancer and sentinel node micrometastasis; too early to abandon axillary clearance. J Clin Pathol 55(12):932–935
78. Mignotte H et al (2002) Axillary lymph-node dissection for positive sentinel nodes in breast cancer patients. Eur J Surg Oncol 28(6):623–626
79. Van Zee KJ (2004) Residual disease in the axilla: to predict or not predict? Breast Dis 15:231–234
80. International Society of, L (2003) The diagnosis and treatment of peripheral lymphedema. Consensus document of the International Society of Lymphology. Lymphology 36(2):84–91
81. Panobianco MS, Mamede MV (2002) Complications and incidents associated with arm edema in the first 3 months after mastectomy. Rev Lat Am Enfermagem 10(4):544–551
82. Brasil.Ministerio da Saude.Secretaria de Atencao da Saude.Instituto Nacional de Cancer. Coordenacao de Prevencoe Vigilancia de, C., Estimativas 2008: Incidància de Cancer no Brasil. Rio de Janeiro:INCA. 2008
83. Cancer of the breast (invasive) – estimated United States cancer prevalence counts a on January 1, 2007 by race/ethnicity, sex and years since diagnosis – Table 4.25. 2015 [cited 2015 March 8]; Available from: http://seer.cancer.gov/archive/csr/1975_2007/results_single/sect_04_table.25.pdf
84. International Data Base (IDB) – world population summary (Access date 11/12/2010). U S Census Bureau, Population Division [cited 2010 December 10]; Available from: http://www.census.gov/ipc/www/idb/worldpopinfo.php
85. Mortimer PS (1998) The pathophysiology of lymphedema. Cancer 83(12 Suppl American):2798–2802
86. Pain SJ et al (2004) Variation in lymphatic function may predispose to development of breast cancer-related lymphoedema. Eur J Surg Oncol 30(5):508–514
87. Bergmann A, Mattos IE, Koifman RJ (2007) Incidencia e Prevalencia de Linfedema apos Tratamento Cirurgico do Cancer de Mama: Revisao de Literatura. Rev Bras Cancerol 53 (4):461–470
88. Edwards TL (2000) Prevalence and aetiology of lymphoedema after breast cancer treatment in southern Tasmania. Aust N Z J Surg 70(6):412–418
89. Kuehn T et al (2000) Long-term morbidity following axillary dissection in breast cancer patients – clinical assessment, significance for life quality and the impact of demographic, oncologic and therapeutic factors. Breast Cancer Res Treat 64(3):275–286
90. Hojris I et al (2000) Late treatment-related morbidity in breast cancer patients randomized to postmastectomy radiotherapy and systemic treatment versus systemic treatment alone. Acta Oncol 39(3):355–372
91. Johansen J et al (2000) Treatment of morbidity associated with the management of the axilla in breast-conserving therapy. Acta Oncol 39(3):349–354
92. Freitas R Jr et al (2001) Lymphedema in breast cancer patients submitted to modified radical mastectomy. Rev Bras Ginecol Obstet 23(4):205–208
93. Ververs JM et al (2001) Risk, severity and predictors of physical and psychological morbidity after axillary lymph node dissection for breast cancer. Eur J Cancer 37(8):991–999
94. Meric F et al (2002) Long-term complications associated with breast-conservation surgery and radiotherapy. Ann Surg Oncol 9(6):543–549
95. Almeida AM et al (2002) Mulheres com cancer de mama: estudo de morbidade. Acta Oncol Bras 22(2):263–269

96. Beaulac SM et al (2002) Lymphedema and quality of life in survivors of early-stage breast cancer. Arch Surg 137(11):1253–1257
97. Rampaul RS et al (2003) Incidence of clinically significant lymphoedema as a complication following surgery for primary operable breast cancer. Eur J Cancer 39(15):2165–2167
98. Deutsch M, Flickinger JC (2003) Arm edema after lumpectomy and breast irradiation. Am J Clin Oncol 26(3):229–231
99. Schijven MP et al (2003) Comparison of morbidity between axillary lymph node dissection and sentinel node biopsy. Eur J Surg Oncol 29(4):341–350
100. Yap KP et al (2003) Factors influencing arm and axillary symptoms after treatment for node negative breast carcinoma. Cancer 97(6):1369–1375
101. Goffman TE et al (2004) Lymphedema of the arm and breast in irradiated breast cancer patients: risks in an era of dramatically changing axillary surgery. Breast J 10(5):405–411
102. Deo SV et al (2004) Prevalence and risk factors for development of lymphedema following breast cancer treatment. Indian J Cancer 41(1):8–12
103. Ozaslan C, Kuru B (2004) Lymphedema after treatment of breast cancer. Am J Surg 187 (1):69–72
104. Armer J et al (2004) Lymphedema following breast cancer treatment, including sentinel lymph node biopsy. Lymphology 37(2):73–91
105. van der Veen P et al (2004) Lymphedema development following breast cancer surgery with full axillary resection. Lymphology 37(4):206–208
106. Bergmann A (2004) Diagnostico de linfedema: analise dos metodos empregados na avaliacao do membro superior apos linfadenectomia axilar para tratamento do cancer de mama. Rev Bras Cancerol 50(4):311–320
107. Isaksson G, Feuk B (2000) Morbidity from axillary treatment in breast cancer – a follow-up study in a district hospital. Acta Oncol 39(3):335–336
108. Sener SF et al (2001) Lymphedema after sentinel lymphadenectomy for breast carcinoma. Cancer 92(4):748–752
109. Duff M et al (2001) Prospective evaluation of the morbidity of axillary clearance for breast cancer. Br J Surg 88(1):114–117
110. Herd-Smith A et al (2001) Prognostic factors for lymphedema after primary treatment of breast carcinoma. Cancer 92(7):1783–1787
111. Swenson KK et al (2002) Comparison of side effects between sentinel lymph node and axillary lymph node dissection for breast cancer. Ann Surg Oncol 9(8):745–753
112. Temple LK et al (2002) Sensory morbidity after sentinel lymph node biopsy and axillary dissection: a prospective study of 233 women. Ann Surg Oncol 9(7):654–662
113. Silberman AW et al (2004) Comparative morbidity of axillary lymph node dissection and the sentinel lymph node technique: implications for patients with breast cancer. Ann Surg 240 (1):1–6
114. Ronka R et al (2005) One-year morbidity after sentinel node biopsy and breast surgery. Breast 14(1):28–36
115. Clark B, Sitzia J, Harlow W (2005) Incidence and risk of arm oedema following treatment for breast cancer: a three-year follow-up study. QJM 98(5):343–348
116. Bergmann A (2005) Incidencia e fatores de risco do linfedema apos tratamento cirurgico para cancer de mama: Estudo de uma coorte hospitalar. Escola Nacional de Saude Piblica, Fundacao Oswaldo Cruz
117. Schrenk P et al (2000) Morbidity following sentinel lymph node biopsy versus axillary lymph node dissection for patients with breast carcinoma. Cancer 88(3):608–614
118. Blanchard DK et al (2003) Relapse and morbidity in patients undergoing sentinel lymph node biopsy alone or with axillary dissection for breast cancer. Arch Surg 138(5):482–487; discussion 487-8
119. Golshan M, Martin WJ, Dowlatshahi K (2003) Sentinel lymph node biopsy lowers the rate of lymphedema when compared with standard axillary lymph node dissection. Am Surg 69 (3):209–211

120. Langer S et al (2004) Lymphatic mapping improves staging and reduces morbidity in women undergoing total mastectomy for breast carcinoma. Am Surg 70(10):881–885
121. Mansel RE et al (2006) Randomized multicenter trial of sentinel node biopsy versus standard axillary treatment in operable breast cancer: the ALMANAC Trial. J Natl Cancer Inst 98 (9):599–609
122. Lucci A et al (2007) Surgical complications associated with sentinel lymph node dissection (SLND) plus axillary lymph node dissection compared with SLND alone in the American College of Surgeons Oncology Group Trial Z0011. J Clin Oncol 25(24):3657–3663
123. Bevilacqua JL et al (2003) A multivariate nomogram to predict likelihood of non-sentinel node metastases in breast cancer patients with positive sentinel nodes. Ann Surg Oncol 10(1): S34–S34
124. Fehr MK, et al (1994) Multivariate analysis of clinicopathological predictors of axillary lymph node metastasis in invasive breast cancer. (Meeting Abstract). Breast Cancer ResTreat 32(Suppl):46
125. Barranger E et al (2005) An axilla scoring system to predict non-sentinel lymph node status in breast cancer patients with sentinel lymph node involvement. Breast Cancer Res Treat 91 (2):113–119
126. Degnim AC et al (2003) Clinicopathologic features of metastasis in nonsentinel lymph nodes of breast carcinoma patients. Cancer 98(11):2307–2315
127. Kohrt WM et al (2004) American College of Sports Medicine Position Stand: physical activity and bone health. Med Sci Sports Exerc 36(11):1985–1996
128. Pal A et al (2008) A model for predicting non-sentinel lymph node metastatic disease when the sentinel lymph node is positive. Br J Surg 95(3):302–309
129. Coutant C et al (2009) Comparison of models to predict nonsentinel lymph node status in breast cancer patients with metastatic sentinel lymph nodes: a prospective multicenter study. J Clin Oncol 27(17):2800–2808
130. Kattan MW et al (2004) A tool for predicting breast carcinoma mortality in women who do not receive adjuvant therapy. Cancer 101(11):2509–2515
131. Degnim AC et al (2005) Nonsentinel node metastasis in breast cancer patients: assessment of an existing and a new predictive nomogram. Am J Surg 190(4):543–550
132. Bevilacqua JL et al (2012) Nomograms for predicting the risk of arm lymphedema after axillary dissection in breast cancer. Ann Surg Oncol 19(8):2580–2589
133. Kohrt HE et al (2008) New models and online calculator for predicting non-sentinel lymph node status in sentinel lymph node positive breast cancer patients. BMC Cancer 8:66
134. Saidi RF et al (2004) Nonsentinel lymph node status after positive sentinel lymph node biopsy in early breast cancer. Am Surg 70(2):101–105; discussion 105

Chapter 23
Data Mining and Mathematical Model Development

Masahiro Sugimoto and Masahiro Takada

Abstract The treatment and diagnosis of breast cancer require difficult decision making based on multidisciplinary fields, such as image, clinical, and pathological findings as well as new diagnostic technologies and molecular biomarkers. Thus, mathematical models that can predict a specific status and outcome of treatment by efficient usage of these big data are required. Successful models with high accuracy and high generalization ability can help promote personalized medicine and provide benefits of medical economy. Here, we introduce the use of advanced computational data mining technologies using artificial intelligence or machine learning and describe two models that we developed to predict pathological complete response of neoadjuvant therapy and lymph node metastasis in patients with primary breast cancer. The development and validation protocols are also discussed.

Keywords Data mining • Machine learning • Prediction model • Neoadjuvant therapy • Lymph node metastasis

23.1 Introduction

The recent rapid advances of computer resources have enabled large-data analyses, e.g., high-throughput analysis of omics data (whole genomes) and high-resolution magnetic resonance imaging [1]. The analysis of medical big data with such high-end technologies will make efficient personalized medicine a reality. These large-data analysis methods use patient information and predict the "future" of the patients, e.g., treatment outcomes and changes in disease status. Multivariate analyses have been utilized up to now. Multiple logistic regression (MLR) and

M. Sugimoto (✉)
Institute for Advanced Biosciences, Keio University Institute for Advanced Biosciences, Keio University, 403-1 Nipponkoku, Daihouji, Tsuruoka, Yamagata 997-0017, Japan

Department of Pathology, Kanagawa Dental College, Post Graduate School, Kanagawa, Japan
e-mail: msugi@sfc.keio.ac.jp

M. Takada
Department of Breast Surgery, Kyoto University Hospital, Kyoto, Japan

M. Toi et al. (eds.), *Personalized Treatment of Breast Cancer*,
DOI 10.1007/978-4-431-55552-0_23

multiple variable regression are generally used for the prediction of binary and continuous outcomes, respectively. Both these methods sum up the odds or contributions of the variables in a linear way. For the treatment and diagnosis of cancers, nomograms of MLR models have been developed. Nomograms were designed to visualize the relationship among variables. The MD Anderson Cancer Center in Houston and the Memorial Sloan Kettering Cancer Center in New York have been involved in developing this tool.

These statistic methods all require independent minimum variable sets as inputs; therefore, only a small number of variables are normally selected as inputs into these models using statistical or empirical approaches, even though various variables are commonly available before any treatments and diagnoses. As a result, the accuracy of the models is usually limited. Nowadays, the more recently developed mathematical modeling methods based on data mining technologies have the ability to deal with a large number of variables that have a complicated structure. However, rigorous validation of the data mining-based model is required, and interpretation of the predictions of the developed model is also necessary.

23.2 Strategy of Development and Validation of Mathematical Models

A variety of machine-learning methods are available [2]; therefore, the selection of a method that is suitable for a given problem is the first important step. Artificial neural networks (ANNs), decision tree (DT), and support vector machines (SVMs) are some of the common available techniques [3, 4]. ANN can discriminate specific data from other data using a nonlinear approach and has been applied to solve complicated problems. However, multi-linearity (or colinearity) among input variables will dramatically reduce the generalization ability of a model developed using ANNs, i.e., the model often performs well only on training datasets and does not generate good predictions on independent datasets. DT offers definite advantages over ANN, because a model developed using DT can generate a treelike structure containing if-then branches and variable nodes, which is visibly interpretable. However, DT uses only a combination of linear discriminations, meaning that it tends to have lower discrimination ability than nonlinear methods. SVM separates two groups of data using kernel functions, which can increase the dimension of the given parameter space. This method does not suffer from the multi-linearity problem and is robust against outliers. However, the prediction performance of SVMs strongly depends on the parameters and kernels, which require rigorous validations. Bayesian network (BN) and classification and regression trees (CART) have been also used in machine-learning models.

The development of a mathematical model for breast cancer diagnosis and treatment would generally start with the development of a database of clinicopathological data, followed by data selection, training of the model, and validation of

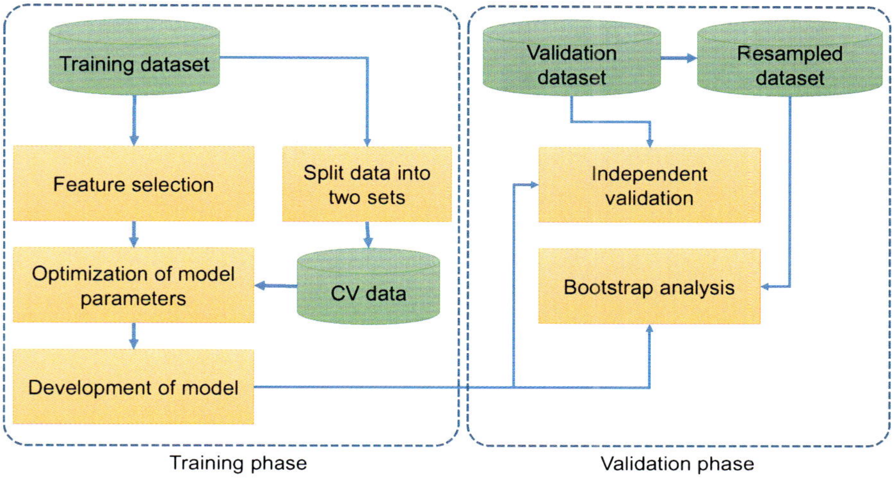

Fig. 23.1 Representative scheme of mathematical model development and validation. The training dataset is used for feature selection and cross validation (CV) to optimize the model parameters. A model is developed using training datasets with optimized parameters and subsequently validated using independent datasets. A validation dataset is usually used for this purpose, and a resampled dataset from the validation dataset is used for bootstrap analysis

the trained model (Fig. 23.1). For the database, quantitative values with no missing values or noise are preferable. Feature selection is usually conducted to select variables that have a predictive ability. For example, if an ANN model is to be used, multi-linearity of the data should be eliminated and an independent variable dataset should be selected. SVM-feature selection (SVM-FS) is commonly used for ranking the predictive ability of the variables without considering the multi-linearity among these variables.

23.3 Models for Breast Cancer Diagnosis and Treatment

Here, two prediction models that use machine-learning methods in breast cancer diagnosis and treatment are described. One model can be used to predict the efficacy of neoadjuvant chemotherapy (NAC) (Fig. 23.2), and the other can be used to predict axillary lymph node (AxLN) metastasis in primary breast cancer (Fig. 23.3).

23.3.1 Prediction of Efficacy of Neoadjuvant Chemotherapy

NAC is administrated before the surgical operation of cancer. This treatment provides several benefits including tumor size reduction, which raise the opportunities

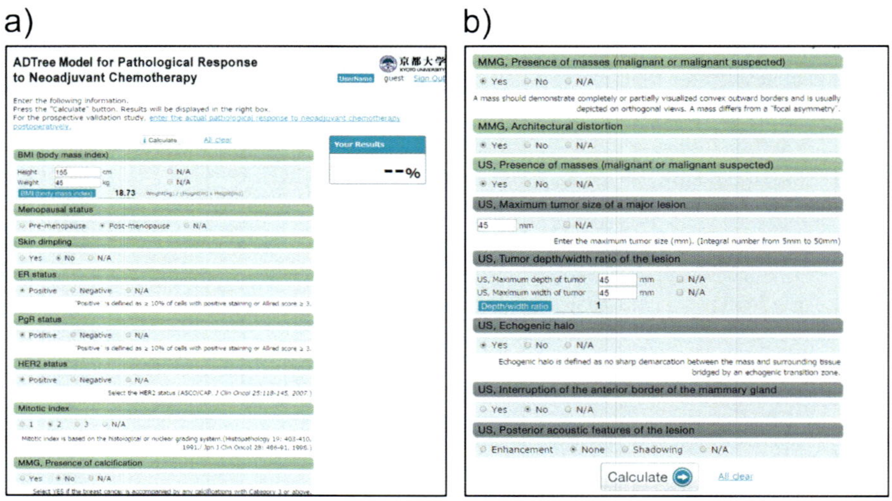

Fig. 23.2 Interface for predicting the pathological complete response to neoadjuvant chemotherapy in primary breast cancer. Panels (**a**, **b**) are the *top* and the *bottom* part of the Web site

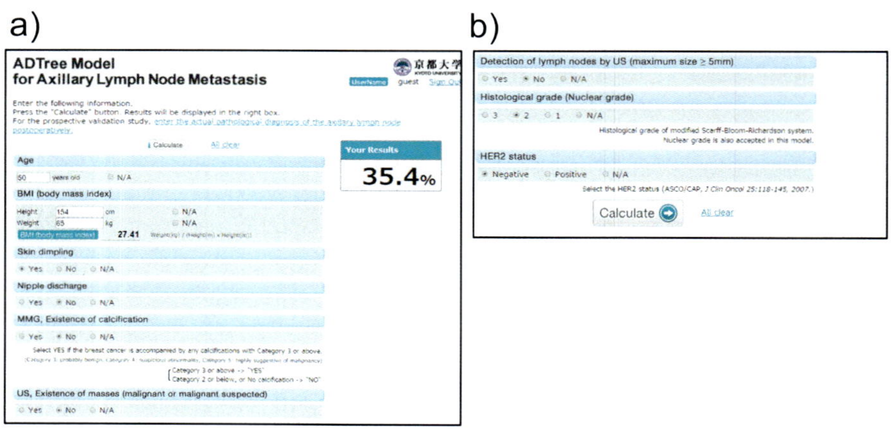

Fig. 23.3 Interface for predicting axillary lymph node metastasis in primary breast cancer. Panels (**a**, **b**) are the *top* and the *bottom* part of the Web site

of breast conservation and reveal the sensitivity of the chemotherapy, which helps clinicians design later adjuvant therapy [5]. Pathological complete response (pCR) is commonly used to evaluate the NAC response as well as a surrogate prognostic indicator in these patients. Predicting the pCR using information collected before NAC can help in the oncologists' decision making. Therefore, we developed a mathematical model to predict pCR after NAC using a relatively large number of variables collected before starting NAC, such as estrogen receptor (ER) status, human epidermal growth factor receptor 2 (HER2/neu) status, histological grade, and proliferative activity [6].

We collected patient data from a number of institutions and split them into two datasets: training datasets ($n = 150$) and a validation dataset ($n = 173$). The training datasets were collected from three institutions from 2005 to 2009. A consecutive dataset of 58 patients was collected from the Tokyo Metropolitan Cancer and Infectious Diseases Center Komagome Hospital. The rest of the data were collected from the Osaka National Hospital and the Tsukuba University Hospital. Among the patients were 89 patients who had participated in the OOTR N003 trial. The validation datasets were collected from the OOTR N003 trial conducted in the Niigata Cancer Center Hospital, National Kyushu Cancer Center, and the Aichi Cancer Center (see [6] for details).

All the patients received the same neoadjuvant protocol, consisting of four courses of FEC (5-fluorouracil 500 mg/m^2, epirubicin 100 mg/m^2, and cyclophosphamide 500 mg/m^2 administered intravenously [IV] every 3 weeks) followed by four courses of docetaxel (75 mg/m^2, IV, every 3 weeks) with or without capecitabine (1650 mg/m^2/day, oral administration, for 14 days every 3 weeks).

We used an alternative decision tree (ADTree) method as the prediction model [7, 8]. To enhance the accuracy and generalization ability of the model, an ensemble technique that used the predictions of multiple mathematical models was employed [9].

For each patient, 28 clinicopathological variables were retrospectively collected. These data included physical findings, information on mammography and ultrasonography images, and histological type, ER status, progesterone receptor (PgR) status, HER2 status, and histological/nuclear grade of needle biopsy specimens [10]. The clinical response was evaluated after both the FEC treatment (i.e., the clinical response after anthracycline) and the taxane-containing regimen (i.e., the clinical response after taxane). The pCR was defined as the absence of residual invasive cancer cells in the breast and axillary lymph nodes (ypT0/is + ypN0).

The ADTree model was trained using cross validation and 15 features were selected. The model predicted the area under the ROC curve (AUC) = 0.766 (95 % confidence interval (CI) 0.671–0.861; P-value = 0.0001) for the training dataset and AUC = 0.787 (95 % CI 0.716–0.858; P-value = 0.0001) for the validation dataset. The similar AUC values for the testing and validation datasets indicated a low possibility of over-fitting.

Because the structure of this model is quite complicated, interpretation based on a visualized model is difficult. Instead, we used an indirect approach to analyze the features of the developed model. We eliminated each of the features from the trained model and then ranked the importance of each feature based on the decrease in prediction accuracy compared with the accuracy of the original model. Clinical features such as ER, HER2, and PgR were ranked in the top 3, and subsequently image findings—such as the halo in ultrasonography images—were ranked. The prediction accuracies of the model for each subtype were evaluated as AUC = 0.779 ($n = 102$; 95 % CI 0.641–0.917; P-value = 0.0059) for luminal type, AUC = 0.718 ($n = 24$; 95 % CI 0.496–0.940; P-value = 0.074) for HER2-positive type, and AUC = 0.531 ($n = 44$; 95 % CI 0.350–0.712; P-value = 0.743) for the triple negative (TN) type. The low prediction ability for the TN subtype indicated that the currently available variable lacked predictivity, probably because of its heterogeneous genetic background [11–13]. To improve the prediction results of this subtype, the development of new biomarkers or diagnosis methods are required.

23.3.2 Prediction of Lymph Node Metastasis

AxLN metastasis is an important prognostic factor in patients with primary breast cancer for predicting survival and for making decisions about the use of chemotherapy [14–16]. Currently, sentinel lymph node (SLN) biopsy is commonly employed to investigate AxLN status, avoiding AxLN dissection. However, SLN biopsy can reveal only 20–30 % positive metastasis, and more invasive, usually two-stage, procedures are needed for accurate determination of AxLN status [14]. A considerable number of patients with node negative require invasive procedure in order to confirm that they do not have a metastasis in their AxLNs. Therefore, it is important to use the available clinicopathological variables for the predicition of AxLN metastasis. To achieve this, we developed a mathematical model using an ADTree method.

A total of 24 clinicopathological variables for primary breast cancer patients who underwent SLN biopsy or AxLN dissection without prior treatment were collected from three institutes (Dataset A from the Tokyo Metropolitan Cancer and Infectious Diseases Center Komagome Hospital, n = 148; Dataset B from the Kyoto University Hospital, n = 143; Dataset C from the Seoul National University Hospital, n = 174). Data A and B were used for variable selection and model training and the developed model was validated using external data C.

The ADTree model used 15 variables and yielded AUC = 0.770 (95 % CI 0.689–0.850) for the model training datasets and AUC = 0.772 (95 % CI 0.689–0.856) for the validation dataset. The bootstrap value of the validation dataset was 0.768 (95 % CI 0.763–0.774). The similar AUC values between the testing and validation datasets indicated the low possibility of over-fitting and high generalization ability of the model.

The model's variables were ranked by eliminating each variable from the original model. Image findings, such as halo, lymph node size, and tumor size, were ranked in the top 3.

23.4 Analysis and Web Interface for Data Mining Models

Clinical data retrospectively collected frequently contained missing data. Therefore, prediction models should be robust against missing values. We compared the decreasing level of the prediction ability of our models and MLR models that were published previously [17]. The options for determining the structure of the ADTree model were boosting and ensemble numbers that corresponded to the size of a tree and the number of trees, respectively. We found that even small ensemble numbers dramatically increased the model's robustness against missing values, indicating that a complex structure using multiple trees may further contribute to this beneficial feature.

A disadvantage of such mathematical methods is the low interpretability of the predictions. Additionally, such models can be used only by oncologists who have good computer skills. On the other hand, Nomograms require no computer skills and show clear relationships among variables and predicted outcomes [18–22]. Therefore, the development of user-friendly interfaces for mathematical models is necessary. We developed a Web interface (Figs. 23.1 and 23.2) for the two prediction models described above (https://www.brca-pm.net/model/entrance.php). To access the interface, users require an account that can be set up by contacting the corresponding author [23]. In the future, we plan to incorporate many different models into one portal site, which will further benefit both patients and oncologists.

Although data mining-based mathematical models using clinicopathological variable have shown enough accuracy compared to gene expression-based models [24], more sophisticated computational methods are required to better use the available clinical information. Several computer companies have begun collaborative studies with the MD Anderson Cancer Center and the Memorial Sloan Kettering Cancer Center to develop a data mining system using a supercomputer. Advanced informatics technologies to maximize the values of medical datasets are required to make full use of the large amounts of accumulated data.

References

1. Savage N (2014) Bioinformatics: big data versus the big C. Nature 509(7502):S66–S67. doi:10.1038/509S66a
2. Mjolsness E, DeCoste D (2001) Machine learning for science: state of the art and future prospects. Science 293(5537):2051–2055. doi:10.1126/science.293.5537.2051
3. Ghavidel AA, Javadikasgari H, Maleki M et al (2014) Two new mathematical models for prediction of early mortality risk in coronary artery bypass graft surgery. J Thorac Cardiovasc Surg 148(4):1291–1298 e1291. doi:10.1016/j.jtcvs.2014.02.028
4. Shouval R, Bondi O, Mishan H et al (2014) Application of machine learning algorithms for clinical predictive modeling: a data-mining approach in SCT. Bone Marrow Transplant 49 (3):332–337. doi:10.1038/bmt.2013.146
5. Mieog JS, van der Hage JA, van de Velde CJ (2007) Preoperative chemotherapy for women with operable breast cancer. Cochrane Database Syst Rev (Online) 2:CD005002. doi:10.1002/14651858.CD005002.pub2
6. Takada M, Sugimoto M, Ohno S et al (2012) Predictions of the pathological response to neoadjuvant chemotherapy in patients with primary breast cancer using a data mining technique. Breast Cancer Res Treat 134(2):661–670. doi:10.1007/s10549-012-2109-2
7. Freund Y, Mason L (1999) The alternating decision tree learning algorithm. In: Proceedings of the sixteenth international conference on machine learning, Bled, Slovenia. pp 124–133

8. Horiguchi K, Toi M, Horiguchi S et al (2010) Predictive value of CD24 and CD44 for neoadjuvant chemotherapy response and prognosis in primary breast cancer patients. J Med Dent Sci 57(2):165–175
9. Che D, Liu Q, Rasheed K et al (2011) Decision tree and ensemble learning algorithms with their applications in bioinformatics. Adv Exp Med Biol 696:191–199. doi:10.1007/978-1-4419-7046-6_19
10. Colleoni M, Viale G, Zahrieh D et al (2008) Expression of ER, PgR, HER1, HER2, and response: a study of preoperative chemotherapy. Ann Oncol 19(3):465–472. doi:10.1093/annonc/mdm509
11. Perou CM (2010) Molecular stratification of triple-negative breast cancers. Oncologist 15 (Suppl 5):39–48. doi:10.1634/theoncologist.2010-S5-39
12. Darb-Esfahani S, Loibl S, Muller BM et al (2009) Identification of biology-based breast cancer types with distinct predictive and prognostic features: role of steroid hormone and HER2 receptor expression in patients treated with neoadjuvant anthracycline/taxane-based chemotherapy. Breast Cancer Res 11(5):R69. doi:10.1186/bcr2363
13. Parker JS, Mullins M, Cheang MC et al (2009) Supervised risk predictor of breast cancer based on intrinsic subtypes. J Clin Oncol 27(8):1160–1167. doi:10.1200/JCO.2008.18.1370
14. Fisher B, Bauer M, Wickerham DL et al (1983) Relation of number of positive axillary nodes to the prognosis of patients with primary breast cancer. An NSABP update. Cancer 52 (9):1551–1557
15. Fitzgibbons PL, Page DL, Weaver D et al (2000) Prognostic factors in breast cancer. College of American Pathologists Consensus Statement 1999. Arch Pathol Lab Med 124(7):966–978
16. Nemoto T, Natarajan N, Bedwani R et al (1983) Breast cancer in the medial half. Results of 1978 National Survey of the American College of Surgeons. Cancer 51(8):1333–1338
17. Sugimoto M, Takada M, Toi M (2013) Comparison of robustness against missing values of alternative decision tree and multiple logistic regression for predicting clinical data in primary breast cancer. Conference proceedings: annual international conference of the IEEE engineering in medicine and biology society IEEE engineering in medicine and biology society annual conference 2013, pp 3054–3057. doi:10.1109/EMBC.2013.6610185
18. Colleoni M, Viale G, Goldhirsch A (2009) Lessons on responsiveness to adjuvant systemic therapies learned from the neoadjuvant setting. Breast 18(Suppl 3):S137–S140. doi:10.1016/S0960-9776(09)70289-9
19. Rouzier R, Pusztai L, Delaloge S et al (2005) Nomograms to predict pathologic complete response and metastasis-free survival after preoperative chemotherapy for breast cancer. J Clin Oncol 23(33):8331–8339. doi:10.1200/JCO.2005.01.2898
20. Bevilacqua JL, Kattan MW, Fey JV et al (2007) Doctor, what are my chances of having a positive sentinel node? A validated nomogram for risk estimation. J Clin Oncol 25 (24):3670–3679
21. Rouzier R, Pusztai L, Garbay JR et al (2006) Development and validation of nomograms for predicting residual tumor size and the probability of successful conservative surgery with neoadjuvant chemotherapy for breast cancer. Cancer 107(7):1459–1466. doi:10.1002/cncr.22177
22. Pal A, Provenzano E, Duffy SW et al (2008) A model for predicting non-sentinel lymph node metastatic disease when the sentinel lymph node is positive. Br J Surg 95(3):302–309. doi:10.1002/bjs.5943
23. Sugimoto M, Takada M, Toi M (2014) Development of Web tools to predict axillary lymph node metastasis and pathological response to neoadjuvant chemotherapy in breast cancer patients. Int J Biol Markers. doi:10.5301/jbm.5000103
24. Fan C, Prat A, Parker JS et al (2011) Building prognostic models for breast cancer patients using clinical variables and hundreds of gene expression signatures. BMC Med Genomics 4:3. doi:10.1186/1755-8794-4-3